Let's talk about the first year of parenting

Let's talk about the first year of parenting

Amy Brown

pinter & martin

Let's talk about the first year of parenting

First published in the UK by Pinter & Martin Ltd 2020

ISBN 978-1-78066-710-2

Also available as an ebook

Edited by Susan Last
Index by Helen Bilton
Proofread by Sarah Dronfield
Design by Blok Graphic

British Library Cataloguing-in-Publication Data
A catalogue record for this book is available from the British Library

Printed in the EU by Hussar

This book has been printed on paper that is sourced and harvested from sustainable forests and is FSC accredited

Pinter & Martin Ltd
6 Effra Parade
London SW2 1PS

pinterandmartin.com

Where to get support – a quick guide

This page is intended to be a guide to finding the support you need quickly and easily, especially if you are feeling a bit overwhelmed and need the support right now. It is not designed to be a comprehensive list of all sources and you will find further links to support embedded in each chapter as you go through. For health issues please contact your midwife, health visitor or GP or ring NHS 111.

Infant feeding support
National Breastfeeding Helpline 0300 100 0212
Association of Breastfeeding Mothers 0300 330 5453
La Leche League 0345 120 2918
National Childbirth Trust (NCT) 0300 330 0700

Mental health support
www.samaritans.org/wales/how-we-can-help/contact-samaritan
www.mind.org.uk/information-support/helplines

Birth trauma support
www.birthtraumaassociation.org.uk

Postnatal depression support
www.pandasfoundation.org.uk

Parenting support
www.family-action.org.uk/what-we-do/children-families

Support for a crying baby
www.cry-sis.org.uk

Your legal rights as a parent
maternityaction.org.uk/get-free-advice

Relationship support
www.relate.org.uk/about-us/contact-us

Domestic abuse support
www.gov.uk/guidance/domestic-abuse-how-to-get-help

Contents

Author's note

This book is designed to support you as a parent whether you are a biological, adoptive, foster, step, or any other type of parent. It is for heterosexual and same-sex couples, single parents, separated parents and more. Grandparents, siblings and friends may also find it useful. It would also be helpful for those caring for a young baby such as a childminder or nanny.

Basically, it's for anyone who is living with and caring for a baby during the first year. It recognises that you probably have your own pattern for who takes on different roles. Maybe you have a 'traditional' set-up where mum stays home and dad goes out to work. Maybe you're on your own. Maybe you're a stay-at-home dad, and mum went back to work two weeks after giving birth. Maybe you both went back to work at two weeks. Maybe you are a same-sex couple and are taking equal roles including both of you breastfeeding. Maybe you gave birth but identify as dad. Maybe you really hate being referred to as 'mum' or 'dad' (sorry!). I very much want this book to be useful in a way that doesn't put people in boxes. However, that makes things a bit complicated when it comes to writing in a way that is inclusive... but also easy to read. I apologise if sometimes the words I use do not fit with your situation or how you identify.

As an academic I like my books to be as evidence-based as possible, drawing on what research studies tell us. A major problem with this is that most of the research done with the parent who didn't give birth assumes that person is a father and male rather than considering the needs of same-sex parents or those who may identify in other ways. Many assume the main person staying home with the baby is a mother. Very few consider the experiences of transgender parents. When looking for evidence I tried to find research that looked at all these different variations of families where at all possible. But there just isn't a lot of published research out there. Many of the ideas that arise from studies with male fathers will be transferable to partners whatever their gender, but of course there will also be many nuances and downright differences. I apologise for the lack of inclusivity in research and promise to ensure my own research is as inclusive as possible in the future.

There are also geographical and cultural differences. I am writing this as someone living in the UK. Much of it will be relevant to parents in other countries, but there will be some major and minor differences when it comes to things like employment law and parental rights. Maternity leave is an obvious example. In the UK we are privileged to have the right to maternity leave for up to a year, and even though statutory maternity pay may not be much, we are in general in a much better position than parents in the US where there is still no statutory right to leave or pay. I recognise that this might be frustrating in places, but I hope that if you're reading this in a different country then the bulk of the book is useful.

All in all, I want this book to be for everyone and I hope it is helpful to you whatever your circumstances.

Introduction

→ Congratulations! You have become a new parent. How do you feel?
Great? Overwhelmed? Terrified? Exhausted – I bet it's exhausted.
Having a new baby changes your life – for the good, the bad and the surreal.
But while everyone around you turns up with tiny socks, demands to hold the
baby and then goes back to their everyday life, who is there to hold and care
for you? Who is there to reassure you what's normal, agree that it's all a bit of a
mess (albeit a very cute one) and point you in the direction of support if you're
struggling?

Becoming a parent isn't just about practically having to care for a baby. It's
so much more than that. In fact, it's recognised as one of the major transitions
in life as you go from caring mainly for yourself to suddenly being responsible
for meeting the needs of a small, wriggly and seemingly insomniac octopus.
Maddie McMahon, in her book *Why Mothering Matters*, describes it as a
metamorphosis and it really is. Looking back in a few years you will see how
much you have changed and just how strong you were, bending and adapting
to the twists and turns and highs and lows of being a new parent. It really is
life-changing. You won't go back to how things were before, or the person you
were. And that's okay. It's only the adverts that tell you that you should somehow get your old life back. It's gone. But I promise you that there is something
much better in its place.

I remember having my first baby, over 14 years ago now. It was such a strange time, filled with a storm of emotions – the good, the bad and the downright ugly. But most of all I remember thinking that no one else could be finding it this tough or feeling this anxious about it all. Everyone else I met at baby groups seemed really happy and like they had it all together. And that was before we had social media with its perfect photos and #SoBlessed hashtags. It wasn't until I made some new friends and opened up to them that I realised everyone was in the same boat. We just didn't talk about it. Until we did. And then we were all hugely relieved that in fact our experiences were normal.

So, if you feel overwhelmed or are worrying about whether how you are feeling is 'right', be reassured that other people are feeling that way too. If you're struggling with anxiety, feeling really low or just on edge and angry, there is support out there. If you're fighting with your partner, know that this is so common that I bet your fights are listed in the relationships chapter, as everyone argues about the same things (even if on social media they're #SoBlessed about their relationship too). If you are aching in places you didn't know you could ache, we can get you stronger again. And if you're staring at your baby wondering why they won't be put down, that is normal too (silver lining: you'll have great arm muscles in a few months).

This book isn't a step-by-step guide to how to care for your baby. It won't tell you how to change a nappy or give them a bath. There are many books out there that cover that, ranging from the broad to the minute detail on what your baby will be doing at 9.27pm on day 127 of their life. This book does cover some of the key challenges of early parenting – feeding, sleep and normal baby behaviour – as these decisions are so closely tied to how confident or happy you might feel as a parent. It will give you the information that you need to make decisions, tell you where to find support and consider ways in which you can look after yourself. There is no one right way to care for your baby, so it covers breast and bottle-feeding, co-sleeping and cots and looks at what we know about routines for young babies and whether they might work.

This book is designed to be an oracle, agony aunt (remember them?) and honest friend all rolled into one, supporting your needs as a parent during the first year and beyond. It is packed with information about stuff that's helpful to know, but more importantly it looks at how you might honestly feel at this time and acknowledges that this obviously matters. Babies are great – they matter very much. But you know who matters just as much? You.

“ Babies are great – they matter very much. But you know who matters just as much? You. ”

"

Part one

Let's talk about the early days of becoming a new parent

"

Let's start how we mean to go on.

This first section is all about you. It focuses on getting the support you need, how to get through those tricky first days and ideas for looking after yourself as your baby gets older. It looks at who you could lean on for support, including organisations that can help with feeding and caring for your baby, your mental health or simply helping you find other parents to connect with.

We also talk about the importance of focusing on your recovery and taking time to rest and have space for yourself. Your baby is ever so important, but you need time to focus on you too. We look at managing visitors, ways people can actually help you and the importance of making a postnatal recovery plan. I know not everyone has a long line of family and friends queuing up to help. You might be the only one of your friends who has had a baby, or you might live a very long way from family. You might be doing this on your own as a single parent or your partner may work away, meaning your day-to-day reality is doing stuff on your own. So we look at ways to help you get a break, even if your baby is coming along with you.

Most of all, this section is to remind you that you matter, and taking time to rest, recover and find some headspace is more than okay. You've got this.

Chapter one

First things first, let's make sure you're supported

$\rightarrow$ This chapter is going to explore the importance of support, how well supported you feel and where to find specific sources of support if you need more. And so many of us do need more support as new parents, as so many of us are now carrying the burden of parenting alone, a long way away from family or in communities with little time for connection. But we were never designed to have babies alone. We were never designed to be the only adults in our babies' lives. We were never designed to have the sole weight of responsibility for shaping a child on just our shoulders. It was meant to be a team effort. But for many of us that is not the case in modern society, and the stresses and strains show.

New parenthood comes as a shock to most of us, and a major reason why is because we aren't part of interwoven, multigenerational communities anymore. We have, on average, started having babies later and later. The majority of women now have years, if not decades at work before they have a first baby. Many of us are now in dual-earner families, reliant on two salaries, or with a female breadwinner; one-third of families in the UK have a woman earning the higher salary.[1] We move for university, jobs or affordable housing. And we're having fewer and fewer babies – half the number that were born in the 'baby boom' period after World War Two.[2]

What does this mean for our experience of having babies?

- Our own baby might be the first newborn baby we have any experience of, or indeed have even held
- We may live a very long way from our family
- Our friends may not have had babies yet, or may plan never to have them
- We are used to having control of our lives, a routine and money
- We don't have everyday experience of seeing babies and how they behave
- We're less likely to be part of a tightknit community in which people support each other

All this means that when we come to have a baby and realise what it entails we don't have an automatic support system around us. Years ago, we would have known more people having babies, our families would have been closer and we'd have grown up around more babies ourselves. That's not to romanticise things – we know many women felt trapped, overwhelmed and lonely despite all of this, with few escape options if things weren't great. But while we have gained many freedoms over the years, when it comes to having a baby we can feel very alone.

It's odd but I feel really lonely

It's strange, isn't it, that you should feel lonely at a time when actually you are never away from someone. But loneliness isn't just about human company – it's about how we engage with others and how they make us feel. It's about genuine connection. You can be in a room full of people and still feel lonely, yet have great connections with other people on the internet who you have never met.

But a lot of new parents, mothers in particular, are really missing those connections. In fact, loneliness has been described as an epidemic among new mothers. For example, a survey by the British Red Cross and The Co-operative in 2018 found that 82% of new mothers under the age of thirty said they felt lonely.[3] And in 2017 a survey by channelmum.com found that more than 90% said they felt lonely, with 54% saying they felt they didn't have any friends. Many tried to hide this, with over a third not even telling their partner how they felt.[4]

When you have a baby, physically speaking you are rarely alone. Yet actually it might be one of the loneliest times in your life. As Leah McClaren wrote in an article on mothering and loneliness: *'Like many new mothers, my first experience of prolonged loneliness coincided with a time in which I was rarely ever on my own, either in public or in private. It's ironic, isn't it, that the most isolated period of my life was spent with the human I loved most in the world literally strapped to my body?*[5] How true are those words? I mean, on the one hand you probably have the most physical contact with someone you will ever have in your life. But on the other? They can't muse about your day, make mundane conversation about last night's telly or comment on the latest Facebook drama.

Maybe you do feel connected to your newborn, but disconnected from everyone else. Until this point, your friendships and your relationship may have been fairly equal. You probably had shared experiences - places you liked to go, things you liked to do, your job or hobbies. These things all help with conversation. But now you've had a major change in your life and suddenly your shared experiences are far fewer. You can't talk about your latest night out, or what happened in the office today. In fact, you don't really think you can muster a straight sentence at all.

This is when the loneliness can really kick in. Maybe you're still in touch with friends. You might see your partner every night. But that emotional connection, that conversation, isn't there. You might feel lonely because you are missing your 'old' life. You miss your old routines with friends, the people you barely spoke to in the gym, or even colleagues who seemed intent on making your life difficult. This can be especially true if you had a very busy or demanding job, or one that put you in contact with lots of people day in, day out.

Don't panic - there are options and we'll look at these in a bit. For now, one really great option is to use video messaging as much as you can. I had to rewrite this paragraph as I'd initially written it before the COVID-19 pandemic. I'd talked about perhaps keeping a video connection going in the day, so you could see people even if you weren't sat talking to them. Or using online video software like Zoom to have quizzes or meet-ups. I'd worried it would feel a bit odd, but now... well, we're used to it, aren't we?

I feel like a failure needing people

Becoming a new parent can make you feel vulnerable, and that perhaps for the first time you are having to rely on other people to cope. This is difficult if you have felt in control and independent for a long time, earning your own money, sorting your own stuff out. And really, really difficult if that independence was your way of emotionally coping with bad stuff that has happened in the past - see, I don't *need* anyone... oh. It can also feel really tricky if you have a long history of being let down by people who were supposed to care for you. Relying on people might make you feel anxious.

But needing other people's support isn't any reflection on you – after all, this isn't just about you suddenly not being able to look after yourself. You have an entire new human being relying on you, and you've just gone through some major physical and emotional changes. Please, cut yourself some slack, at least for the next few months or so!

'I was really shocked at how dependent I was on other people. I wasn't expecting to 'need' people. I struggled with how dependent I was on my mum and my husband to do jobs that I felt I should be doing but didn't have the inclination to do or couldn't find the time for.'

Ami

The feeling of hating needing others is not only common, but actually has a fancy name – counter-dependency. It's the opposite of co-dependency, or relying too much on others, which you might have heard about. People who feel this way are very scared by the idea of relying on others, don't trust them, don't like asking for help and will try to keep their distance to avoid being too close and intimate with people. It's ironically sometimes linked to a fear of being rejected or abandoned, due to low self-esteem or worry you're not good enough. You make sure you do the rejecting/abandoning/not getting too close first. It often stems from a childhood that taught you to be very independent, either deliberately or through neglect. Maybe you spent a lot of time on your own, or maybe you couldn't find anyone to reliably meet your needs. Maybe you were criticised by those you loved as not being good enough or not coping well with things (despite actually coping very well indeed).

In very serious cases, support in the form of counselling may be needed to support you to work through past experiences. Counter-dependency – feeling reluctant to seek support, and that you should be able to cope on your own – is a really common feature of postnatal depression (more about this in Chapter 15). Whether this feeling leads to postnatal depression, or whether postnatal depression causes this feeling is not clear, but either way, seeking support (the irony, I know) and talking through how you feel with someone is a key first step towards starting to feel better.[6]

If you are worried about being a burden on others, or feel that you should be coping, stop! It's not just okay to need support right now – you *deserve* support right now. Support is a really important part of making sure you are healthy and well enough to care for your baby. It's like putting petrol in a car so you can drive down the road – or indeed making sure you get enough energy from your food to be able to function. I wouldn't say it's non-negotiable, as of course you can technically still cope without support, but it makes things easier. A lot easier.

So getting support is worth it then?

Yes. Absolutely! Copious research has shown that practical and social support makes life a whole lot easier as a new parent. However, as with everything, what that individual support might look like depends on you and your family and your own needs and preferences. You might find that your family and close circle offer enough support, or you might find that parenting discussions are placed in the 'do not discuss over dinner category', alongside politics, money and family skeletons in the closet. You might feel excited at the idea of going along to a new parents' support group, or you might hide under the bed at the very thought. So what might different forms of support look like?

1. Finding other new parents

Sometimes the support you need might just be finding other like-minded people. Perhaps you're the first or only new parent in your friendship group, or all your parent friends live a long way away. Of course, you can still meet up with your 'old' pre-baby friends, but sometimes they might just not get it. And they probably don't want to spend their Sunday mornings in a soft play centre. And if they are awake at 3am it's probably not for the same reason as you.

Of course, just because you've had a baby recently doesn't mean you are going to be instant friends with everyone else who has also procreated. It might mean a bit of 'shopping around' and meeting lots of new people before you click with someone. As with any friendship it's about finding stuff in common, whether that's something to do with your baby, a shared hobby, similar work or just a general outlook on life.

If you have a look online, or ask your health professional, there should be lots of local groups that you can pop along to. Perhaps baby massage, rhyme time or messy play sessions (yes, even for babies). All of these centre around stuff to do with your baby, and that's great for them, but really they're also about you and getting you in contact with other local parents. I've always thought, especially when babies are tiny and don't really mind what they do, that they should make these things more parent-friendly. Why isn't there a new parents' cocktail hour, for example, or an afternoon tea party or binge-watching box sets club? Many cinemas do have baby-friendly showings for exhausted new parents, but you're not really encouraged to chat your way through those. And actually, there are also growing numbers of fitness and exercise classes aimed at new parents if you have the energy to spare (more on these in Chapter 23).

You might prefer online options for meeting other parents – Mumsnet, Netmums and BabyCentre are all long-established communities with online forums on different topics. And they're not just for mothers either. There are plenty of men posting on there now, although there are also specific boards for dads. These websites also have 'meet up' boards where you can find local

"You can't talk about your latest night out, or what happened in the office today. In fact, you don't really think you can muster a straight sentence at all."

parents and get together if you prefer. Social media sites can also be brilliant – you can try a number and see what works for you.

There are also apps designed to put you in touch with other parents. Mush, for example, has an app that works a bit like a dating service for finding new friends in your area letsmush.com/the-app. For dads there is the 'This dad can' website www.thisdadcan.co.uk/connect, alongside the broader but very well evaluated 'Men's shed' project, which is a series of projects around the UK where men can get out and socialise, often doing something practical menssheds.org.uk. Again, stick to what works for you and don't be afraid to just lurk or indeed delete something if it's not your style.

There are also numerous drop-in groups, peer support groups and postnatal clubs run by the major parenting and breastfeeding organisations which serve as a handy way to meet new people. More on these in the sections that follow – I've put them under separate headings for organisational purposes, but that doesn't mean they are just about feeding or baby care.

Sometimes you don't need a group of people. You might feel too knackered to even think about interacting face-to-face, and if you're an introvert what you might actually crave is just some time alone. This is where parenting blogs, particularly those on social media, can really come in useful, as they can help you feel that you're not alone in your thoughts, even if you might be physically alone (and possibly quite happy about that). Many are active communities where articles are shared and discussions happen – and you might well end up meeting other local parents and becoming friends in 'real life'.

2. Professional support in caring for your baby

You may also want to find some practical support in helping you care for your baby. There are some really great organisations that provide free and paid-for support across the realms of new parenting. Many run face-to-face groups too, so you can learn and meet new people at the same time. Knowing where to find that support is the first step. Some of the best places to start include:

The NCT: The NCT (you might know this as the National Childbirth Trust) www.nct.org.uk. As well as antenatal classes, the NCT run postnatal courses, activities and meet-ups around the country (including virtual ones due to the COVID-19 pandemic, which may well continue). You can also get involved in campaigns, volunteering and even training if you'd like to. Their website is also a great source of information about caring for your baby.

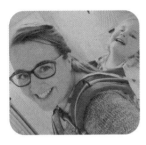

A spotlight on parenting blogs

Claire Hackett, founder of the Mummy McMumface Facebook page, talks about why she set up her parenting blog and her top tips for coping as a new parent.

Tell us about Mummy McMumface – why did you set it up?

I set up my Mummy McMumface Facebook page in March 2017. It's a bit of a lazy blog: I like just posting directly onto Facebook and getting the interaction with the people that read it. At this stage, my third baby, Nina, was three months old. However, the story began before that.

After my second child was born, in late 2013, I demented myself trying to uphold the standards I set for myself. I found it so hard to keep up with the parenting practices I had used with my eldest and struggled massively with that. On top of that, my social media had me believing that everyone else was doing better than me (which was, of course, utter nonsense).

Eventually I took a social media sabbatical which let me get perspective. Upon my return, I posted things on my own timeline relaying the bonkers stuff that would happen, such as my middle child taking a dump on the back doormat. I wanted to let other friends know that we didn't all have our shit together and people seemed to respond to it.

After a while, with the encouragement of good friends whose opinions I valued, I started the blog. My aim is still to show that not everyone has their shit together. I figure if I am feeling or experiencing something, the chances of me being the only one are fairly remote, and maybe it will help those other people to know that they aren't alone. When I got private messages from local mums after one of my first posts saying how amazing it was to hear someone else say what they were feeling, I thought there must be something in it.

The other aim is to inform. One of the things I struggled with as a new mum was knowing who to listen to – so much advice was conflicting. Discovering evidence-based information and how to use it was a huge turning point for me in my parenting journey.

However, as a breastfeeding mum and a breastfeeding supporter and advocate, I have also been extremely frustrated by the obstacles to honest conversations and information-sharing around breastfeeding. 'Making people feel bad' was to be avoided at all costs. So I want to share the information and have the conversations.

All while hopefully having a bit of craic!

I think motherhood is tough and supporting women has become my passion. I am in the process of launching a social enterprise, 'The Sisterhood of Motherhood', to enable women to access timely and appropriate support, be that seeing an IBCLC, a women's health physio or accessing hypnobirthing. After years of volunteering, I agree with Milli Hill that it is a feminist issue: mainly women volunteers are propping up a service for women. I want to see the women that give of their time and expertise knowing, and getting paid, what they're worth, and the social enterprise will also address that.

What would you say to new parents who are feeling frazzled?

1. Manage your expectations

All that fourth trimester stuff – read that. Understand what the womb-to-world adjustment will be like for your baby, and hopefully it will help you to realise that your baby isn't broken, or manipulative. You are their oasis of familiarity and safety. They know your smell, your heartbeat, the sound and vibration of your voice. Your baby will want to be close to you, and you to your baby. Understanding why will hopefully help you relax into it and shut out the voices telling you otherwise.

2. Be Elsa: let it goooo

Ok, you can't let it all go. But when it feels like everything is getting on top of you, take a minute. Think about what you can let go. Baby needs fed – you kinda need to do that. You really want a shower. The dishes need done. You haven't cleaned the poo off the couch yet. People have been texting and you need to reply.

STOP. Breathe. 'It's funny how some distance makes everything seem small...' What on that list really, actually, needs done? How much of it could you let go? Put it on a list for tomorrow. Or pass it to your partner or visitors. Which leads me to...

3. Ask for, and accept, help

I know, I know. You want to make sure everyone knows that You Have Got This. Being a mummy means doing it all yourself, doesn't it? People will think you aren't coping otherwise... not a good mummy. Except: NOPE. We all need help. We are not meant to do this alone. And apart from that, you have basically just run a marathon then been handed a baby and not had any sleep. Your body has done a lot. You are physically and emotionally adjusting. Let people tidy up. Let them leave you foil-wrapped lasagnes that you can freeze for later. Let your mother-in-law send you to bed between breastfeeds, and cook you a full meat, veg and gravy dinner for when you wake up (thanks, Maura!).

4. Don't try to return to 'normal'

Yes, it is important to still be, and feel like, you. But normal, aka your pre-baby life, is... not over, but transformed. Like a caterpillar. Still essentially the same but totally different at the same time. You can torture yourself trying to re-capture things that just can't be recaptured. Including, but not limited to, your jeans. Embrace those maternity leggings and soft nursing bras. When the time is right you will recognise the caterpillar parts of you in the butterfly.

However, I will add one caveat: mental health. It is normal to feel wibbly af-ter having a baby. Hormones are disruptive mofos at the best of times, but after birth they are rampaging through you. Add in a lack of sleep and of course you are going to have weepy/angry/wtf moments. However, if something doesn't seem 'normal' for you, please speak to someone. It has been estimated that one in five women in the UK will experience some form of mental health condition during pregnancy or the first year after birth. There is support there, through the NHS and lots of wonderful voluntary and charitable organisations.

5. Find your tribe

Yep, total cliché. But of everything, this had the biggest impact on my experi-ence of motherhood. When you feel raw, unsure of everything, in a body that feels unfamiliar, trying to keep this tiny human you love more than chocolate cake alive, having other people who can look at you and say 'I know. I get it' and you know they truly do, is invaluable. The collective wisdom of women is also important and when you have found your tribe, you can share information, dis-cuss it, argue about it, all the while safe in knowing that it will not shake your friendship. The Sisterhood of Motherhood.

6. Dry shampoo and moist toilet wipes

You are welcome.

Best Beginnings: Best Beginnings is a charity that seeks to empower new parents. They have a great website full of information about parenting, but they are most famous for their Baby Buddy app **www.bestbeginnings.org.uk**. You can download it for free and it covers lots of different aspects of caring for your baby.

Home-Start: Home-Start is a local community network of trained volunteers and expert supporters who help families with young children who are going through challenging times. If you are struggling, maybe with things such as postnatal depression, isolation, physical health issues or bereavement you may be able to access the support of a volunteer who can offer around two hours' support in your home each week. You can get in touch with your local Home-Start via the website or ask your health visitor for more information **www. home-start.org.uk**.

Sure Start: Sure Start is a council-run initiative that works in communities to offer support to parents who need it most. They are often based in areas that haven't had a lot of investment or do not have a lot of money, aiming to offer lots of opportunities to families in terms of meet-ups, baby massage and play sessions, and parenting and mental health support. The scheme has helped a lot of families. The best way to get in touch and explore what you might be able to access is through your health visitor or local council.

3. Infant feeding support

There are lots of options available if you need infant feeding support (more details in the infant feeding chapters later on). Your first port of call could be a health professional, but there are also lots of other places where you might find help and connection with other parents.

For example, the main breastfeeding charities all run breastfeeding helplines (although this name is a little misleading, as they will happily support you with formula and bottle-feeding queries too, as well as introducing solids). Don't be afraid to get in contact with any question related to feeding your baby or how you feel about it. If you look up their websites there is more information, including details of email, online chat and face-to-face support (drop-in groups or one-to-one).

- National Breastfeeding Helpline 0300 100 0212 **www.nationalbreastfeedinghelpline.org.uk**
- Association of Breastfeeding Mothers 0300 330 5453 **www.abm.me.uk**
- La Leche League 0345 120 2918 **www.laleche.org.uk**
- National Childbirth Trust (NCT) 0300 330 0700 **www.nct.org.uk**
- The Breastfeeding Network supporter line in Bengali and Sylheti: 0300 456 2421

A spotlight on social media breastfeeding support: The Breastfeeding Yummy Mummies (BFYM) Facebook support group

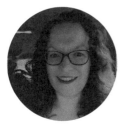

Hayley Carter (founder): I started the group Breastfeeding Yummy Mummies in March 2011 upon completion of my NHS Breastfeeding Peer Supporter training. My youngest child was just four months old and I wanted a place where my friends could come together to share breastfeeding experiences and seek support. At this time we were spread across the UK, so seeing each other face-to-face wasn't an option.

With a background in neonatal and maternity care, it has always been important to me that mothers have up-to-date, evidence-based information to help them make the best decisions for their babies and families. With that in mind, we always defer to current NHS guidance on matters affecting breastfeeding and infant safety.

The initial group members asked if they could add other friends to the group and that's how we started to grow. We soon became international and now have over 48,000 members across more than 60 countries. It quickly became clear that I would need support to maintain the group and its ethos, so I am proud to have a team of over 40 admins and moderators. Every admin and moderator is trained in infant feeding peer support as a minimum. In addition to this, many have careers in health, such as neonatal care, midwifery, nursing and health visiting and we also have two IBCLCs. This is incredibly important for the integrity of our support and for women to have trust in our group. I am extremely proud of what we have created and the support we provide to our members. I hope we can continue to support many new families in the future.

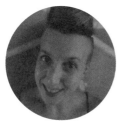

Charlotte Treitl (admin): I became an admin for BFYM about three years ago, not long after I qualified as a breastfeeding peer supporter. Facebook groups, including BFYM, were the primary source of support for me when breastfeeding became unbearable, and it was these incredible women, strangers to me, who were able to connect me to people locally who could help me with my feeding issues. It was these women I turned to when I decided to leave an abusive relationship. It was these women who sat with me in my pain and grief, day and night, as I struggled to progress through my breastfeeding journey, healing from postnatal depression and rebuilding my life. It was this community that rallied together and cheered me on at each milestone, while I established myself within a local community of breastfeeding mothers.

Supporting mums online is challenging, because you don't pick up nuances of tone or body language, and you can't reach out a gentle hand or pass them a tissue. The process of completing a feeding assessment can seem a bit more rigid because of the questions, so you have to be mindful more than ever of language and phrasing, and often spend lots of time really coaxing out the information you need to help support appropriately, by building a good rapport. The fact that BFYM is a fully evidence-based group enables us to provide support and information that empowers women to make the best decisions for themselves, and this key message remains undiluted.

I am so proud of the community we have here. Especially in difficult times or in areas where face-to-face support is scarce or non-existent, women turn to each other online to get the help they need, and I feel privileged to be entrusted to support them to continue to breastfeed, or to safely stop breastfeeding, or to hold space for them as they grieve the end of breastfeeding. Our team works together, learns from each other, and always strives to do better. To know there is this giant invisible web of kindness just waiting to hold you through your struggle is truly inspiring.

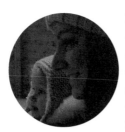 **Dawn Bond (member):** BFYM both made and saved our breastfeeding journey, repeatedly. I learned a great deal during pregnancy by reading all the evidence-based advice as other mums were given support. When I had my baby, BFYM answered my every question, supported my every wobble and met my every need. Without the group, I would have given up long ago, but here we are still going at two years! The support was invaluable and I made friends along the way. I couldn't have done it without the group and I will forever be grateful. They even inspired me to become a breastfeeding peer supporter myself. I owe our breastfeeding journey to BFYM.

Find them at **www.facebook.com/groups/BFYummyMummy**

Many of the breastfeeding organisations run peer-support groups, where breastfeeding mothers meet regularly for feeding and all-round support from trained supporters. There are also lots of local peer-support groups run by health boards, often with a health professional who oversees things. You don't have to have a problem to visit, and you don't actually have to say anything once you're there if you're too exhausted! You will find many a woman propped up in a corner, drinking tea and just feeding her baby. Many of the groups also have an online version to continue the conversation and support around the clock (someone is always awake at 3am). Ask your health professional for a list of local groups or search online.

" You will find many a woman propped up in a corner, drinking tea and just feeding her baby. "

There are also some amazing peer-support groups online and on social media. It's best to check to make sure that they are run by moderators who have training in infant feeding so you know the information and support you are getting will be evidence-based and useful. Some great Facebook support groups include:

- Breastfeeding Yummy Mummies
- Breastfeeding Younger Babies and Beyond
- Breastfeeding Twins and Triplets
- Can I breastfeed in it?

4. Mental health support

One in five of us will need support with our mental health in any given year. Never be afraid to reach out for more support (also, see Part 3). Ask your health visitor for more information on local mental health peer-support groups in your local area, where you can talk to other parents and those who have experienced difficulties in the past. This support has been shown to have positive impacts on wellbeing, but it's important to find a group that works well for you. In particular, it's important to find a group where your cultural and language needs are taken into consideration and you feel comfortable.[7]

- The PANDAS (Pre And Postnatal Depression and Support) website offers a free helpline and email support alongside support groups on Facebook. They also offer some face-to-face group support in the community. All details can be found on their website: **www.pandasfoundation.org.uk**.
- The Village is a great group on Facebook founded by psychologist Dr Emma Svanberg. Based on the wisdom that it takes a village to raise a child, the group is a supportive place to talk about the stresses and strains of being a parent. It recognises how, despite being surrounded by people all the

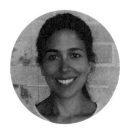

Spotlight on the Nest Club, an expert team across birth, nutrition, fitness, baby care, mental health, work and more

Meera Khanna – Founder and Director of the Nest Club
www.thenestclub.co.uk or www.instagram.com/thenestclub

What is the Nest Club?

The Nest Club is all about connecting the dots between pregnancy and parenthood. It offers expert, empowering, straight-talking antenatal education and connects parents with the postnatal care they need when baby comes along. Designed by the superstars of midwifery, obstetrics, health and wellness, it has been created for life today.

Why did you set it up?

Having experienced my own exhaustion, anxiety and despair, often thought to be just 'side effects' of motherhood, during what is meant to be one of the biggest and most exciting adventures in life, I decided there must be a better way to prepare parents for the reality of having a baby, and support them when baby comes along.

We are often sold a 'fantastical' idea of birth in antenatal education, and there is very little, if any, discussion of what comes after birth. Many women in the UK leave hospital after birth in as little as six hours and are expected to 'soldier on' with no support, so it's really no surprise that new parents often feel misled, abandoned, dismissed and broken in the first year with a new baby.

It's our mission to positively transform the approach to postnatal care and support in the UK so that recovery from birth is swifter and the experience of early parenthood is more joyful. We believe that straight talking, expert information is vital so that parents-to-be understand their rights and options. One size doesn't fit all, learning self-care is as important as baby care and crucially, we need to talk about what comes after birth in a frank and honest way: recovery from birth, mental health, pelvic floor, relationships, sex, fertility and all the sticky stuff in between. We offer local face-to-face courses, online courses and connect parents with the support that's right for them in the postnatal period.

time, parenthood can often be lonely. It offers solidarity and support from other parents, moderated by a team of volunteers. You can find it at **www.facebook.com/groups/visforvillage**.

- For broader mental health support the charity Mind has a number of articles including support for parenting when experiencing mental health issues. You can find lots of information about local support groups, their online community and helpline at **www.mind.org.uk/information-support**.
- You can find a list of local qualified counsellors on the British Association for Counselling and Psychotherapy website **www.bacp.co.uk**.

5. Tailoring a package of support online

The internet has really helped advance the support that is available for new parents, not just by provision of information and ideas, but by helping bring experts who share an ethos of parent-centred care together in one place. With a few clicks you can find and vet practitioners and mix and match yourself a package of support according to what you need and want.

However, the internet can be a bit of a jungle. Always make sure people are who they say they are – do a bit of background digging, ask for qualifications and ask around among friends for recommendations and reviews. Never be afraid to ask questions of someone before you part with money – a decent practitioner won't mind and will expect it!

There are so many options for information and support as a new parent. Don't be afraid to get in touch with any of these services, and remember, it's okay to try a few different things to find what works best for you.

What about hiring a doula?

When we talk about the importance of support in the early weeks after birth, some people will have a network of family and friends around them who might be able to provide the support they need. Others won't, either because of distance, not having the kind of relationships in which that is possible, or because they simply don't exist at all. One really great option in this situation is to consider whether hiring a doula to support you would help. Or, perhaps you do have plenty of support around you, but you would like more or different support from someone who really understands what it's like to have a new baby and how to care for a new family. Doulas are also (usually) outside of your family, so are able to focus on you and care for you without being part of any wider family politics or considerations.

You might automatically think of birth when it comes to getting support from a doula and perhaps you have already worked closely with one. If you haven't had support previously, or just think of them in a birth context, the brilliant news is that a) postpartum doulas who support you through the days,

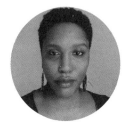

Why you might benefit from a postnatal doula

Anna Horn is a London-based postnatal doula and breastfeeding specialist with a background in maternal health research. She is one half of Every Woman Doula where she specialises in supporting vulnerable families with breastfeeding. See www.everywomandoula.co and www.annahorn.co

Birth is the day that all new parents await. How we birth our babies has an immediate and long-term impact on the health and lives of families. However, preparation for the birth and not the postnatal period is like planning for the wedding without a thought about the marriage.

Anna Horn Postnatal Doula Services arose from my own experience after the birth of my daughter. As a relatively recent immigrant to the UK, I found being away from my family and familiar customs very difficult as a new mother. My husband had to return to work very quickly and though there were visitors and support groups, I often had days when I felt isolated. My instinct was to keep my baby close, to nurse often and rest, all while recovering – leaving very little time for much else. Much like labour and birth, I needed someone who was focussed on me, my needs and what I wanted for my baby as we adjusted to life as a family. From limited paternal leave to a lack of postnatal services and living far from relatives, in many ways society leaves new families feeling vulnerable while adjusting to life with a new baby. Two and a half years later I trained to become a postnatal doula.

A postnatal doula offers practical and emotional support to families after childbirth. Every doula will arrange with the family what kind of support is needed and for how long, though usually it's about the first six weeks after birth. Doulas do not provide medical advice, but are very skilled within our remit. Services may include: infant feeding support, newborn care, cooking meals, light housework, helping with older siblings and providing companionship to a new mum. Some postnatal doulas may specialise in skills such as baby-wearing, rebozo massage, yoga and breastfeeding support. There are as many different types of doulas as there are families, so new parents are bound to find a match.

Research has demonstrated how having a doula leads to positive birth outcomes for both mothers and babies. In my experience as a postnatal doula, new parents seem to appreciate support, evidence-based information and a listening ear so that they can focus on providing love and care to their new baby. In my practice I enjoy offering very skilled breastfeeding support, cooking comfort foods and listening with an open heart to the stories of new mothers.

weeks and months after childbirth exist, and b) research and anecdotes agree about how invaluable they can be.

What do postnatal doulas do? It might be quicker to write about what they *don't* do! One study exploring mothers' perceptions of postpartum doula care found benefits to working with a doula across 11 different types of care:[8]

- Emotional support: working through birth stories, talking about experiences of being a mother and help with identifying support networks
- Physical comfort: help with breastfeeding, healing from birth, or help with finding more support for physical issues
- Self-care: helping the mother to look after herself, including sleep, nutrition and exercise alongside supporting her mental health
- Infant care: support with sleep, nutrition, safety and development
- Information: helping parents identify high-quality information and learning related to their baby
- Advocacy: supporting the family when engaging with others, i.e. medical professionals
- Referral: supporting the mother in seeking support from others, i.e. financial support or healthcare
- Partner/father support: supporting the needs of the partner and helping them support the mother
- Support mother/father with infant: teaching skills such as soothing the baby or gentle play
- Support mother/father with sibling care: helping with issues that might arise in older children on becoming a sibling, i.e. jealousy or bed-wetting
- Household organisation: support with light housekeeping, making snacks or making things otherwise comfortable

Working with a doula, you can discuss what a postnatal care package might look like. It might literally be about coming around regularly for a supportive chat. It might be more. You might have specific needs or things you want to work through. You might want support for just a few weeks, or for longer.

Research has also shown that having a doula can help with breastfeeding and infant care[9] and leave mothers feeling less anxious, more confident and more connected to others.[10] However, the impact of postnatal doula care is hugely under-researched. Given what we know about the importance of new parents feeling supported during the postpartum period, it would hardly be a surprise if more research showed more benefits.

Some places where you might find a local doula include Doula UK **doula.org. uk**, Abuela Doulas UK **abueladoulas.co.uk/your-abuela,** or through searching online. Ask lots of questions about a doula's approach and training and look for reviews and recommendations. Anyone worth their salt will be more than happy for you to do this.

Chapter two

Managing the early days

So, you're home from the hospital or birth centre, or perhaps you gave birth at home, and now everyone's gone. Maybe you are sat there just staring at your new baby as your new normal slowly dawns on you. What's next?

If you're at this stage, or reading this while planning ahead, take time to pause and think about what you ideally want to happen at this time. Do you want to jump straight into things, seeing people and being busy? Or do you feel you would benefit from time to rest, recover and get to know your tiny new person? Hint: the latter, whether you take it to mean full-on nesting with your baby or simply taking things at your own pace, can be really valuable and something that is etched into traditions and rituals in many cultures around the world. Carving out time for yourself, so you can be in charge of this special but strange period, is important. At some point soon – whether that is in the coming weeks or months – life is slowly going to return to normal, albeit a new normal, with your small person in it.

With this in mind, there are two important things to remember:

1. Your recovery comes first – you are in charge here and you matter too

2. It is absolutely okay to take time to look after yourself and get to know your baby – you are not being weird or selfish, and in most of the world this is the norm

Yes – you probably do have people clamouring to come and meet your new baby. And you can understand why. Babies, especially brand-new freshly birthed babies, are just delicious. The smell of their heads. Their tiny hands. How they fit so snugly into your one arm. It's understandable that everyone wants to turn up and get a piece of that and celebrate a new life.

But... and it's a big but. Think about what the two most important people here ideally need – you, who have grown and birthed your baby, and your baby. What do they need and want? Thinking about that from the perspective of your baby, who do they actually want to spend time with right now? The answer is you. You are their reassurance and familiarity. You are the one who smells right and tastes right. Your heartbeat and voice take them back to the womb and comfort them. And from your perspective, well – you've just had a baby. Yes, you may feel fine. You may feel elated and as if you can take on the world, albeit a little gingerly. Or you may feel far from that – shocked by birth, exhausted and stunned, and physically like you've been taken apart. Indeed, you might feel all those things at once – and more.

In many cultures around the world this time after birth is sacred and prioritised as a time of rest and recovery. Mother and baby are seen as a unit and the focus is on helping them both heal and recover from birth, with those around them coming together to support them as a unit (rather than just visit for a cuddle with the baby). There are often rituals and traditions in place for welcoming the new baby, which are often centred around strengthening the mother and making her and her baby feel special, connected and part of the community.

But in countries such as the UK, we have lost sight of these traditions and instead have the opposite: pressure to get back to normal. We see social media posts about mums out and about in the early days with everyone praising them and calling them superwoman. Maybe they are happy. Maybe it was just a quick trip out. And if that's what they wanted, then great. But many new mothers would much rather be at home, in bed, cuddling their baby or getting some rest. And that's okay too. In fact, it's more than okay! You have just grown and birthed an entire new human being. It's okay to simply say no to the pressure to be out there, sharing your baby with everyone else.

I'm not saying you should lock your door and refuse to talk to anyone or ever leave the house again (although equally if you want to do that, crack on). But think about what works for you. You and your baby and your partner if you have one are the most important people – you're a new little family. It is okay to put yourself first and to look after yourself, and to expect support and care from those who love you. This is not being selfish, or a diva, or high-

maintenance, or whatever else we label women who simply take time to care for themselves and think about their own needs. And you're certainly not a 'failure' for not being out and about showing your baby off.

But how can you make this happen, in a culture that is so focused on 'getting back out there'? This chapter looks at ways you can manage and think about these early days and weeks of life with your new baby that put you at the centre, including:

- What can we learn from different cultures?
- Planning a babymoon
- Making a postnatal recovery plan
- Dealing with visitors
- How people can help, including gifts that help you

The next chapters will then expand on this information – what to expect for your baby's development and needs, and supporting your own physical recovery and mental health.

While we're here: a short word on the second night

For some reason, the second night phenomenon is missing from many baby care books. If you're past the second night you might be reading this in hindsight and thinking '*ohhhhh, right*', but if you haven't got there yet, be reassured that your baby being much more unsettled on the second night than the first is usually absolutely normal. And it has no bearing on what your baby will be like in future.

Lots of new parents find that when their baby is first born they are still quite sleepy. They may feed fairly frequently, but immediately fall back to sleep. They may well be content to lie in their Moses basket or crib. Many people think that this is because they are recovering from the stress of being born and are tired out. It may even be an evolutionary thing to help mums rest for at least a short time after giving birth.

Then comes the second night – for many, the first night at home – and suddenly your baby starts crying lots, feeding lots and generally won't be put down. This is the point at which many new parents freak

'We had a really good birth and when she was born she was quiet and settled and I was smug that I'd created this really content baby. Then the second night hit and it was like I'd taken the wrong baby home. She screamed and cried unless I was holding her and it felt like she fed constantly. I rang a friend in tears who explained the second night to me and not to panic, but what if I hadn't phoned her? I tell everyone about it now.'

Tess

out, wondering what on earth they have done and worrying it will always be like this, while panicking about how to soothe their baby.

Think of this from your baby's perspective. Until now they have been inside you – snug, warm and with an unlimited supply of food on tap. Then birth happened, with a load of hormones and being squeezed, before they were born into a big, bright and noisy world. After a brief phase of being a bit stunned and exhausted, they suddenly realise that the constant source of everything they need has disappeared, and they aren't overly happy about that.

Breastfeeding lots and lots on that second night is not necessarily a sign that something is wrong. More details on this later, in Chapter 9, but essentially once your baby is born it is their job to kick-start your milk supply. The more they feed the more milk you start to produce, so this sudden very frequent feeding is most likely a result of that. They are not starving – they have laid down fat during pregnancy to manage the change from the first milk you produce to having a full milk supply. Have a look at Chapter 9 for checklists for making sure they are getting enough milk at this stage and making sure they are latched on comfortably and clearly feeding, and always check with your health professional if you are worried, but more frequent feeding in itself is very normal on the second night – and it is a pattern you will see again later when your baby has growth spurts and is trying to stimulate your milk supply.

The very best thing you can do to manage the second night is to recognise that this is about them needing to reclaim your warmth and comfort and that holding them and keeping them close will reassure them that you are there. This will not last forever! Hold them close to you so they can feel your heartbeat. Strip off and have some skin-to-skin time (covering them with a light blanket unless it's really warm). If you're breastfeeding, feed them as often as they want – breastfeeding is about the milk, of course, but it's also about your baby increasing your milk supply and finding comfort. Talk to your baby in a reassuring voice – they will be able to recognise it, as they could hear it when you were pregnant (babies can hear from around 20 weeks of pregnancy). Another tip is to take off any mittens you have put on them – let them feel you, or get their hands in their mouth – the contact seems to soothe them.

What can we learn about postnatal recovery from cultures around the world?

Different cultures around the world have different rituals and traditions when it comes to caring for a mother and baby after birth. One of the commonalities between them is that the period of rest and recuperation typically lasts around six weeks or 40 days, maybe a little less. The individual traditions, beliefs and support practices may differ, and are interwoven with religion and local culture, but a review of different practices from around the world found four important themes:[1]

1. Organised support

Support is given to the new mother, typically by other women – family, friends and others in the community. Older, respected women are often at the heart of this, and it might include providing support through cooking, doing chores and caring practically for mother and baby and perhaps other children.

2. A period of rest

The key bit here is that the mother is 'prohibited' from doing housework! Yes, you must not be up and about cleaning stuff and picking up after people for three to five weeks after having your baby. Family, the community and your partner do it instead. Sometimes more emphasis is put on this for your first baby. There is a belief that if you don't have this period of rest you will become unwell and age quickly – in Vietnamese culture, for example, wrinkles are believed to come from not being cared for properly during this time. In Cambodian culture you may develop 'pruey cet', which translates as a 'sad heart'. Symptoms are similar to what we would recognise as postnatal depression: unhappiness, anger and anxiety. We know that postnatal depression is more common when women are not supported and cared for. Many of these rituals from around the world make complete sense: they nurture and nourish new mothers, reducing their risk of postnatal illness and exhaustion. If only they were more common in Westernised cultures.

3. Diet

Many cultures around the world have specific foods and meals that are recommended for postnatal women, all of which seem to aim to restore certain nutrients, provide energy and be comforting. One broad concept often seen in Chinese and parts of African and Latin American culture is whether a food is considered 'hot or cold', not in the sense of temperature, but in terms of the perceived properties of the food. During pregnancy you are viewed as being 'hot' and postnatally you are viewed as being 'cold', and therefore the diet focuses on hot foods that are designed to warm you back up again. These foods are typically high in protein and energy, such as nuts or ghee, which of course would help give new mothers energy.

Foods containing lots of herbs and spices, particularly oregano, ginger, turmeric and cumin are also believed to nurture the mother. Research increasingly shows that these herbs and spices may help to protect our immune system, particularly in terms of reducing inflammation.[2] New motherhood brings a lot of stress to the body – the stress of birth, learning to care for a baby and exhaustion – which can increase inflammation.[3] Therefore, anything that brings down stress and inflammation will be beneficial.

Other foods aim to improve milk supply. In Hindu culture, for example, a mother is offered special foods such as dried fish, dahl and aubergine, which are believed to increase the quantity and quality of her milk. Whether these specifically work to increase milk supply, or just increase energy and wellbeing in the mother, indirectly boosting her milk supply, is unclear.[4]

It is important to remember that we shouldn't necessarily romanticise or adopt traditional post-birth practices. They do need to be seen in the context of the history of the culture. Confinement to the home and the involvement of family is not always positive, and can be downright harmful in cases of abuse and control. Feeding rituals that involve not breastfeeding babies in the days after birth can also negatively affect breastmilk supply. And of course, you cannot simply pick and choose customs from other cultures without thinking about how the world has generally treated those who follow the traditions in their own culture, and what it might mean from a religious or spiritual perspective for the Western world to rock up, steal those ideas and recreate them in a general way, potentially misappropriating and destroying wisdom developed across generations. What we can take from traditions, however, is the ethos – to nurture, care and involve our new mothers and babies in communities and to celebrate and look after them. The focus is on rest, recuperation and getting to know your baby while those around you care for you.

4. Hygiene and physical warmth

There are a number of different practices around bathing, sex and engagement with the mother in the weeks after birth that on the one hand look derogative, but may actually be about supporting the mother to rest. For example, in some cultures you do not invite postnatal women to visit your home, cook for you or do household chores. In others you must not be visited by men for a week or so after having your baby.

Sex is often included as not being conducive to rest in many cultures, with women being advised not to take part for three to 13 weeks after birth. Some cultures suggest that women are 'unclean' or 'polluted' after birth, and men are instructed not to have sex with them. Although this is stigmatising, and obviously complex, I wonder how much it is to do with protecting women who live in countries where males are more dominant?

Across cultures women are warned not to have cold showers or baths because it may lead to ill health. Some traditions prescribe warm baths, steam baths or sitz baths. Others encourage the mother into hot or steamy environments, possibly to help sweat out water retention. Massage also features heavily. Binding of the mother's abdomen is thought to support her recovery.

The central role and value of the mother

In all of this, a key feature of postnatal care around the world is that the mother is at the centre. Traditions and rituals are based around her. She is given time to heal and recover. The community cares enough to give her their time, love and resources. All of the elements discussed above, and this strong emphasis on maternal care, are thought to be why postnatal depression is not as common in some other cultures (although certainly not all, and in fact it may just be labelled and treated differently). You can certainly see why, in cultures where women are valued, surrounded by others and cared for, giving them time to rest, their mental health would be better![5]

What might postnatal recovery look like for you?

Not everyone wants the same type of postnatal recovery. Your ideal will be based on your needs and preferences and what support can practically be put in place. Maybe you are really extroverted and thrive on other people's company and energy... or maybe you reenergise best alone. Maybe you are at your best when in your own home, alone with time to just be... or maybe you thrive on getting out and about. Maybe you have family you adore and will help you... or maybe you'd rather chew off your right arm than have family round.

What you can implement will depend on the resources you have around you. It's all very well to look at the Goan practice of regular massages and think 'I'd like that please', but of course you need someone to give it. So think about what you might like to happen, and consider how variations of it might work in your circumstances. You could suggest a gift certificate for a massage as a postnatal present. Your partner could brush up their massage skills, or a friend or doula might know how to do a head massage. Or you could take some time to relax with some oils yourself. Self-massage can be very healing.

Try having a babymoon

No, not the travel industry version, which is promoted as an expensive holiday before having a baby (it's possibly too late for you to do this, although if you have chance, crack on), but the one where you have your own private little holiday with your baby... in your own bed.

The idea of a babymoon is basically to lock your front door (apart from when accepting takeaways and helpful gifts) and concentrate on you and your new baby, doing whatever it takes to help you feel rejuvenated and restored (or at least a little bit). It could last a day or a week or whatever. Now I know this isn't for everyone. You might be an outdoors-loving extrovert who shudders at the very idea, but at least give it some thought. It's about protected time, a slow pace and getting to know your baby. You might make it work for you just by declaring afternoons to be babymoon time.

What might a babymoon look like?

- You getting lots of rest, perhaps in bed or on your sofa or in your garden if it's sunny – wherever you feel comfortable
- Lots of skin-to-skin with your baby, getting to know one another – you might find that with the calm slow pace they spend lots of time asleep on you

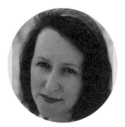

The importance of postnatal care and making a postnatal recovery plan

Sophie Messager, antenatal educator, doula and author of *Why Postnatal Recovery Matters*.

How did you become particularly interested in postnatal recovery?
I was a biology research scientist for 20 years. What led me to choose this first career was intense curiosity. This is still an inherent part of me, so when I retrained as an antenatal educator and doula, I found myself reading avidly around the topic of how we can best support women after they have had a baby and asking questions of all the pregnant and new mothers I met. One particular topic that piqued my curiosity was the way we treat mothers after birth.

After training in a traditional postnatal massage technique known as 'closing the bones', which involved the use of a scarf to rock and bind the new mother's pelvis, I started asking every mother I met, especially if they weren't from the UK, if there was something similar in their culture. I was amazed to find that similar practices (in particular the use of wrapping during the postpartum) were present on every continent and that these practices were all designed to support the mother and aid her recovery both physically and emotionally. This led me to read more and more, both to support my practice as a doula and to write my book.

In your conversations and reading about cultural practices around the world, what particularly struck you in terms of comparisons to the UK?
I found that in most cultures, the new mother is dispensed from doing any work or chores for about a month after the birth, and that family and the community rallies round to ensure this happens. The new mother does nothing but rest and get to know her new baby. She is fed nourishing foods, and the household is entirely taken care of. But most importantly she is never alone and is surrounded by experienced mothers who help her build her confidence. This seemed so different to many new mothers' experiences in the UK today, but actually my research revealed that such practices used to be the norm in the UK too.

Do you think this period of rest and care is important?
Absolutely! As a doula and antenatal educator, I have been dismayed by what I see happen to new mothers in the UK. What do we get here? Two weeks' paternity leave and then you're on your own, trying to meet your own needs,

those of your newborn, and those of everyone else in your household. Not only are new mothers not receiving any practical support, but they are also under immense pressure to 'return to normal' as soon as possible, and even shamed for failing to do so. It is very telling that almost every present a new mother receives is for the baby. This led me to want to start a campaign to revive postpartum care in the UK.

The lack of care is not only damaging to new mothers and society as a whole, it's frankly ridiculous when you look at the tremendous changes that happen to a mother's body when she grows and births a baby, and then needs to undergo these changes in reverse. It's crazy that there is no process in place to help support her recovery. Heck, even marathon runners take a week or two of R&R after a big event! If men gave birth, there would be a Cambridge professor of postpartum science, as well as specialist postpartum physiotherapy treatment available as standard for all on the NHS.

This is why I wrote my book – to encourage the return to a more supportive postpartum culture, and making it feasible in a culture that doesn't include extended families.

What would be your message to pregnant and new mothers (and those that support them) who are reading this?

I suggest that pregnant women plan for the postpartum and write a postnatal recovery plan, so that they have support in place and can have a more positive experience. The plan might include what I think of as the four tenets of postpartum recovery: rest, food, bodywork and social support. Under each of these headings you can plan things like what you would like to see happen, who will help, how you will get rest and where you might get food from and so on.

What might a postpartum recovery plan look like? What sorts of things might people include?

You might write your plan as a bullet point list, or you might find it easier to write it as a mind map or spidergram. Here are some ideas you might like to include and discuss with those who might support you.

Rest

- Help with the household (chores, cooking, cleaning, other children). Make a list of potential helpers. In particular sit down with your partner and separately write a list of all the chores and who normally does them.
- Visitors. List them/how to manage them so they do not interfere with rest (and also explain your expectations: visitors should come to support you rather than expecting to be entertained). Suggest they bring you a casserole, or help by doing the dishes.

- Naps/sleep when the baby sleeps/early nights/sleep with your baby.
- Relaxation: techniques and apps.

Food
- Batch cook and freeze.
- List who can make/bring you some/meal deliveries from friends.
- Deliveries (supermarkets, takeaway meals, frozen, fresh, meal boxes).
- Stock up on nutritious non-perishable snacks.
- Use a sling so you have your hands free to fix yourself some food if alone.

Bodywork
- Postnatal massages or 'closing the bones' ceremony.
- Seeing specialist manual therapists such as osteopaths, chiropractors, and physiotherapists.
- Wrapping your pelvis/abdomen with a scarf or velcro wrap.
- Keeping warm.

Social support
- Friends, family, neighbours. Make sure the people who help you are supportive and not judgy.
- Hired help (doulas, nannies, cleaners...).
- Online support (social media groups, WhatsApp groups...).

Remember that your list is flexible. You can add things to it or change your mind depending on your birth and how you feel after having your baby.

- Quiet thinking time, or talking to your partner about your experiences so far, or chatting by text with friends while you relax – again, whatever works for you
- Lots of binge-watching TV, listening to audio books, or reading (one-handed)
- Your partner being in charge of meals, lots of easy-to-eat nutritious snacks or family and friends organising a meal rota
- Perhaps a visit from a massage therapist or reflexologist, or your partner brushing up on their skills

Babymoons are often recommended if you are having difficulty getting to grips with breastfeeding (see Chapter 9). Spending just a couple of days without lots of clothes on, keeping your baby skin-to-skin and focusing on your rest and recovery can really help boost your milk supply while you both get the hang of it.

What about visitors?

It's only natural that once your baby is here and you are settled at home people close to you are going to want to visit and see the baby. There are certainly no hard and fast rules, or one best way that will suit everyone, but thinking about what you want (and being open to that changing, perhaps daily!) can help manage other people's expectations.

Some top tips:

- It is absolutely fine to 'manage expectations' and suggest specific times that people arrive and leave. There is no need to explain this, but if you're someone who needs to, no one will argue if you tell them you've been up all night, are in pain or are struggling after a difficult birth.
- Remember that you are the one who has just had a baby and you are recovering. Think like a 'hospital patient', especially if you haven't had a straightforward delivery (or even if you have). Would you be jumping up and down making cups of tea and running round after visitors if you'd just had any other kind of operation? No. So sit down. A perfectly reasonable follow up to asking someone if they would like a cup of tea is to give them instructions on where to find the kettle and whether you want milk or sugar.
- If visitors ask 'Is there anything I can do to help?' don't be a martyr and say no. Have a list ready: the washing up, feeding or walking the dog, hanging some clothes out to dry – and don't be afraid to use it. Likewise, if anyone asks if there's 'Anything you need me to bring?' – tell them! In fact, don't hesitate to suggest these things before they ask. If they want to see the baby, they can pop into the shops on the way, or do the washing up for 10 minutes while they're with you, can't they (assuming they are healthy and able-bodied)? For a fuller list, see the 'Ways people can help' section coming up.
- Ask for the baby back whenever you want – especially if you are breastfeeding. Visitors are probably going to want to hold your baby. It's absolutely fine to say no to this in the first place – or you may be grateful to get your arms back for even a moment. But if your baby starts wanting to feed, or you simply want them back, say so. It's really important, especially in the early days if you're breastfeeding, to feed your baby whenever they want feeding – and for this not to be delayed by your mother-in-law refusing to give the baby back.
- Conversely, maybe you really welcome someone holding the baby for you or even taking them out for a short walk while you have a nap. Visitors can wear a baby in a sling too. Don't feel you have to personally 'host' your guests if you'd rather take the opportunity to catch up on sleep or just stare into space for a bit.
- Think about how soon you want visitors after the birth. Maybe you will welcome everyone as soon as possible. Maybe you will have close family briefly after the birth and then a few days to yourself. Maybe you would prefer to wait a few days to settle in to being a new little family.

- Don't be afraid to have certain rules for one person and different ones for another. Some people you might have happily stay all day while you lounge about half-dressed, but others you might want out the door after 20 minutes. Some people will be overbearing, while others will quietly look after you.
- Remember you can change your mind at any time. You may be bouncing around on top of the world after having your baby... or things might not have gone to plan and you are feeling very vulnerable – physically, emotionally or both. This may mean you welcome the whole neighbourhood with open arms, or it might mean you feel like seeing barely anyone at all. And that can change from day to day.
- If you have a partner, put them in charge of visitors. They can be a bouncer, throwing people out when they overstay their welcome or stopping them from coming in the first place if you simply don't want them to, or there is a reason they shouldn't, such as they're unwell (yes, really, some people will try this).
- Make the most of technology. If you don't feel like you can face people in real life, think about whether they can video call, either to chat to you or simply stare at the baby.

We talk a lot about too many visitors after the birth, but it may be that you end up feeling that you aren't really seeing anyone. Some people will not want to intrude, or will want to wait for an invitation from you, and crossed wires can leave you all alone and wondering where everyone went. Others may assume you will be inundated with visits from close family, not realising that maybe you aren't that close to your family, either physically or emotionally. Don't be afraid to tell people you need company.

What about baby gifts?

This is one that will naturally divide opinion. Some may feel that a gift is a gift chosen by the giver. Some may prefer no gifts. Some may be more comfortable asking for specific things. If you are happy asking for specific things, have a think about what you might actually want. There are all sorts of gift registries you can set up, or you can simply share ideas with family and friends.

One key thing to think about is how useful the gifts you are requesting will be. Tiny babies grow quickly. You might be someone who likes pretty things and a bunch of flowers is a huge pick-me-up. Or you might have hayfever and much prefer nutritious (or not so nutritious) snacks. Remember it's okay to ask for gifts that suit *you*. Your baby is tiny and will have no idea about gifts for a very long time. It's okay to ask for stuff that helps you temporarily, like food or a cleaning service. It doesn't have to be things that you have to treasure forever. In fact, stuff that gets you through the early days and weeks can be the best gifts someone can ever give you *and* your baby. I find it very strange that everyone turns up with gifts for the baby – who spends their life being pampered and cared for! – when it's the mother or the parents who have had their life turned upside down and could do with all the support and care possible. Let's try and start a revolution: baby gifts are for those caring for the baby.

Here are some suggestions for the most useful and least useful gifts, based on a highly scientific marketing research exercise (I asked on Facebook). Feel free to disagree – see 'the great muslin cloth debate' that ensued, described below. The list can basically be summarised as 'food and care good', 'gimmicky stuff bad'.

Brilliantly useful

- An insulated mug so hot drinks don't go cold
- Luxury (or sensitive) hand wash and cream as you'll wash your hands more
- An extendable fork (so you can hold baby and reach food)
- A sling of the mother's choosing
- Nappies and wipes (especially larger sizes or cloth if parents prefer that)
- A meal delivery service – or delivered meals you can pop in the oven
- Supermarket or takeaway vouchers
- Snacks – healthy and otherwise, especially stuff she couldn't eat in pregnancy
- Cleaning – a paid-for service or someone gives their time to you regularly
- Books and DVDs (or a Netflix subscription)
- A voucher for a postnatal doula or lactation consultant

Thrown in the back of the cupboard

- Things with 'my baby's first' on it that were impractical
- Pamper stuff that takes a long time (when she doesn't have any)
- Snow suits (appears to depend on your climate!)
- Top and tail bowl
- Tiny baby clothes that they grow out of immediately or are impractical
- Flowers (depending on how many you get), especially if allergic
- Photo frames
- Any 'big' things that might not be used, e.g. changing table, cot
- Teddies, comforters or other toys that just won't get used
- Bottles (if she's breastfeeding)
- Presents for older children that require her assistance

The great muslin cloth debate

Alongside these great and not-so-great gift suggestions, an entire discussion was had on the benefit of muslin cloths (that was *not* how I envisaged my Saturday afternoon going!). For me (and many others) you can never have too many of these wondrous things. Others were confused and never used them. The key variable seemed to be how much your baby was sick or drooled. Lovely. However, the general consensus was that they made a lovely gift because of their potential use for a million and one other things, including:

- To stop baby sick getting on your clothes
- Wipe up any spill from your baby
- Use underneath them when changing if changing mat is cold
- Drape them strategically if you're feeling a bit self-conscious breastfeeding
- If you are breastfeeding and have a fast milk flow, or dribbly baby, tuck them over your lowered bra cup to prevent it getting soggy
- Use them as a lightweight cover in a pram (never drape anything over a pram or buggy to protect from the sun, as this can lead to very high temperatures underneath)
- They can even be used as an emergency piece of clothing or a nappy if your baby has had a nappy explosion when out
- A cool swaddle
- A light protection when they're sleeping on you and you're trying to eat over their head
- Useful for wiping up spills with older children

Ways in which people can give their time

Some people will be unable to buy a gift for you but may want to help in other ways. Others might want to give their time rather than buy something that might not be used. Here is a list of suggestions to use if anyone asks 'Can I help?' or 'What would you most like as a present?':

- Cooking meals or setting up a meal donation rota
- Housework: washing up, cleaning, sorting out dirty clothes, changing beds, dealing with all the flowers people have inevitably sent you
- Going to the shops or arranging deliveries for you (and putting it away!)
- If you can't drive yet, driving you to appointments or just getting you out of the house
- Coming to appointments and advocating for you
- Looking after older children or pets
- Popping your baby in a sling and holding them while you nap
- Helping with inevitable paperwork or finding out information
- Sitting and listening, or just being with you with no expectation of conversation
- Giving you a shoulder massage, foot rub or pedicure
- Returning gifts for you
- Organising other people to do these things

It's okay to put yourself first. Never forget that or let anyone else tell you otherwise.

Chapter three

Looking after yourself once everything goes back to 'normal'

→ We looked at the idea of postnatal recovery in the last chapter – specifically making a plan and taking time to rest and recover after the birth. But gradually you will heal, your baby will grow and the visitors and rush of the newborn phase will melt away.

This doesn't mean that things become a walk in the park for you, and the rest of your leave or time with your baby is an extended holiday. You're still adjusting to being a new parent, probably not getting a lot of sleep, feeding seemingly all the time and generally feeling as if all of your energy and time is spent caring for someone else rather than being able to focus on your own needs. Time to yourself might seem like a distant memory. New and growing babies are exhausting and there always seems to be something that needs to be done.

However, if at all possible, try and carve out some time to focus on yourself for a bit. It's the old analogy of putting on your oxygen mask first on a plane before helping others because you're no use to them if you're collapsed in a heap on the floor. And more importantly – you don't *deserve* to be collapsed in a heap on the floor – you are important too.

47

Rest? I feel like I don't get anything done all day?!

This is another really common feeling, especially if you had a fast-paced lifestyle or job before you had a baby. It's exacerbated by the media screaming at us that we should be 'getting our lives back' and acting like nothing has changed (even though you now have a tiny new person depending on you). People play along on social media, posting their best bits: trips out, upcycling, sourdough – ignoring the days when they were collapsed, quietly crying, on the sofa.

Suddenly it feels like you're not 'accomplishing' anything at all. I mean, what changes during the course of the day? What did you produce? What goals did you meet? Well, nothing much really... apart from keeping a whole brand new human being alive all day! Be kind to yourself. You are absolutely 'getting something done' – you are getting *so* much done. And if you had the time to stop and make a diary of it you would see it. And if you didn't do it, you would all *really* notice straightaway.

Babies take up a lot of time. They need someone else to meet or help them meet all their needs. You're feeding and soothing. Cleaning and changing. Rocking and swaying. Throughout the day and night, alongside all the other things that need to be done to keep life ticking over. Buying the nappies. Planning the shopping. Keeping things going. Even when they're sleeping you often have to hold them. And that's before we even get to all the additional thinking, planning and general worrying. And you're doing it all on fractured sleep.

All these things are so important. The fact that you can't leave a baby at home all day on their own should tell us that! The problem is not that you don't 'do' anything, but rather that society, for some ridiculous reason, doesn't seem to *value* the things you do. They're not part of paid employment, and therefore aren't counted in productivity and the increasing wealth of the country. I bet if they were, mothers would be seen as vital. Instead we are often unseen and undervalued.

If you added up what it would cost to employ someone to do what you are doing, day in, day out, you'd get a very different perspective. A nanny costs £10–£15 an hour. Multiply that by 24 hours a day, seven days a week, 52 weeks of the year and you've got a 'salary' of £80,000–£120,000 a year. But a nanny wouldn't be expected to do everything that you do – they don't sort out your car insurance, or remember your family's birthdays. In fact, estimates of what a full-time stay-at-home parent is worth to a family come in at around £160,000 a year! No, that's not a typo – it's what it would cost to pay someone else to do all the stuff you do.[1] And that's before you add in any production of breastmilk. Norway actually includes breastfeeding in its gross domestic product, valuing it at around $907 million USD.[2]

Of course, caring for a baby can't be reduced to figures. It's not a job in the traditional sense, in that you love and are biologically programmed to care for your baby. But it does show the unpaid value of the 'work', and therefore the importance of looking after the 'staff' (that's you). I'm saying that tongue-in-cheek, but seriously, think of some of the perks employees of good organisations get – time off, healthcare, gym passes and even massages – because their employer recognises the importance of healthy and happy (aka productive) employees. Why not pretend you're a brilliant boss and invest in your 'company'!

So never feel guilty about not doing enough. You are doing more than enough. If you want to read more, Naomi Stadlen has written a beautiful short book called *What mothers do: especially when it looks like nothing.* I really recommend it.

> 'I remember feeling guilty and frustrated that I wasn't "doing" anything useful/productive. I hear a lot of new mothers say this, and usually reframe it by saying that they are keeping a vulnerable new human being alive all by themselves, and that's the most important task there is.'
>
> <u>Sophie</u>

Self-care?

You'll see a lot of articles written about the concept of self-care for new parents. On the one hand, this is great: permission to take time to put yourself first and look after your needs. Brilliant. This is really important. However, on the other hand I am wary of the phrase, as it can make it seem as though it is *your* responsibility to make sure you look after yourself and therefore your fault if you don't, without recognising that there are a million and one different reasons why new parents might *not* be able to take the time and space to focus on self-care. Thinking back to the cultural traditions we looked at in the last chapter, the onus isn't on the mother to go out and find care or look after herself, it's about everyone else supporting her. And that to me is just as important as the support they give – it's the fact that *someone else* has taken the time to look after you that matters.

'Self-care' also seems to suggest that if only you would take the time to have a massage or whatever, all your other problems would just disappear. It subtly tells us that a massage, a walk in the sunshine or a pedicure can fix the real problem – a lack of support, a lack of community and a lack of value in society because you're not making money. No amount of sunshine is going to fix the fact that you're sleep-deprived and no one is there to help.

There is also an underlying suggestion that it is up to you to make time for self-care on top of everything else you have to manage. You're exhausted, you're physically recovering, you're juggling everything... and now you have to organise a massage, when it's all the steps involved in organising the massage that mean you need it in the first place! You need to find a place, find a time, find the money, make an appointment, sort out who will have the baby, maybe express milk, travel... it's exhausting. What you really need is for someone to organise a massage at your house at a time when you will be relaxed and come and hold the baby for you while it happens. But instead of encouraging that, society just tells you that you 'need to look after yourself'. All this is brilliantly summed up by Erin Pepler in her article for *Today's Parent* 'The pressure for moms to prioritize self-care is a bunch of BS'.[3]

So firstly, communicate what you need to those around you. When people ask what they can do to help, tell them. Tell your partner what you need, whether they ask or not. There is a great line in Michelle Obama's documentary *Becoming* (do watch it if you can) when she says that she learned as a new mother not to get angry at Barack for going to the gym when their babies were small, but instead work out how she was going to go too. To generalise for a moment, men are much better at taking time for themselves when babies are small. Don't get angry, get equal and get that time for yourself too.

Secondly, you're going to need to put some plans in place to make sure it happens. In reality, without a major cultural revolution, a lot of new parents will find that after the early days and weeks have passed, unless they explicitly make time for themselves and ask others for support it won't happen. Although we need to keep fighting for the world where it does, for now we need a compromise. Ask for help. Work out how it can happen. Never feel guilty for asking, but equally never feel guilty for not being able to do it. If you don't have time for yourself, it's other people's fault, or society's fault. Not yours. We should be nurturing our new parents, not leaving them to fight for any downtime at all.

So, take the time to think about what you need and would like. What would help you feel human again? What support might you need to make that happen? This will look different for everyone, based on their own circumstances, needs and desires. But here are some things to think about:

1. What might space for you look like?
Sometimes, all you need is a bit of space to feel like you again. What that space is will completely depend on you and what makes you feel rejuvenated. What gives you energy? Who gives you energy? Where gives you energy?

- Will you be doing something? Do you get energy from a set activity and sense of purposefulness? Or do you get energy from doing absolutely nothing? Can you relax if you do nothing? Or do you need something to occupy your mind or body? Is sleep a priority, or doing something that reminds you of yourself?
- Will you be around other people? You might feel like you need time on your own in relative silence to relax and reenergise. Others might find that they thrive being around other people, as long as the weight of just being their

baby's parent is lifted.

- Will you be around your baby? You might feel that you need to be separated to regain energy. Or you might feel that you can't relax when away from them, that you can't be separated for long, or you have no one who will take them. If so, where could you go where someone else could hold the baby or take care of you?
- How long will you need? Do you need short bursts every day? Or do you prefer a longer session less often?

Sorry, that was a lot of questions for an exhausted brain, wasn't it? But they are questions you might like to think about. There is no right answer for everyone – just a right answer for you. And even that might change from day to day or as your baby grows. You might need a mixture of all of the above.

2. Carve out time for yourself

Obviously the most practical challenge to overcome when you have a new baby is making sure they are taken care of while you have time for yourself. How could that work?

- Talk to your partner so that you both have protected time to do whatever you want. This time should, as far as possible, be equal – although you may negotiate between yourselves that some things take longer than others or one of you is happy with a little less time as long as your needs are being met. Maybe you need regular shorter bursts and they need a long single burst. More on this in the relationships chapter, but ideally you would have a pattern in which both of you get some time alone to do (within reason!) what you want. This can be a challenging conversation, especially if your partner thinks their commute is close to hell and you think it sounds like a relative spa break. Keep talking.
- Take up friends' and family's offers of help. This obviously works better if you are close by. But how will you make it work? Will they come to you while you go out? Hold the baby while you have a nap or walk? You go to them for a change of scene and time off from being the one in charge (and a nap)? Meet for a coffee with the understanding that they will jiggle the baby while you drink yours hot?
- If neither of the above work, how about finding support elsewhere? Can you work with a doula, so they watch or cuddle or sling your baby while you have a bath or nap? Could you pay for some childcare support? A morning a week at a childminder or with a childcare student? Yes it costs money, but if you can afford it, see it as an investment in your health and your family. Rest is important. Alternatively, do you know anyone in your neighbourhood who you trust and would love to spend a few hours with your baby even if you're close by? A responsible teen? An older person

without grandchildren nearby? If you have little money to spare, is there another way you could support each other – doing shopping, baking, dog walking, having your partner be a handyperson (not for gendered reasons, but more time reasons – if, for example, you're breastfeeding, it's difficult to fix someone else's dripping tap at the same time).

- Another solution is to team up with friends with small children so that you watch theirs and they watch yours. You might all stay in the same house, and one of you has a bath or nap or whatever. Or one of you goes out. Or one of you takes the other's baby out for a walk in the pram or sling.

3. It doesn't have to be time away from your baby if you don't want that

'I felt a lot of pressure to leave my baby before I was ready. "It's good for you" they said. Nothing about it felt good. I cried all the way to the gym, burst into tears during the class, left to go collect him and didn't leave him again until I was ready. He was four months at the time and I didn't leave him again until he was closer to 10/11 months.' <u>Ami</u>

As we've said, it may be that for whatever reason you don't feel you can be away from your baby, or don't have anyone suitable to take care of them. You do not have to justify this. Maybe you feel less anxious with your baby close. Maybe they feed lots. Maybe it's not your baby that you find difficult, but more the lack of adult company. There are still many ways you can get a break – or at least a change of scene (never underestimate the power of that) – while your baby is still with you.

'The friends I made at Australian Breastfeeding Association meetups helped me understand that I didn't have to leave my baby behind to get that headspace/time to relax. We would gather at one or other of our homes, day after day and just not be alone. We would bring our washing and do it all together and often one of us would make or prep dinner for the two or three families of the mums gathered to take home. Older kids would play together. It was incredibly normalizing of the chaos that is parenting in the newborn trenches.' <u>Nina Jane</u>

'I adored going to La Leche League meetings. There was always a mum of an older baby or a baby-obsessed home-schooled preteen or a Leader there who would take my baby and bounce them so I could sink into the couch and just absorb what was going on at the meeting.' <u>Ruth</u>

You could also take a different approach, by looking at what day-to-day tasks other people could support you with (or you could just ignore them completely – I'm convinced once you have one layer of dust it doesn't grow *that* much). If you know your baby tends to sleep for a few hours straight in the evening, but you don't really benefit because you're running round cleaning or cooking or whatever, could anyone support you by doing those things so you get some free time? Options might include:

- Your partner taking on a bigger share of household stuff because you're the one feeding the baby or up more in the night or not getting any headspace.
- Friends or family having a cleaning or cooking rota for you.
- Hiring help (paid over the living wage) to support you. This makes a great gift or way of practically helping a new family that lives a distance away. Make use of local teenagers who are keen to earn money.
- Sharing batch cooking with a friend with a new baby. You each cook large portions and help fill up each other's freezer.
- Finding a good, healthy takeaway delivery or meals delivery service.

What might self-care look like?

So you've worked out *how* self-care might happen, but then the big question is what might it actually look like? It is likely that you would benefit from care that supports you both physically and emotionally. Think back to before you had your baby (yes, I know it feels like a lifetime ago). What did you enjoy doing? What relaxed you? The same things may or may not work so well now, or it may be a while before you can do them – like taking off for a long weekend in some distant city, or going on a rock-climbing expedition. Again, take time to listen to yourself and what your body needs.

You might know exactly what you need, but if not, here is a list of ideas from other new parents. Often it might not be the thing you are doing that matters most, but the fact that you are doing it at all.

1. *Box sets, or favourite programmes that I'd watch when they slept. I'd refer to them as 'my programme'. For instance, if my child didn't sleep for a day I'd moan that I didn't get a chance to watch 'my programme' that day. What it meant was I didn't get a chance that day to switch off and not worry if my child was about to jump off anything etc. When they were asleep I could zone into another world. I'm sure reading does that for many too.* Sophie

2. *Husband taking baby when they woke first thing after a feed so I could have an hour of sleep, literally a life saver!* Clare

3. *Thirty minutes alone for a hot bath and a cup of tea (while in that bath!) is phenomenal.* Asha

4. *Any exercise that made me sweat and worked my muscles. It felt like I was using my body for me again and showing it could do something else other than feed and carry a baby.* Jodie

5. *Weird to some people but I found it relaxing to wash, hang, fold and prep nappies (cloth nappies). Also sort of felt like I did it for the baby... I suppose it's some sort of mindfulness?* Claudia

6. *I NEEDED to go to our local farmers' market for one hour every Saturday morning. I would go buy broccoli, sit with a coffee and my notebook and write out all my whinges. I realised pretty soon that if I missed that Saturday hour (visitors, illness, hubby's work etc), I'd get really very depressed from Tues/Wed the next week. I started to view it as 'my work', a necessity that everyone had to work around in order for me to survive.* Johanna

7. *Walking. Two littlies in the double pram, one blissful half-hour of silence, and we'd get home and nobody would have trashed the house. It was like a reset button. I also remember one epic excursion to the museum. I took them swimming in the morning, to get them nice and tired, and then I walked the pram around the museum until both were asleep (they were 10 months and 2.5 years) and then the moment they had both nodded off, I raced into the museum to see this exhibition. Went through the whole thing rocking the pram to keep them asleep. It was a memorable day not because of the exhibition itself, although Queen Victoria's undercrackers were very interesting, but because the whole day was about putting my needs first.* Kath

8. *I love knitting. I just really, really love it. Nothing gives me more pleasure than knitting something for my babies. The counting and steady rhythm works wonders for clearing my head and it means that I actually sit still. It gives me a sense of achievement that I don't get with the endless task of running a household and I feel immense pride when people compliment my children's clothes. Because I'm knitting for them I don't feel guilt or like I should be doing something more productive with my time. I can just be.* Ami

For some more ideas, the *Little Book of Self-care for New Mums* by Becky Hands and Alex Strickland is a lovely book with lots of ideas for looking after yourself physically and emotionally in the months after birth.

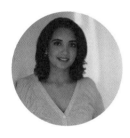

How to take care of yourself when you're short on time and energy

Avni Trivedi is a women's health and paediatric osteopath and birth doula. She can be found at www.avni-touch.com.

It goes without saying that your physical and mental health are vital, especially in the early weeks of motherhood. But it's easier said than done isn't it? How are you supposed to tend to your baby, take care of yourself and all the chores and responsibilities in your life? Enjoy every moment and sleep while the baby sleeps, do your pelvic floor exercises and be a picture of 'having it all'?!

What's true is that your physical and mental health is vital, and that this is a time with conflicting priorities, where resources may be feeling rather thin. The fourth trimester is an extension of pregnancy and is often rushed through or not recognised.

In my work as a women's health and paediatric osteopath, I am lucky to have the time to listen to clients and hear about their personal situation. Some struggle to feed themselves the right foods as by the time they have prepared a meal, the baby needs a feed or change. Others find it hard to do something for themselves, as they feel guilty and think they should put all their attention into their newborn. I do my best to offer solutions that will work for their situation.

I created an approach called 'The Intuitive Way to Wellness' to help people to connect with their body in ways that feel good and don't take up time or energy. The feel-good, self-care aspect is necessary because we aren't robots who can be programmed to eat the right foods and move in an aligned way. I focus on the aspects that make us feel connected to ourselves, in the fullness of who we are. The things that give us joy and calm. And that starts by listening to ourselves as the body knows what's right for us.

Here are five tips to take care of yourself when you're short on time and energy:

- Turn everyday activities into a self-care ritual. That might mean a cup of tea while sitting and doing nothing else, or making shower-time feel decadent.

- Express your emotions each day. Have a good cry, dance and move or journal to let go of the emotions that build each day. You'll feel lighter in yourself.
- Connect with your senses. An essential oil diffuser can instantly change your mood, such as peppermint to feel more awake and cedar wood to feel more steady. Fresh mint or ginger tea for your taste buds, and soothing music for your ears.
- Ask for and accept help. You don't have to be the one that does everything. Perhaps your partner can place jugs of water around your home so you're always in reach of a drink, or run you a bath so the only thing you have to do is get in. Loved ones can prepare easy-to-heat meals or take your baby for a walk while you have a quiet moment. Or a postnatal doula or food delivery service can support you in the early weeks.
- Rest even if you don't think you need to. We don't value rest enough, as it's not as seen as productive. Even five minutes of lying on your bed, sofa or floor with your eyes closed and your hands free will give your nervous system a moment to breathe.

If you're interested in the Intuitive Way to Wellness: www.avni-touch.com/the-intuitive-way-to-wellness
Speak From the Body podcast: podcasts.apple.com/gb/podcast/speak-from-the-body/id1473722377

What about being creative?

There is lots of research to show how restorative being creative can be.[4] Whether that is making art, music, singing, writing... whatever. Art uses the body and mind in a way that is gentle and calming. It can actually help you focus on what you want, rather than your mind whirring – some people find that they can concentrate better on what people are saying if they knit (at least that's what they tell me when they do it during my talks!).

You don't need experience of doing art to benefit, or any great talent. It's about time to yourself and being creative, not winning the Turner prize. Look around in your local area – I bet there are all sorts of classes or sessions you could try, either with or without your baby. Jewellery-making, weaving, painting... there will be something to suit you. For inspiration see our spotlight on creative journaling on the next page.

Key message? Oh, it's the same as the last chapter – remember you matter too.

Further reading

Some books your might enjoy about taking care of yourself include:

- *Why Postnatal Recovery Matters* - Sophie Messager
- *The Fourth Trimester: A Postpartum Guide to Healing Your Body, Balancing Your Emotions, and Restoring Your Vitality* - Kimberly Ann Johnson
- *Life After Birth: A Parent's Holistic Guide for Thriving in the Fourth Trimester* - Diane Speier

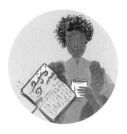

Spotlight on creative journaling: the Maternal Journal movement

Laura Godfrey-Isaacs is a mother of two daughters, an artist and midwife. She's gone through many experiences as a mother that include miscarriage, premature birth, and a baby separated from her in the neonatal unit. She has also learned so much through supporting her younger daughter, who is deaf and has specific learning difficulties. As a practising midwife in London, she meets people on a daily basis who are finding pregnancy, birth and building families challenging, particularly if they have a history of mental health issues.

Sam McGowan has one young son and was pregnant when she took a pilot workshop organised by Laura. She loved the concept and immediately felt the benefits. With a background as a content producer working on global creative campaigns to support women and girls and human rights, she felt inspired to join the team and help others create their own Maternal Journal.

What is Maternal Journal?

Maternal Journal is an award-winning, growing community movement that uses creative journaling to explore thoughts, feelings and experiences through pregnancy, birth and beyond. It was set up by two mothers, Laura – an artist and practising midwife – and Sam, a communications specialist, and works in collaborations with mothers, visual artists, poets, writers and performers.

There is a website full of advice, guidance, and creative prompts to support journaling and creativity for improved maternal mental health and wellbeing. Creative prompts, guides, artwork and more are posted regularly on social media for extra support. Everything is grounded in the tradition and legacy of women's journaling and its powerful potential as a feminist practice to address the changes, challenges and joys of birth, mothering and being a parent.

How do you think it helps parents?

Journaling is known for its positive effect on mental health and wellbeing. It can help us explore and better understand the thoughts, emotions and expectations around birth and parenting that we don't always get the chance to think about. Lots of support for new mothers comes as practical parenting advice; instead, Maternal Journal focuses very much on the mother or birth parent's overall wellbeing.

Maternal Journal supports people to journal either within a group, by themselves or both. Journaling groups are like traditional women's making circles; they create a safe space to connect over shared emotions and experiences. It's a comfortable and empowering environment. Journaling by yourself can give you better control over how you feel by working things out on paper (or a screen). Meaningful connections are made over shared experiences in Maternal Journal groups and the online community.

What sort of experiences have participants used in their journal and how?
People have created journal entries about postnatal depression, miscarriage, health anxieties, loneliness and the pressures of building a family as well as capturing joyful moments and memories using anything from painting and poetry to sketches and collage.

What would you say to someone wanting to start their own journal?
It's about you. How you feel and what you want to explore. Everything you need to get started is on our website, including journaling guides, top tips, ideas for books and blogs to read, and a full toolkit for setting up a group. The Maternal Journal team is also on hand for any questions and support. You will be part of a growing community of more than 50 Maternal Journal groups and many mothers and birth parents around the world, creating and connecting through shared maternal experiences.

You can find out more by visiting www.maternaljournal.org
The *Maternal Journal* book will be published in 2021.

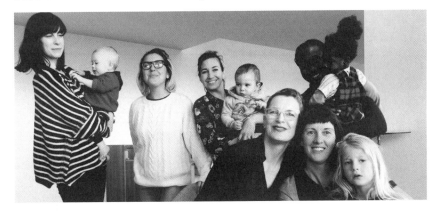

"

Part two

Let's talk about caring for your baby

"

This section considers some of the key information and questions you might have about caring for your baby.

It's not meant to be a definitive 'how to' guide – there are plenty of other books that consider baby care and development. It's not going to tell you how to change a nappy or bath your baby as they're quite straightforward things. A lot of stuff you can just google. This book is about you, how you feel and what support you need. But of course you and your baby come as a package at the moment, and there is some information that will help you that you might not find in other books.

Specifically, this section looks at three main things: your baby's behaviour and development, feeding your baby, and sleep. It covers what's normal, common queries you might have and where to get support (both in practical terms and with how you are feeling about these things). It also gives you lots of links and recommended reading so you can find more details if you need them, but sometimes a few simple points can be enough, especially when you're exhausted.

I've included these three things because they are the hot topics of baby care that seem to provoke debate, result in all sorts of advice being offered and can be really closely tied to your wellbeing. It's not just about whether you decide to breastfeed or not, or co-sleep or not, or put your baby in a routine or wear them in a sling. Sometimes these decisions aren't straightforward and can be a source of contention and long-lasting feelings. So having a good understanding of what to do and where to find support can really help give you the best shot at things turning out how you want them to.

Unfortunately, you'll probably encounter quite a lot of misinformation about things like how breastfeeding works or the safety of different sleeping arrangements. People love to give their opinion, which isn't always evidence-based, and the internet has a lot of confusing nonsense on it. What I've tried to do in this section is tell you what the evidence says and leave you to make a decision that is right for your family. There is no one right way, despite a lot of books promising quick solutions. Here we'll look at what is normal and point you in the direction of where to get support to cope with that. It is a judgement-free zone.

A short note here before we continue: learning to deal with other people's advice

Ah, babies. They definitely bring out the 'expert' in other people. You're probably going to find that everyone has an opinion on how you should hold/feed/care for your baby, based on their own experiences, that one time they held a baby or something they read on the internet. Sometimes this can be very helpful indeed. Other times it can be downright infuriating. Remember:

1. Their advice is usually more about them than it is about you. Especially if they had their baby some time ago, and things have changed, then they might be telling you what they were told was best for their baby. It might be confusing or unsettling for them to see things being done differently now. They may still worry whether they did it 'right', or carry scars from people telling them they should have done things differently (ironic, I know). It's very reassuring when people we like do things the way we like, and some people will therefore – consciously or subconsciously – be trying to get you to do the same as them.

2. If they love you then they likely have your best interests at heart. If they see you exhausted and struggling, then they might think they're helping by suggesting a bottle/routine/sleep training even if it's not something you want to do. They may not have thought that you doing things your way is important to you, and think they are helping. Try and remember this even if you want to throttle them.

3. You do not need to take advice. You can thank people for giving it and leave it at that. Sometimes you might encounter people who then get annoyed with you (see point one) and withdraw all further offers of support. Given that their support hasn't necessarily been useful, this is not the threat they might think it is.

4. Find your people and listen to them. Whether that's a feeding support group, a professional or a group of friends who always have your back, whatever decisions you make. Let them tell you that you're doing a great job, and everyone struggles. Never underestimate how much having someone reassuring you that you are doing the right thing can help, even if you know they might be doing so because they do the same thing (see point one - complicated, isn't it!)

5. Tell people that sometimes all you want is for someone to say 'Wow, it's tough isn't it,' or 'That's crap,' rather than find a practical solution or tell you how to do things. They might not realise what you need (i.e. to moan without consequence) and think they have to fix it. Again, they think they're helping.

Saying all of that, you'll probably encounter numerous irritating people - family, friends and complete strangers (and sometimes sadly the occasional misinformed health professional) - who give you downright daft advice. For these situations we have a handy bingo card. I'm not sure what you win... Photocopy it and keep it on the fridge or mantelpiece and theatrically stop and cross one off whenever you get a match.

It never did you any harm	Should he really be feeding again?	He should be in a routine	Why aren't you listening to my advice?
Things were different in my day	He should be sleeping through by now	Rod for your own back!	You're spoiling that baby
You just slept all day	A dummy will solve that	Should you be holding him like that?	In my day babies didn't need all this attention
If you're not going to listen, I'm not going to help	You need to leave him with me	You're too attached to that baby	Isn't he too cold / hot?
You need to let him cry	Is he good?	You'll never get him out of your bed!	He's manipulating you!

Good luck: believe in the evidence and yourself, and do what is right for you.

Chapter four

Caring for your small baby mammal

→ *I remember being surprised at how much I needed to tend to the baby. I think TV and movies contributed to that a lot. When the birth of a baby is depicted in a show they're usually more of a plot point that sits quietly in a bassinet in the corner, only making noise when it contributes to the storyline. Babies aren't like that in real life. Your life revolves around them rather than them conveniently slotting into your life as you already know it. I was pretty self-centred before having kids (as most people are). I really wasn't prepared for how much that needed to change in order to provide for a baby. Before my first arrived I remember having a disagreement with my husband and my mother-in-law about wanting to get tickets to a big concert that was set for about a month after I gave birth. I genuinely thought I would pop out a baby and still be able to carry on life pretty much as normal. It's really not like that. The life as you know it will be gone. I think it's normal to grieve the loss of your old life while still being incredibly grateful for the new changes that come with having a baby.* Emma

Understanding how your baby is growing, changing and developing is not only interesting, but can also help explain their behaviour. Although this won't change the behaviour, there is something comforting about knowing that it is normal and will change as they grow. When you understand what their brain is doing, or how their physical development is adapting, you can understand why they suddenly won't let you put them down or are getting frustrated. Okay, so it's not a full night's sleep for you, but it at least stops you thinking your baby is broken.

Here are five key lessons about what is normal for your baby:

Lesson one: Remember your baby is just a tiny mammal

And an underdeveloped mammal at that. I remember being 18 and in a developmental psychology lecture when we were told that really, for the best chance of survival, babies should be born at 18 months old: able to walk, speak, and feed themselves (well, put food in their mouth, not pop to Tesco, rustle up a three-course dinner and do the washing up).

Of course, given the size of a toddler and the size of the human pelvis, that would be unfeasible to say the least, so babies are born sooner. This means, however, that most of their first year is devoted to brain development and getting the hang of key skills like holding their head up and eventually being able to move around. Other baby mammals, such as giraffes or cows, can walk and feed themselves soon after birth and spend most of their early months growing bigger. Of course, human brains are also more complex (we have rational thought, more developed language skills and can think in abstract terms about the future and so on) and babies need time to develop their brains too.

Not to freak you out or anything, but this means that your small person is pretty much totally dependent on you (and anyone else who cares for them). Unlike a baby giraffe, they can't walk, feed themselves or run away from danger. So they need to be *absolutely sure* that you are going to care for them and help them out a bit. When they cry it's not because they're manipulating you, but because they can't do things for themselves. When they don't want to be put down, it's because they're afraid of being left alone. When they feed all night, it's because they're growing so quickly.

It's not wrong (or unusual) to start to find this frustrating over time. But evolutionary psychologists believe that, just like many newborn animals, babies are designed to draw our attention to them to make sure we care for them. Large eyes relative to their body means they are endearing, and we're programmed to want to respond. Some believe that the timing of babies starting to smile in reaction to people they recognise and things they find stimulating (usually at around six weeks of age) is another way of bonding you together. There is even research that shows that your own baby's cry is particularly distressing and provokes a primitive response in you to go to them. All in all this means you probably won't leave them in a bush somewhere when they've been crying for hours – well played, Mother Nature.

Lesson two: Responding to your baby's needs helps them thrive

Some people might tell you that if you respond to all your baby's needs you'll spoil them, or teach them that things will always be that way. Or maybe that your baby needs to learn to be independent and do things themselves or they'll need you to do it for them forever.

Hmmm. Want to know the secret to having a confident, independent and thriving child?

It's actually by responding to those needs. We all learn about the world through our experiences. We learn how things work, how to behave and who to trust. Trust is really important. When we have positive interactions with people we learn that the world is (mainly) a good place and we have the confidence to go out and meet more people and explore.[1]

The same is true for your baby. When you meet your baby's needs in a way that is appropriate (i.e. what they need), timely (i.e. within a reasonable time) and gently (i.e. in a caring and responsive way) then they learn that they are loved and cared for and that when they need something you will be there for them. This means they're more likely to grow into capable, confident and caring adults.[2]

Remember that what is important is your *overall pattern* of engagement with your baby, i.e. how you respond most of the time. We all have moments when we just can't bring ourselves to get up again and see to our baby who is crying at night, so we lie there for a bit hoping that maybe... maybe this will be the time they decide to self-settle. Or we put a grizzly baby in a pram or the car and take them for a walk/drive in the hope they'll sleep rather than trying to cuddle or soothe them. Or we utter a few choice words because they cry every time we put them down. All this is normal – we're human.

Lesson three: Remember, crying is your baby's means of communicating

Crying is a very normal thing for your baby – it's how they communicate with you. It doesn't necessarily mean that something is awfully wrong, but simply that they need your help with something or need you to hold them because it's all a bit much (a feeling we probably know far too well as adults!).

Reasons why your baby might be crying include:

- They are hungry
- They need a nappy change
- They got scared by something
- They're too cold or too hot

- They're too tired
- They're frustrated
- They can't reach something they want
- They just want a cuddle
- They just want you
- They don't even know what they want
- The state of the world and politics

At first your baby's cries might all sound the same, but over time you will probably learn to understand what they might want. You'll learn that one cry is definitely a hungry one, another a sleepy one and another a grizzly 'just hold me' one. As they get older you'll learn the 'I'm bored' one and the 'I just fell over' shriek. This is backed up by science – researchers have actually spent time looking at the pitch and duration of cries and matching them to babies' needs.[3]

A really common time for babies to cry is late afternoon and early evening. Something seems to happen then, and it's often called the 'witching hour' even though it can last more than an hour! It is probably because this time of the day is really busy and you're a bit more tired. Maybe you're trying to cook dinner and your partner or other children are home and it's all a bit frazzled and babies pick up on that. Most babies, if you just give in and respond to them, will settle. They want comfort and that comfort is you. They want to be held and rocked and if you are breastfeeding they will probably want to feed on and off a lot (more on this in Chapter 9). It's exhausting but normal and the best way to fix it is just to try and soothe them.

The main thing to remember is that – especially for a very young baby – crying is just their way of communicating. They are incapable of planning it and doing it to wind you up. They can't 'manipulate you' as some people might tell you, and by responding to them you aren't 'creating a rod for your own back' but instead making them feel their needs are heard and met. A baby cries because they need something. You might not necessarily agree that they need it, but they *really* believe that they do. And responding to them helps them feel safe and secure and relieved that they're not alone. Responding to them doesn't make them more dependent as they grow up, it actually makes them more independent and confident, and a whole load of evidence backs that up.[4]

I want to emphasise again that it's the overall pattern of responding that counts. Your baby will be just fine if you need to leave them to cry for a moment because you're at a critical point trying to cook dinner and you can see they're not in danger. Or because you really need to go to the bathroom.[5]

The fact that this is normal doesn't mean it's easy. It's difficult to consistently respond to someone who just screams at you. You're probably exhausted and fed up of having someone need you all the time, and you could really use some sleep. You might be angry at your baby, or frustrated, or feel totally overwhelmed. And your arms really hurt. As long as these are just thoughts, it's all normal. They will pass. And your baby *will* change as they get older. Crying, at least the type where nothing seems to work to soothe your baby, is usually at its worst at around six weeks and starts to get better by around 3-4 months.[6] However, they will still cry if they have other needs.

My baby seems inconsolable - is something wrong?

As you get to know your baby you will start to recognise their cries and what is normal for them. Sometimes though a cry might be more important. Usually, if you respond to your baby's cry of communication with whatever they need – a nappy change, cuddle or feed or whatever – it will stop. And those early evening crying sessions will start abating as they get older.

But sometimes it doesn't seem like you can do anything to stop your baby crying, or they seem more frantic than usual. If your baby suddenly starts acting this way do seek medical advice, particularly if they seem out of sorts in any other way – lethargic, limp or hot. They may be unwell. Speak to your GP or call 111.

If you are breastfeeding and your baby suddenly becomes more unsettled you might wonder if it was something you ate. There is a lot of debate about whether babies can react to foods in milk, and there are a lot of vocal opinions online, some of them from sources with financial interests in diagnosing allergies. If you are worried about this, talk to a health professional or seek advice from one of the breastfeeding organisations. Although babies can sometimes respond to things you've eaten, it is more unusual than we might be led to think, and it can be difficult and inconclusive to just cut foods out of your diet.

If your baby is reacting to something you have eaten, it is unlikely that crying will be the only sign. They will probably have symptoms such as vomiting/bringing up milk a lot, a rash or red itchy eyes, being very gassy, having green, mucousy or bloody stools, or being congested. They will often seem uncomfortable, and their sleep will be even more disrupted than usual. They may also have lower weight gain as they might not be absorbing milk effectively. If your baby does show these signs, do think about whether you have eaten anything different and have a chat to your health professional, especially if they seem to be in pain or have bloody stools. To read more it's best to look at information from one of the trusted breastfeeding organisations rather than industry-funded pages. La Leche League has a great article here: **www.laleche.org.uk/allergies**.

What about colic?

You might wonder whether your baby has 'colic' if they cry a lot. Colic has several specific behaviours: the cry is high-pitched, babies will pull up their knees, maybe arch their back, clench their fists and their tummy will be hard. Around a quarter of babies regularly have these symptoms, but it is more likely in babies that are formula fed or if someone in your house smokes.

Babies with colic often have these symptoms in the evening. It's important not to confuse this with the common unsettled baby crying that occurs. If your baby is showing signs of colic they really will look as though they are in pain rather than being unsettled.

What can you do about it if your baby seems to have colic? Lots has been tried, but not a lot has actually been shown to work. One reason for this is that colic often seems to go away by about 3-5 months. So if you design research poorly and test something over time... you might conclude it had worked when actually it had just passed, regardless of the intervention. There is a big industry out there trying to sell you stuff, and to some extent trying some of the 'probably won't work but is harmless' things might actually make things better as it feels as if you're doing *something*.

It is possible that if your baby is showing these signs and particularly if they are formula fed, that they *might* be symptoms of cows' milk protein allergy, lactose intolerance or other gut problems. Speak to your health visitor and GP if you suspect this, but make sure they do a full assessment of other signs of intolerance rather than diagnosing it from crying alone.

Some things you might like to try include:

- Infacol or Dentinox - drops which try to reduce the surface tension of bubbles of gas trapped in liquid so they join together.
- Colief or Lactaid - lactase drops, which help break down lactose in the milk if your baby is struggling to process lactase.
- Gripe water claims to neutralise acid in your baby's tummy and break down air bubbles, but as far as we know there is no evidence for that.
- Other herbal remedies claim all sorts of things with no evidence - it might just be that they taste nice and distract your baby.
- Hold your baby upright, with their tummy pressed against you, so they have their head on your shoulder.
- Try and work out where any gas might be coming from - are they gulping it down when crying, or if you're breastfeeding might it be the latch?

Some might suggest that you try giving your baby probiotics to improve colic. A recent Cochrane review suggested that there was no clear evidence that these worked any better than a placebo.[7] Although, quite a bit of research in this area is poorly designed, as I mentioned above, so one study found improvements in both the probiotics group *and* the placebo group because colic symptoms resolved naturally over time.[8]

Shel Banks, an IBCLC (International Board Certified Lactation Consultant - the highest qualification we have in infant feeding) and expert in infant colic has a great Facebook live hosted by BabyEm (an organisation that provides training for health professionals) that's well worth a watch **www.facebook.com/ babyemltd/videos/live-with-ibclc-shel-banks-talking-about-colic-reflux-and-infant-allergies/844689979204853**.

Lesson four: Skin-to-skin is not just for after birth

When you were pregnant you were hopefully told about the benefits of having skin-to-skin contact with your baby after birth, where you held your naked baby on your naked chest. It helped calm them and you, by making them feel close and secure and increasing your levels of oxytocin – the hormone of love, calm and bonding. There are lots of reasons why skin-to-skin is great, but the best news of all is that it isn't only beneficial straight after birth, but for a long time afterwards. Skin-to-skin can help turn your baby from a fraught little crying bundle to a calm one within a few minutes and is very much encouraged. The same principles apply as they would have after birth. The main idea is to have as much of their skin touching yours as possible, though if you want to err on the side of caution you can keep a nappy on! Skin-to-skin can be helpful particularly in the fourth trimester as it has a direct physical impact on babies, calming them in many ways. Research has shown that it:[9]

- Reduces crying
- Keeps babies in a calmer, more alert state
- Helps regulate their temperature – if they are too hot they will cool down, and vice versa. This can help if they have a temperature
- Stabilises their breathing, heart rate and blood sugar rates
- Calms you by increasing those oxytocin levels
- Helps with breastfeeding as they are close by and calmer
- Generally helps ease their transition into this loud and bright world – keeping them close to your heart, close to your skin and close to the smell they find so familiar.

Some ideas for skin-to-skin could be:

- Going to bed with your baby
- Popping them down your top
- Wearing them skin-to-skin in a sling
- Having a bath together
- Sitting on the sofa with not many clothes on

Remember skin-to-skin works for anyone – your partner can do it, or whoever you like really. Babies apparently don't mind chest hair. And research shows that it can help increase levels of oxytocin and dopamine in fathers, increasing their connection to their baby and making them feel calmer. I know of no research with female partners or other family members, but logic suggests similar results would occur.[10]

Lesson five – buy a good sling (or several)

Carrying your baby in a sling or other piece of material is a practice seen throughout history and around the world. There are some beautiful images at this website: wrapyourbaby.com/cultural-babywearing. I particularly like the historical Welsh photos of babies being carried in the Welsh nursing shawl – known as *siol fagu* – not just by their mother but by grandparents, siblings and men in the family too, at carrymycariad.wordpress.com/tag/wales.

Carrying our babies close to us is normal. It would have developed as a means of both protection and comfort. We are one of two broad types of mammal – the ones that carry our babies and keep them close, rather than the other type that tends to leave them in a burrow or nest and come back later. This is in part due to how easily and quickly our milk is digested compared to some other mammals – it is not very high in fat, so babies need to feed often. Or perhaps our milk developed this way to make sure we weren't left down burrows, as we had relatively little ability to hide, run or defend ourselves.[11]

We are also more closely related to primates than to any other mammal – and as you will know, primates also carry their babies, often with them clinging on as they move around as they have fur that enables that. Humans (well most of them) are decidedly less furry, so we developed a method that left our hands and arms free so we could more easily move around – the sling.

There are many reasons why having a sling can be really useful:

1. It frees up your arms and hands
You can get on with other things or simply give your arms a rest from carrying your baby (how can something so small seem to weigh so much?). Although the increase in arm definition and strength is a great thing, sometimes you just need a break.

2. It helps reduce the likelihood of your baby developing a 'flat head' (plagiocephaly)
Carrying your baby helps support a healthy head shape as they are more upright and the back of their head is not flat against a surface. Since guidance has stressed the importance of putting babies on their back to sleep, there has been a rise in plagiocephaly, particularly if babies also spend a lot of their awake time lying on their backs on playmats and in prams. Having them upright reduces that pressure on the back of their heads.

3. It helps recreate the womb
A good sling really does help recreate the womb for a baby. This is particularly true for tiny babies who can be wrapped up in supportive slings where their whole body is cradled – rather than older babies who are interested in

everything and have their head out looking around. Babies get huge comfort from this, and a great article by Claire Niala called 'Why African Babies Don't Cry' describes how the way of caring for babies in her native Kenya was hugely different to that in the UK. She talked about how in Kenya mothers seemed to wrap their baby up so snugly and securely that you could almost not see them. They were carried around most of the day, fed when they needed feeding and each need was met as it developed, meaning babies rarely cried as they were comforted and secure, or, as she describes it *'cocooned from the stresses of the outside world'.*[12]

4. It stops them crying
Research now shows that babies cry less on average when they are regularly carried in a sling. In one study, carrying babies for three hours a day reduced crying by nearly half. In another study, mothers were asked to pick up, sit with, and stand with their babies and it was found that when the mother stood up, their baby became stiller, quieter and their heart rate decreased. The same effect was not seen when just picking her baby up – she had to be standing up and moving. Similar effects have been seen in other mammals, suggesting a shared protective response.[13] The authors suggested that babies may feel closer and safer in a position where they can feel they are being held and moved. If you think about it from an evolutionary perspective, a baby who was still and alone would have been at risk of being eaten. It also keeps them close to your heartbeat, warm and secure – it's no surprise really that they cry less.

5. They are more stable
Research has also shown that many of the benefits of skin-to-skin contact can be observed when you carry your baby close – after all, they are there next to your heart, held in your arms and can hear your voice and smell your skin. So babies who are carried have lower heart rates and better temperature regulation. They are also more likely to spend time in a state known as 'quiet alertness', in which they are calm but awake and taking everything in. This is an optimal state for learning new things.[14]

Remember that all these benefits apply to other people too – partners and family can carry your baby in a sling. It can be a really useful way for other people to calm and relax your baby while you get a break.

Choosing a sling
There are many different types of sling in different patterns and colours. Seasoned sling users will tell you that buying them can be addictive! It's important to make sure the sling is the right size and shape for your baby. Unfortunately the cheaper slings that are sold in shops (or that you might be given as a gift) might not be the most suitable, so it's worth doing some

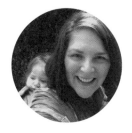

How babywearing supports your baby's early communication development

Marissa Webb, specialist speech and language therapist and director of the Orchid Practice
theorchidpractice.co.uk

I am an enthusiastic babywearer. I fell into it almost by accident. I found babywearing because my oldest son was colicky, which meant his tummy was uncomfortable a lot of the time and he preferred to be upright and on my chest constantly. Babywearing was the solution for us.

However, we got so much more out of it that I never even realised at the time. It was only later on, when I became a more experienced babywearer with my middle son, that I began doing research into the connection between babywearing and communication. Babywearing has many benefits including comforting and bonding, creating a secure attachment, and increasing social interaction. Many of these benefits are foundational to the development of early communication skills, and they have lasting positive effects.

How does babywearing impact early communication development? There are three main ways:

1. Closeness

It's no secret that babies love to be held close. They enjoy the comforting touch and warmth of being held. While a baby is being carried, either in arms or worn in a sling, they are elevated to the level of the adult's face and even when worn on the adult's back they are in close proximity, meaning they can see what the adult sees. This establishes the opportunity for developing joint attention, meaning that since the baby and adult can see the same things, they can engage in a joint activity more easily. It is also much easier for the adult to notice and respond to feeding cues and generally respond to the baby's needs, which the baby will be able to communicate through crying, facial expressions or noises, which are the early forms of initiating communication. When we respond to a baby's needs, they learn that they can have an impact on another person, which is a fundamental to communication. We communicate to get our needs met.

2. Face-to-face

Having baby and adult face-to-face means there are so many opportunities to engage in eye contact, and the baby is able to see the adult's facial expressions and therefore spends lots of time watching and learning about non-verbal communication. Communication is actually around 80% non-verbal, so this is a really fundamental skill, and babies have all the time in the world to enjoy being face-to-face. It also creates more opportunity for children to hear and learn new words and watch mouth movements during talking or singing, which is preparation for future speech development. Babies and toddlers develop speech sounds by watching, listening and imitating, and being face-to-face means they can watch, copy and engage in a verbal or non-verbal exchange much more often.

3. A better view

A baby being carried is up high, so not only can they see more, but they are also able to interact with more people. The baby becomes involved in all of the adult's conversations and is therefore given increased opportunity for conversation, by both the adult carrying them and other people who they can also see up close. I went out the other evening to a social event with my baby in a sling and he had so much fun being involved in every conversation I had, as people were able to look straight into his eyes and interact with him on a much more personal level. He absolutely loved it! Also, for a carried baby the view changes all the time and they can see so much more, giving them the opportunity to explore many different things, both near and far.

Babywearing is a great way to start encouraging early communication development and is beneficial for all children, including those with additional needs, providing comfort and promoting secure attachment. It's an enjoyable experience and a wonderful way to spend time with your child as you explore the world together. It also has a positive impact on emotional wellbeing and can have a lasting impact on adult–child relationships.

research into what might work best for you.

The main thing you need to think about is how a sling supports your baby's spine and hips. Lots of baby carriers put a baby in an upright position or spread their hips out – which is not a natural position for them until they are older and walking. Instead a sling, especially for a young baby, needs to hold them in a natural tucked-up position, which means their spine should be gently curved with their legs in an M-shaped squat, rather than dangling down like you see in some carriers. Their knees should be higher than their hips and bottom.

A good acronym to check your baby's position is 'TICKS'. Your baby should be:

- Tight
- In view at all times
- Close enough to kiss
- Keep chin off the chest
- Supported back

This can be a bit tricky to get your head around, but luckily sling enthusiasts have created 'slingmeet', which are groups that meet around the country to share information on slings and often loan them out to try before you spend a lot of money on one. There are more details on the Slingmeet Facebook page **www.facebook.com/slingmeet**. For detailed diagrams and information have a look at Dr Rosie Knowles's website Carrying Matters: **www.carryingmatters. co.uk.** You could also check out Rosie's book *Why Babywearing Matters*.

Embracing the concept of the fourth trimester

You might have heard people talk about the idea of a 'fourth trimester', but what exactly does that mean? Basically, during pregnancy your baby had their every need met. It was warm and muffled, they had food and drink on tap, and they were gently swayed as they curled themselves up as you walked around. And then suddenly they were born and it was bright, noisy and cold (and probably raining) and people expected them to put clothes on and lie in a crib.

This is all a bit of a shock, and babies usually protest about it. It's only natural that they would prefer to stay close to you – you're warm, there's food about and they can hear the familiar sound of a beating heart. This is where the concept of seeing the first three months of life as another trimester of pregnancy comes in. It's not a novel idea – if you look to our history, and many cultures around the world, when babies are born they aren't cleaned up, dressed and placed in a crib. Instead they're carried in a sling for most of the time, making a more gradual transition from womb to world.

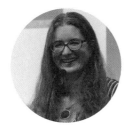

The importance of the fourth trimester

Karen Hall, NCT breastfeeding counsellor, has spent the last 10 years immersed in supporting new mothers. She also produces The Motherworldly podcast www.motherworldly.com

What do we mean when we talk about babies being in the fourth trimester?
The fourth trimester refers to the first three months of life with your new baby, when you and they are adjusting to the world with them in it. Their needs are high, and you've got a lot to learn about how to meet them.

Close your eyes for a moment and imagine the life your baby led when you were pregnant, swaying gently in the cosy hug of their mother's body, dim lighting, familiar comforting sounds, perfectly modulated warmth, and a continuous supply of nutrients. It's like a five-star spa break, the perfect primordial soup in which the baby grows and develops, already making connections to the familiar sounds and movements of the outside world. A world which they will be encountering soon, and which may come as a shock to someone with no concept of time or, let's face it, anything other than the agreeable environment that they have known for some months.

Humans have evolved to have babies with large brains; about 30% of the size of the adult brain, and ready to explode into rapid growth in the weeks and months after birth, and requiring a relatively large head in which to contain all that genius. So the theory of the fourth trimester tells us that our babies are born 'too soon'. That is to say, they are usually born exactly when they are supposed to be born, but they are physiologically under-developed compared with the young of other mammals. A foal, for example, can stand up and walk minutes after birth, which is necessary from a survival point of view, because the newborn foal would be easy prey if it were immobile.

So what do our human babies need, from a survival point of view? Cast your mind back to the continual comfort of your baby's womb world, and ask yourself, what might they feel in the first minutes of life? Mild surprise, to say the very least. This world is brighter, colder, and the noises are unfamiliar. The food supply has been cut off. And your baby cannot make rational sense of any of this. So what does he or she need at that moment, and for the next few weeks of life? They need to feel safe. They need to be held close where they can hear the familiar music of your heartbeat, feel the warmth of your arms, anticipate the comfort of the next feed, and be gently rocked, just as they are used to, by the movements of an adult body. They need you.

What is normal behaviour for many babies at this time?

The evolution of our social world has far outstripped the evolution of our babies' brains. That means that their fundamental expectation is that their survival needs will be met, and all their behaviour is adapted to that expectation. Our babies are cute and soft and vulnerable-looking, to provoke a protective response in their caregivers. If looking cute isn't enough, they have a range of sounds, from appealing little gurgles and snuffles, to heart-wrenching howls that may leave you desperately trying everything on the list of reasons why babies cry to make it stop. Everything your baby does at this stage is completely reasonable from the perspective of a small creature trying to ensure its own survival, but may bring challenges for the adults responsible for that survival at the same time as coping with their own physical recovery, hormones, lack of sleep, and great social and emotional change.

Many parents describe their newborn baby as 'unsettled'. Of course the range of unsettledness is huge, and one family may find normal what another family finds intolerable. Perhaps they have spent a lot of time with younger family members, or have friends with new babies, and so have a good idea of what to expect. But many of us come to parenthood having rarely even held a newborn before in our lives, and this little bundle of relentless need, no matter how cute and appealing, can be hard to figure out.

It's normal for babies not to like being put down in a cot or Moses basket. Remember the wonderful world of the womb? When a baby is held in a parent's arms, they are experiencing the familiar sounds and smells and movements, and they feel safe. When they are put down, the temperature drops, the sounds recede, and the world is strangely still. This is weird for the baby, and if they are still in a light stage of sleep, they may well wake and feel distressed. So it's also normal for babies to sleep more soundly when they're held. You absolutely cannot spoil a newborn baby with too much love, so sleeping on a parent is one way for the other parent to get some rest. Some families choose to bring their baby into their own bed for sleep, and find that this increases the restfulness of everyone's night. If you decide to do this, make sure you are aware of safer co-sleeping guidelines.

It is normal for babies to wake up at night, usually two or three times, and usually for a feed. Babies have short sleep cycles (about 45 minutes, compared with an adult's 90-minute cycle), and spend more time in light sleep, from which they are easily woken. In fact, most people wake up several times a night, briefly check that all is well, and fall back to sleep with no trouble – unless all is not well. For your baby, not knowing where you are means that all is not well, and so they are much less likely to settle back to sleep, until they have been reassured by you. Often this will involve feeding or rocking, creating those safe and reassuring womb-like associations that help your baby to settle.

It is normal for babies to feed very frequently (often 12 or more times in 24 hours), and when they ask for a feed, they are asking for so much more than food. For adults, feeding is about more than just nutrition; it's temperature regulation (a cool refreshing drink, a warming mug of tea), comfort, and any kind of social occasion from a quick gossip at the water cooler to a long romantic dinner. And adults are sometimes known to eat something just because it's there! For babies, it's temperature regulation, comfort, and social occasions including a quick check-in with someone you love, or a long evening at the bar with great company and delicious snacks. On a technical level, the newborn digestive system works best with frequent small feeds, whether they are breastfed, bottle-fed, or both. For the breastfeeding mother, those frequent small feeds stimulate the hormone release that builds her milk supply.

It's normal for babies to cry, but they will tend to cry less if they are held more. Crying ensures that you won't accidentally leave them outside the cave or on the roof of the car, in terrible danger. Our babies are the descendants of thousands of generations of excellent and successful criers. And it's normal that sometimes there is no apparent reason for the crying, and nothing consistently helps; sometimes this is categorised as 'colic', when a baby cries for more than three hours a day, more than three days a week. It is common in the fourth trimester, and usually passes by itself after a few weeks.

And finally, it is normal for babies to expel copious quantities of bodily fluids. In fact, lots of wee and poo is a good sign that your baby is feeding well, so expect to be changing plenty of nappies (or rope someone else in to do it for you). Poo changes in the first few days, from sticky black newborn meconium, to a day or two of greenish splodges, until the more mature breastmilk after a few days usually results in lots of soft, yellowish, yoghurty poo; or browner poo for a baby getting more formula milk. Hallelujah! Every poo is a sign your baby is doing well. The other common bodily fluid that you may expect to see is vomit: some babies sick up a little bit after every feed, and some occasionally bring back what looks like an entire day's worth of milk in one go. The range of normal again is huge, and you will start to get to know what to expect from your own baby. If they are sick a lot but otherwise seem well, then there is probably nothing to worry about, but if you are concerned then do speak to your midwife or health visitor, or a breastfeeding counsellor.

All babies will be different, but what advice do you give to parents about how to respond to their baby during this time?
Parents often worry that giving their babies too much attention will spoil them. Sometimes they are advised against responding to their babies by older family members, childless friends, and complete strangers that they meet in shops, as though too much love and attention were the worst thing you could do for a child, when in fact the opposite is the case. In their pamphlet 'Building a Happy Baby', UNICEF recommends keeping your baby close and responding to them with love, which helps them to grow into happy, secure children, and confident adults. When your baby is distressed, and you soothe them, they are learning that soothing is a possibility. The more this happens, the more they are able to learn to do this for themselves.

Responding to your baby's cues for attention, feeding, and comfort, helps to build a trusting relationship between you and your baby. As your baby grows, their need for such rapid response and close attention will decrease, and your parenting will evolve; so the way you respond to your newborn is likely to be different from the way you respond to them as a toddler or teenager. I would recommend getting those cuddles in now, before they can be responded to with an eyeroll and sarcasm.

What do you tell new parents that you support who are feeling overwhelmed by the fourth trimester?

It's all very well to say that all of this is normal survival behaviour, and all newborns have been like this since the dawn of man, but that doesn't mean it isn't challenging for 21st-century parents, who have led busy and exciting lives, which have suddenly been disrupted by this new little human. However much you have read, watched, listened and learned at your antenatal classes, it is very hard to grasp the reality of life with a newborn until you're in the driving seat, usually without an instructor beside you. It's normal to feel a bit overwhelmed some or even most of the time.

The fourth trimester is a period of adjustment and realignment of priorities. It's not just your baby who is getting used to life in the world; you have been through many changes and challenges too. New parents experience a lot of pressures, particularly in an age of social media, when the constant and competitive display of images frequently reminds you of the many ways in which you are apparently failing. The Duchess of Cambridge appeared gracefully at the door of the hospital, perfectly made up and wearing heels. You don't have to do this. You don't even have to get dressed. During the coronavirus lockdown, parents frequently reported that one silver lining was being able to rest and get to know their baby.

Some things that parents find helpful are:

- Restrict the number of visitors, or channel some of those early visits to video call so that you don't have to get out of your pyjamas (or your bed), keep the house clean, or make cups of tea.
- Don't expect too much of yourself too soon: it takes weeks to learn a new role. Set small goals, and celebrate achieving them.
- Look after your own mental health, eat well, get some exercise, and take time for yourself sometimes.
- Follow your instincts. You know your baby better than anyone.
- If you want your baby to sleep in your bed, check the guidelines, but you don't have to justify your decision (about this or anything) to anyone.
- A sling is a good investment, whether around the house, or out and about. Babies who are carried tend to settle in the sling and cry less; and you have two free hands. But don't use them for housework.

Chapter five

Understanding your baby's development and needs as they grow

→ Babies grow and develop rapidly in the first year of life. They go from pretty helpless creatures who can't really even hold their heads up, to ones that on average can waddle around and yell random words at you. I won't lie - every stage has its exciting points, along with its frustrating ones. Understanding your baby's perspective, needs and physical abilities at each of these points is really useful because it helps you understand what is normal, which is reassuring (although it doesn't make you feel any less exhausted).

This chapter presents a handy summary of what you can expect from your baby in terms of physical and social development and sleep and growth during the first year. More in-depth information on feeding, sleep and growth follows in the next few chapters. Remember this is a rough guide. Some babies will do things more quickly, and some at a more leisurely pace. That's fine. If you have twins or triplets (or more) they may develop at different rates. That's also fine.

These stages and milestones will also likely be different if your baby was born prematurely, has a developmental disability or has a serious illness. If any of these apply you may or may not want to read through this next section - you may want to jump ahead to the next sections where we will look at what might differ and how you might feel.

Your newborn

Your baby's physical development

Your baby has just spent nine months growing in the womb where their every need was met. They may still be curled up, preferring to sleep in a frog-legged position on you. They will have very little control over their body, particularly their relatively large and heavy head, which is why it needs carefully supporting. During the first few days newborns are slowly adapting to an outside world of brightness and louder sounds.

Newborns have an inbuilt series of reflexes that are there to protect them. Reflexes are completely involuntary movements. Your baby doesn't think about doing them, or have the limb control necessary to perform them on demand. They are, however, a sign that everything is working well, and your midwife will probably check them. Many of the reflexes are likely leftover survival mechanisms from millions of years ago when babies would have had to cling to their mothers. Again, remember that your baby is really a tiny mammal (just a bit less hairy), and think about how many of our closest mammalian relatives carry their babies.[1] Reflexes include:

- **The Moro reflex.** Often known as the startle reflex. Babies will startle, often in response to a noise, and throw out their arms and legs and their head back as if they were about to cling to something. Their fingers will flare and then bunch back into fists. This is probably left over from when our ancestors carried babies in a way where the baby clung to the mother (like you would see apes carrying their babies now). Babies can startle themselves – some have been known to startle themselves by their own particularly loud bowel movements.
- **The rooting reflex.** It is in a baby's best interest to be able to find a nipple easily. If you stroke your baby's cheek, they will naturally turn in that direction, opening and closing their mouth as they search for the nipple.
- **The sucking reflex.** If you put something in a baby's mouth so it touches the roof of their mouth, they will start to suck. Stick to nipples, bottle teats and dummies (depending on your preference) rather than anything else! Some babies will quickly find their finger to suck.
- **The walking/stepping reflex.** Babies cannot walk until around 12 months, but if you hold a newborn baby up, supporting their weight, and put their feet on a flat surface, they will move their feet so it looks like they are attempting to walk.
- **The tonic reflex.** If a baby has their head turned to one side, they naturally

stretch the arm on that side out and bring the opposite one in bent to their chest – looking a bit like superman.

- **The grasp reflex.** Put something in a baby's hand, like your finger, and they'll clasp their fingers around it. Their grip is so strong that you could lift them into a sitting position, or even up in the air. Obviously don't do this in case they let go, but this is most likely a leftover evolutionary reflex to help the baby cling to their mother. Pro tip: suggest people stick a £20 note in there then claim the baby won't give it back.

Your baby's social development

Although your baby may not be physically developed in terms of movement, their senses, particularly in terms of smell, taste and sound, are pretty well developed at birth. For example, there is lots of research to suggest that babies can recognise their mother's voice. Babies' hearing starts to develop in the womb from around 20 weeks of pregnancy. Although it will be muffled, they will be able to hear things going on around them – you might have felt them startle in the womb if a door was slammed or a dog barked loudly. So they are most likely to recognise their mother's voice as a) it's the closest to them and b) they go everywhere their mother goes so hear it the most frequently.

Your baby's sense of smell also starts to develop early in pregnancy and they can taste and smell the amniotic fluid in the womb. It is one of their most heightened senses when they are born as it helps them locate the breast. They will quickly learn the smell of those holding them frequently, especially if you hold them close to your skin. Breastmilk has a similar smell to amniotic fluid, so they will also be able to recognise the familiar smell if they are breastfeeding.

Even at this age, babies can recognise faces – not necessarily individual ones (although some studies suggest they may recognise their mother within a few days), but rather human face shapes. There were lots of studies in the 1980s and 1990s that basically involved showing babies either a piece of paper with random shapes on it or a piece with blocks for eyes, nose and mouth. The babies preferred looking at the face shapes.

Your baby wouldn't be able to recognise you from a distance though. At birth their range of vision is about 8–12 inches, which incidentally is about the distance they are from their mother's eyes during breastfeeding. If you are bottle-feeding, hold them close to you with their head at breast height so they can look more easily into your eyes.

Your baby's sleep

Newborn babies sleep a lot – up to 18 hours or even more. It's exhausting being born and growing and stuff. They'll probably only be awake for an hour or so between their main blocks of sleep, if that. When they are awake they mainly feed before nodding off again. However, much of their sleep will be quite light. They will wriggle and grunt and probably wake up the second you try to put them down as they want to stay close to you.

Although newborns sleep a lot, they will probably only sleep for 1–4 hours at a time. It's important to keep an eye on this and check they are not sleeping for too long. If they are regularly sleeping for more than four hours at a time and not waking to feed it could be a sign that they are not getting enough milk and may be becoming lethargic. If this is happening check the number of wet and dirty nappies they should be having to see if they are getting enough milk.

Your baby's growth

Your baby is actually designed to be able to lose a little bit of weight in the days after birth as they get to grips with feeding. Around 5–7% in the first few days is normal (although a little more can be normal in breastfed babies), after which time they'll start putting it on again. During pregnancy, particularly during those last weeks, they will have laid down fat that will support them if you are breastfeeding as it takes a few days for your milk to fully 'come in'. Newborn babies have very small tummies and therefore will want to feed frequently. Frequent feeding also signals to your body to start producing more milk if you are breastfeeding. More on this in the feeding chapter.

What this means for you

The early days can be a whirlwind of recovering from the birth and getting to know your new baby and new life. It's normal to feel a huge mix of emotions including feeling overwhelmed and even having moments of panic about what you have done. Be kind to yourself – this is a big transition. For more details on normal emotions at this time, have a look at Chapter 13.

Don't be afraid to ask your midwife as many questions as you need to, especially when it comes to feeding if you are breastfeeding. It's okay to feel nervous or as if you don't know what you're doing. Most new parents feel that way.

The newborn days are short. Do what makes you feel good. Spend all day staring at your baby or napping. The time will pass in the blink of an eye.

Newborn nappies

One way to check whether your baby is taking in enough milk is to look at their nappies. Babies should have at least 1–2 wet nappies per day in the first 1–2 days. By days 3–4, your baby should have three or more wet nappies per day, and by days 5–6, five or more. Once your baby is a week old they should be having six or more. To tell what a wet nappy should feel like, try putting two to four tablespoons of water into a nappy and feeling the difference. This is what wet nappies should be like by day three onwards. Before this they should be wet, but may feel a bit lighter.

In terms of bowel movements, on the first or second day your baby should have their first bowel movement. This will be thick, black and sticky - kind of tar-like. Over the next few days they will move through shades of green until by day five they should be mustard-coloured. It should be looser in consistency by day three. By day three they should be having at least two dirty nappies per 24 hours. In terms of amount, this should be more than a 2p coin. Sometimes babies move through this more quickly - especially if they are feeding lots. Earlier is nothing to worry about.

The NCT has produced a handy visual guide (I know, you never thought you'd spend your days looking at something like this, did you?). You can find it here: **www.nct.org.uk/baby-toddler/nappies-and-poo/newborn-baby-poo-nappies-what-expect**. Charlotte Treitl, also known as the Milk Rebel, has also put together an amazing project on Facebook called the 'baby poo gallery', which has photos of different types of baby poo, looking at what is normal and not, for you to peruse. Really useful viewing... just maybe not before breakfast! **www.facebook.com/babypoogallery**

If your baby isn't having this many wet and dirty nappies and is sleeping a lot, please check with your health professional as soon as possible. They will probably weigh your baby and if you are breastfeeding look for signs of effective milk transfer. More on this in the feeding section in Chapter 9.

0–3 months old

Your baby's physical development

The early months are all about your baby gaining control over their body. They'll be learning to support their own head and eventually turn it to look at things. By about eight weeks they'll realise that their arms and legs are actually attached to them and under their control. Expect lots of staring at their hands at this point, followed by them slowly realising that if they reach out a hand and touch something, they can make it move. This is a great time for a reclining chair with an arch of toys they can hit.

In terms of eyesight, they can see colours and shapes but not lots of detail. They may enjoy looking at books even though they're not really able to understand what they're seeing other than the shape or colour.

Your baby's social development

Socially, it's at around six weeks that your baby will start to smile in response to familiar or pleasurable things. They'll recognise your face and smell and be most likely to smile for those close to them – although some will happily smile for the postman and not you.

They'll also be starting to make simple sounds like cooing, which is both lovely to listen to and makes a great change from crying. Their main form of communication will still be crying though, but their different types of cry will probably be clearer. They may start to recognise your voice and calm when they hear it.

Your baby's sleep

Babies sleep a lot at this stage, even if it doesn't feel like it. You'll probably notice they are more alert than they were during the first week or so of life. Roughly, they will sleep around 14–18 hours a day, and they will probably like doing that either on you or close to you. They'll probably wake up every 2–3 hours or so if they're properly asleep rather than dozing. They may be awake for 1–2 hours in between each bout of sleep. As they get closer to three months old they'll gradually start falling into a pattern of sleeping more at night and being more awake in the day.

Your baby's growth

Lots of babies have big growth spurts at around three and six weeks and again at around 12 weeks, when they often look noticeably bigger after a few days! During a growth spurt they may feed a lot more and also wake up more. It's really common to worry that suddenly you don't have enough milk if you're breastfeeding or your baby's sleep has gone haywire. Don't panic, it will likely settle down again in a few days' time.

What this means for you

Those early smiles and coos can feel like a lifeline after weeks of sleepless nights; it can feel as if you're getting a little reward for all the caring effort you've put in. You are also probably getting better at telling what your baby's cries might mean in terms of being hungry, tired, and so on, but it can still feel frustrating when sometimes they can't just let you know what's wrong.

Your baby is still pretty helpless at manoeuvring their own body, and you might find they get frustrated easily if they're not being held. This is under-standable really. If you could see interesting colours and shapes around you, but couldn't do much more than turn your head (if you're lucky), then you'd probably get a bit fed up too.

Babies spend a lot of time supposedly asleep, but based on all that stuff around feeling more comfortable when they are close to you, they're probably going to want to be held while they do it. There are some gentle ways you can encourage them to start realising the difference between night and day (more on this in Chapter 12), but really in these first few months you will be fighting against nature and their instinct. It's easier to accept they'll need a lot of cuddles and comfort and

" They *will* become more independent as time goes on, even if it doesn't seem like it right now. "

think about things like buying a sling to free up your hands. They *will* become more independent as time goes on, even if it doesn't seem like it right now. A partner or friend or family member can really help at this stage by cuddling them for you while you nap/drink coffee/do whatever your wildest current desires may be.

4-6 months old

Your baby's physical development

This is the time when you suddenly start seeing changes in your baby's physical development. During this period, they will probably start to sit more upright, supported by you (for example, on your lap) so they can look around. By six months they may even be sitting unsupported on the floor if you put them to sit that way - but they probably can't get themselves into a sitting position. Always put cushions behind them if they're sitting up alone - they have a tendency to suddenly tumble backwards.

Your baby will probably start rolling over, including at night. Don't worry about this - there's no need to put them back on their back if they roll over themselves. But it is time to start moving them out of their Moses basket if they still sleep (or fit!) in one, as they could push themselves up and fall out.

Babies will also start developing some of the physical skills they need for starting solid foods at this time (but don't start until around six months). This includes having better co-ordination so they can put things in their mouth, and they love exploring things such as toys in this way. As long as these are safe, suitable for babies and clean, let them explore - it's how they learn about objects and the world.

Your baby's social development

This is a lovely time for language development. Babies can suddenly see much better and really study the faces of those around them. As they can sit up they can really look around the room and be entertained.

They will probably start to laugh at funny faces or things they find amusing. They can make all sorts of different sounds like squeals and grunts. They will likely have a conversation with you - not about the weather or the global state of politics, but if you speak to them and pause they will make sounds back at you. They may not be able to directly copy sounds yet, but this 'conversation' (in a language which used to be known as 'motherese', now 'parentese') is a really important stage in helping them start to form sounds and learn about communication.

Babies can enjoy books from birth, soothed by the sound of your voice. But now is a great time to share books regularly with them. They can see more clearly and identify shapes so will enjoy things like books that have mirrors in them, or different faces, shapes and colours. The 'That's Not My...' books are short board books with lots of textures, colours and sensory experiences and are great at this age. There are some excellent spoof ones too (*That's Not My Husband...* etc.).

Your baby's sleep

Most babies this age are still waking up at least once or twice a night and at this point what you feed them has no impact on their sleep. They're just waking for other reasons, such as being cold, or needing a nappy change.

At around four months your baby has a huge growth and development spurt as they get used to all this physical change. This typically means they wake up more and feed more at night, especially if breastfed. It's common to worry that your baby's sleep has gone to pot and that they will never sleep again. Some people worry that it's a sign babies need solid foods. It's not – and if they were waking because they were hungry, then giving them more milk would work better than typical weaning fruit and veg foods. They're waking because so much is changing in their brain and they need some more milk to help with all that growing. The good news is that babies do start to sleep more again after a couple of weeks or so (and giving them solids makes no difference to how quickly they do this).

Your baby's growth

As above, that growth spurt is a big one. Research shows that your baby can literally grow 1–2.5cm overnight or in a few days.[2] That doesn't sound that much, but an inch on someone 25 inches long is quite an increase – the equivalent of an average adult gaining 2.5–3 inches overnight.

By around 4–6 months your baby will likely have doubled their birth weight, but things will start to slow down from around now. Look at the curves on the growth charts in your baby measurement book. They are not straight linear lines but curves. Imagine if we carried on doubling our weight every six months or so...! Some parents worry that slowing growth is a sign that their baby is not getting enough milk or needs solids. The important thing is to check whether your baby is roughly following their growth curve line, rather than thinking about how much weight they are putting on compared to the early weeks.

What this means for you

Things are changing. Your baby is becoming more mobile and might suddenly not seem like a tiny baby anymore. They might be frustrated in their attempts to move or try and sit up. Or want you to hold them upright so they can see the world. Suddenly it feels like they need more engagement. Luckily their ability to laugh and make sounds back at you helps – it's probably an evolutionary tool to stop you leaving them in a bush somewhere.

The four-month growth spurt is absolutely exhausting and can feel like it never ends. Get as much sleep and rest as you can, be kind to yourself and remember it will pass! Have a look at the sleep section in a few chapters' time. There are lots of ideas for helping your baby sleep a little better, but if you can try and remember it's a developmental phase. What you feed them won't make any difference to their sleep, despite what people tell you. If you're feeling alone, google 'four-month sleep regression hell' – there are *so* many articles and threads on parenting forums about it. It may help you realise a) you are not alone and b) it really does pass.

7-12 months old

Your baby's physical development

This is another time of rapid change for your baby. During this time, probably between 6 and 10 months, they'll become mobile, although there's no set way they will do this. Some babies will start to crawl first (maybe backwards or like a crab). Some will shuffle around on their bum (because they want to carry something with them too – probably snacks). They may also be making steps towards walking – perhaps starting to pull themselves up and even move around like that, holding onto things. Babies take their first steps on average at around a year, but it's not as if they all suddenly get to their feet on the morning of their first birthday. The typical range is about 9-18 months, and it's only after this that you might need to check with your health visitor if your little one isn't walking. Some babies love being able to run about the place. Others quite happily sit on their bum waiting for stuff to be brought to them. Who can blame them?

Your baby's social development

Another big change is in language development. Your baby will start to echo sounds back to you and use gestures such as pointing or clapping. They may point at something, such as the cat, and make a sound that is something like 'cat' but not quite. As babies reach the end of the first year they will probably say their first recognisable word, but again it might be up to around 18 months. First words are usually things that are common in their everyday lives. Mumma (or mummum or mamma or similar) and dadda are the most likely. Dadda

" Get as much sleep and rest as you can, be kind to yourself and remember it will pass!"

often comes before mumma because the letter d is easier to form and say than the letter m. Typical. They may also learn to shriek or scream loudly (at awkward times). Delightful. But, oh... that laugh.

Babies often start to understand simple language before they can say words. At around nine months you might find they can understand 'no' or words like 'bye bye' or realise the cat is a cat. I remember my daughter being a bit of a late talker – she'd hardly say a word, but if you asked her to fetch something, she'd do it. She clearly understood what items were and the instruction.

Now is a great time to really foster a love of reading and books. You might find your baby recognises books and may even have ones they prefer. They will be more interactive, pointing and grabbing at pictures, and may be able to 'point to the cat' and other things they recognise on the page. As they approach 12 months they may even be able to make a 'ca' sound, copying you.

Between 7 and 12 months babies also become a lot more aware of people around them. Suddenly becoming anxious when you leave them is normal, even if they have been quite happy before. This is known as separation anxiety and is a completely normal stage, and doesn't mean anything is wrong. With reassurance and consistency, it will likely start to ease. Basically, babies develop a sense of what is known as 'object permanency' at around this time, meaning they can remember people and objects when they're out of sight. Before this babies might cry because they were alone, but not necessarily because they missed a specific person or thing. Now, they can remember you clearly when you leave them (yay!) but this also means they can remember you clearly when you leave them and get upset (boo!).

Separation anxiety can be tough, but some ways to deal with it include starting off with short separations so your baby learns that you come back. Be as smiley and happy as possible when you leave or pick them up. You can try leaving something comforting that reminds them of you or a favourite toy. It will pass. You might also find that your baby seems fine when you leave and then immediately bursts into tears when you pick them up. Don't take this as an insult, see it that your baby was managing to be okay without you, but once they saw you they remembered you were gone and are now actually pleased to see you, even if it doesn't look like it. Remember to try and smile and cuddle and reassure them. All this is normal – it's a positive thing really. Your baby likes being with you.

You will probably also find that your baby becomes a bit wary with strangers, for example not wanting to have people they don't know hold them, or crying if a stranger stops to talk to you in the street. Again, this is a really normal stage and doesn't mean your baby hates people. It's thought to be a normal evolutionary protective mechanism. Your baby is mobile now and could crawl off. You wouldn't want them crawling off into the forest after people they don't know.

Your baby's sleep

Sleep *might* be getting a bit better, although babies this age are still more likely to wake once or twice a night (or sometimes more) than they are to sleep through. Research shows that only around 20% of babies consistently sleep through the night at this stage, although sleep periods do usually start to increase.

You might have decided to move your baby to their own room. It can take a while to learn to settle there alone, so expect your baby to need you a little more. Some people find their baby sleeps a bit better in their own room, while others find they are more unsettled. It's just a case of thinking about why your baby might be acting this way. Changes in sleep location, especially if you're now sleeping alone, unsettle adults – so why wouldn't they unsettle babies too?

You might also find that when your baby starts eating solid foods their sleep becomes a bit disturbed. Again, it's because it's a new thing and things are changing, which seems to disrupt their sleep. Also, it can take time for their digestive system to get used to solid food, which again can make them a bit more unsettled. This should soon pass – if your baby seems to be having any continued reaction to food speak to your health visitor or GP.

Look at the chapter on sleep for some ideas for helping to soothe your baby. As they are older and more aware, things like a gentle bedtime routine, favourite toy or even the cover of a favourite bedtime book may help them settle for sleep.

Your baby's growth

Growth continues to slow from 7–12 months. While babies double their birth weight in the first six months, gaining on average around 3–4kg, they'll gain more like 2–3kg in the second six months. Growth spurts will probably be less frequent. You can expect one at around nine months.

If your baby's growth starts to falter, make sure you are not giving them too many solid foods compared to milk. Have a look at Chapter 11 on introducing solid foods, and remember that introduction should be gradual, with milk (which has more calories than many weaning foods) still the main part of their diet. Adding in low-calorie but bulky foods too quickly can mean your baby doesn't get enough energy.

What this means for you

It's a time of big change. Your baby has gone from just making sounds, to maybe saying their first word, and from maybe needing help to sit up, to pulling themselves up and even walking. It's normal to feel both excited and a bit sad about this. Your baby has changed and is growing stronger and more independent, but you might miss those early months when they were so tiny. It's normal to feel all the emotions at once.

You may have also gone back to work and be juggling that with broken nights. You may have settled your baby into childcare and be focusing on making sure they're alright when really you need support too. Again, it's okay to have mixed emotions! Be kind to yourself.

When you have twins, triplets or more!

If you have twins, triplets or even more you might wonder whether their development will follow that of singleton babies. There is no evidence to suggest that their physical development will be much different, although if your babies were born very early or were low birth weight, they may take a little longer (have a look at the next chapter on premature babies). Given that most multiple births happen a little earlier than singleton pregnancies, it's a good idea to take into account that they have additional growing and development to do that they would usually do in the womb. However, milestones for babies are never about them doing something on a set date – there is always a window of time when you can reasonably expect them to do something. You only need to worry if they are not doing things after that window has passed. Most health professionals also say you should take off the weeks that they were premature to get a more realistic expectation of their development. As always, talk to your health visitor or GP if you are unsure.

One area where twins can take a little longer is in their language development. There are a number of ideas about why this happens, including the fact that you naturally can't spend as much one-on-one time with each baby as you can when you just have one. You might also be speaking to both of them, but you can only look at one: eye contact and facial expressions help babies to learn. Twins also spend more time engaging and interacting with each other, meaning they develop their own means of communication.

Some things you can do to encourage speech development in twins or triplets is to try to spend some one-on-one time each day where you focus on each baby separately. Read each baby a story separately, or sing to them, making eye contact. If you have a partner or visitors, encourage them to take a baby and talk or sing to them. Try to make sure they are surrounded by as many words as possible during the day, by talking to them while you're walking around or making dinner. Try not to have too much background noise. But don't worry – most twins catch up perfectly fine. It's about giving them more opportunity rather than panicking.

Whether your babies will develop at the same rate as *each other* is another question! If your babies are not identical, they may well do things at slightly different times or in a slightly different order, but most identical twins or triplets do things at the same time. But don't forget that they are still different babies and they may do things differently.

You can find out more about twin development and common questions on the Twins Trust website **twinstrust.org/let-us-help/parenting/under-1s.html**.

A final note and where to read more

Finally, remember that this is just a rough guide. Try not to get sucked into daft competitive parenting competitions, where your friend desperately tries to balance her four-month-old baby upright for four seconds to claim he's advanced, and you respond by trying to show off your little one's latest trick. If your baby isn't looking like they will meet milestones by the end of the age range, speak to your health visitor and they can explore whether it's anything to worry about. Some babies just prefer to watch the world go by (or are secretly plotting) and others are more inquisitive. Remember, Einstein didn't speak properly until he was four! If your baby does need further support there are lots of services out there to help.

There are some great books that go into your baby's development and changes in much more detail. If you want to read more I recommend:

- *The Wonder Weeks* - Xaviera Plas-plooij
- *What to Expect the First Year* - Heidi Murkoff
- *First-time Parent* - Lucy Atkins

Chapter six

When your baby is premature or sick

→ Having a premature or sick baby (or babies) is a huge shock, even if you knew from earlier in your pregnancy that it was likely to happen. There are so many things to get your head around, from them perhaps being in special care and you not being able to take them home immediately, to feeding them, and their longer-term growth and development. Life is unlikely to look like you imagined it would after birth. It may be a while before your baby even looks like the babies in the magazines – instead, they might be surrounded by wires, scary-looking equipment and beeps... with other people taking care of them.

It is normal to experience a whole range of emotions – and they may not necessarily go away as your baby gets bigger and stronger. You might be in shock, be angry, feel guilty, be worried or feel nothing at all. All of these are absolutely normal reactions, as is cycling rapidly between these emotions or indeed feeling them all at once. Don't let anyone tell you how you should feel, or expect yourself to feel a certain way. You feel how you feel and that's okay.

Looking after yourself

Remember in the midst of all of the chaos, that you matter. Perhaps you might have forgotten about yourself, or feel too overwhelmed or selfish to sometimes put yourself first. First, stop that. Your health matters. Your mental health matters. But if you can't accept that, put yourself first sometimes for the sake of your baby. You know that bit on the plane where they tell you to put your own oxygen mask on first before helping others because you're no use to anyone if you're collapsed in a heap?

This means spending as much time with your baby as is right for you. Maybe you feel like you should sit next to your baby every second that you can. If that is what you want, then ask friends or family to do everything they can to help make things easier for you. For some ideas if you're stuck, see below.

But if you feel you need a break – take a break! Your baby will be well looked after. If going home for a shower or sleep or out for a walk to get some fresh air or exercise, or even doing whatever makes you happy no matter how 'frivolous' is what you need – do it! If it makes you feel rested or happier (even for a brief moment) then it is worth it.

Take up all offers of help. Don't be British and respond with 'I'm fine, don't worry, but thanks for asking!' if people ask you what they can do. You're not being a burden on them (and if you are – they asked for it!). Lots of people like being able to help others, especially in this sort of situation. It helps them feel useful. Maybe they feel that they are giving back after having had a similar experience themselves.

If you can't think of anything you want them to do, here are some ideas:

- Drive you to and from hospital, especially if you can't drive or parking charges are high
- Make you meals and snacks
- Wash your clothes or clean your house
- Bring you things to the hospital/take them away again
- Put together a 'survival bag' for you of clean clothes, deodorant and other toiletries, something to do, something to eat...
- Sit with you if you're able to have visitors, or come to meet you in the hospital grounds or canteen for a walk
- Video call you when you're sat alone in the hospital
- Look after older children
- Support your partner with meals/cleaning/whatever – anything that enables your partner to give their energy to supporting you

My baby doesn't feel like mine

This is a common emotion and one that I think many new parents experience regardless of the situation. Even after a straightforward, full-term birth everyone feels a bit disconcerted by the idea that this baby is now yours to care

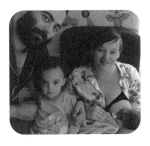

Our premature baby Samuel

Alyssia and Mike Edwards, parents to
Samuel who was born unexpectedly at 31
weeks.

Alyssia

Our first baby was a missed miscarriage, our second was born perfect at 38
weeks weighing 5lb 10oz, and as soon as I found out I was expecting again my
midwife had me listed as high risk due to my previous baby's low birth weight.
My pregnancy wasn't straightforward and I was at risk of miscarriage until 23
weeks when the heavy bleeding I'd been having suddenly stopped. Everything
then seemed normal and we were finally able to enjoy the pregnancy and
let our daughter get excited about being a big sister. The hardest thing was
constantly telling my two-year-old the baby in my tummy was poorly, just in
case something went wrong.

I had a reduction in movements at 30+2 weeks and I was admitted to
hospital, where it took over an hour to get the 'required movements'. A student
midwife assessed me and commented on how low down and engaged the baby
was. I remember hearing her saying to the other midwife 'Should we examine
mum just in case?' The midwife replied 'No, it's just because it's baby two, they
know where to go'. At 31+1 I couldn't sleep, the baby was right up in my ribs and
in my bladder at the same time, so much so that I went straight to antenatal at
9am for a check-up. They checked and dismissed everything – baby was moving
– but that wasn't my concern. I had some pink discharge and pain all down my
back and one side which they said was my SPD (symphysis pubis dysfunction).
They did bloods, said my cervix was closed and sent me home at 1pm.

After getting home I nursed my two-year-old for her nap and got in the bath.
I then knew it was labour because I couldn't move to get out. Panicking, I called
my husband who helped me dress and got us all to the hospital. I then walked
from the car to reception, where I could no longer walk and needed to push.
Amazingly I stayed calm and waited for a wheelchair, just focusing on the keeping baby in as I knew he would need help. We went straight to antenatal where I
saw the same midwife who asked me how I was. I was losing it slightly, saying 'I
need to push, baby's coming!' She replied 'Okay, it's alright, you're early yet, let's
examine you'. I got told to stand up and get on the bed and my waters went.

Two pushes later my little man arrived, screaming, in my knickers as we
could not get me undressed fast enough! He weighed an impressive 3lb 8oz, was
born after two minutes of second-stage labour and smashed every milestone!

Hearing his cry was magical, but my daughter Molly, who was with my husband Mike, had seen it all and got upset. Mike and Molly went to the waiting room while the medical staff tried (and failed) to deliver the placenta. It clearly knew it was too soon!

This is when I wobbled a lot: no matter what I said no one would tell me how my baby was. The midwife had cut the cord straight away and wrapped him in plastic and took him to a table to work on. Then SCBU (special care baby unit) came to collect him and only then did a nurse finally say to me that he was stable but needed some help, so they were taking him to HDU (high dependency unit) and I could see him as soon as I was ready. That turned out to be almost five hours later as I had to have surgery to remove the placenta. My baby was transferred the next morning to a NICU (neonatal intensive care unit) elsewhere, as our local hospital doesn't usually take babies born before 32 weeks.

How did you feel?

I was absolutely terrified, I felt guilty that I'd failed him. No one knows why he came early; my placenta was healthy as was the cord. For the few days he was in NICU I was lucky enough to be on antibiotics for the surgery and had a bed there to stay nearer to him as he was a half-hour drive from home.

The only thing I could do that they couldn't was provide him with milk. I went to the extreme and by day four I was getting 100ml out of each breast at every pump with the borrowed hospital-grade breast pump. The hospital gave me some wonderful reading material: a book about the terminology they use, the process and how best to support him including a milking schedule. This helped me a lot, it felt like I'd been given some control over it all.

The hospital encouraged me from the beginning to do my baby's care (top-to-toe washes and nappies), which made him feel more like mine. It's such a hard thing to explain, but I often felt like it wasn't real, that I was having an out-of-body experience. I was often on wards where women had their baby with them. This was when my mental health started to take a hit, as I was also concerned that I'd never left my two-year-old before and now I was away from her overnight.

When we moved back to the local hospital I started coping a little more with the premature-mum life. I'd have breakfast at home with my little girl and then head to the hospital to give my boy his cuddles and later on his breakfast and then stay till 3pm and head back for tea and bedtime with my girl. It was the hardest time of our lives, mentally, physically and emotionally. I was expressing every three hours on the dot, I was constantly going between my two babies and feeling like I was failing them both.

What helped you cope?

If you're anything like me, asking for help does not come easily. However, asking is a necessity as it is the most stressful rollercoaster and having that extra support is priceless.

Things that helped included the books they provided, and the equipment SCBU allowed us to borrow: the hospital-grade breast pump is an amazing machine and eased my worry as I could not express more than 30ml with my first with a generic hand pump. Having a routine for us all helped as well, as unfortunately as we had booked my husband's paternity leave based on Sam's due date, he went back to work after one (very luckily booked!) week off. This meant I had Molly and visiting Sam to juggle, but thankfully Molly was able to go to her grandparents while I was with Sam.

Our extended family rallied around us. Those who were too far away to visit and help sent Molly post: my mum would send treats and colouring in to keep her entertained. When Molly was with her grandparents they would send me messages about how she was which also helped.

I kept a journal of all Sam's firsts and how I was feeling. I also made sure that no matter how exhausted I felt, I made the time I was with Molly quality time. I took her in to see her brother as much as I could. It's hard for a two-year-old to understand that they can't run about and shout, so we used the unit's little family room and Mike and I would swap between us with Sam.

What did you find most difficult?

Asking permission to hold/touch my own baby. It's for their safety and I fully understand that, but it made it feel as if he was not mine. I also really struggled with cleanliness, not because I wasn't clean, but because I'd walk in with my hoodie zipped right up and then only that T-shirt was allowed to be anywhere near Sam. I remember once I had to go to the ward to see a doctor as Sam and I had thrush, Sam orally and myself in my breast. When I went I obviously had to show my breast and then I had a panic attack that I may have got germs from one place and taken them back to Sam. This is also, in hindsight, where I wish I'd asked for support from staff, but because they were there for my baby, I wouldn't talk to them about my needs as they were busy enough. I should have spoken to my health visitor. It's easier said than done and that's why I felt it was difficult.

What would you tell other parents in this situation?

Talk! Ask questions. So many times the nurses would just say something and I'd nod like I understood and then google it. This is literally the worst thing you can do. Sam had a brain scan and they discovered a cyst. The doctor was so blasé and said 'Yes he has a cyst, it may be bad or it may be nothing. Okay, thanks, see you soon.' I googled it and it linked me to cerebral palsy and I broke down. The guilt just flooded over me and I remember crumbling in on myself, holding him saying 'I'm sorry, I'm so sorry' over and over.

When his nurse noticed she came straight over and after chatting she then went off and called a doctor who turned out to be the neonatal brain doctor for the unit and he came in after his shift had finished to talk me through Sam's scans and explain that the position of his cyst was optimistic because it's not anywhere

where it may cause lasting damage. He also pointed out that they routinely scan neonates but not newborns, so there may be more cases of cysts like this that are just not documented. This was a turning point for me and why I urge you to ask questions. Staff are there to support you in supporting your baby. If I'd asked initially, I wouldn't have been so upset.

Also remember to look after yourself. It's so so easy to forget about it. I would also recommend speaking about any concerns/issues with your health visitor or GP, as I felt okay after taking Sam home, but my anxiety and depression spiralled later and the worse it got the harder it was to admit it. The support for mums and families isn't very obvious but they will help you, and I urge you to seek it. I still cannot walk into a hospital without my anxiety skyrocketing and being anywhere near antenatal or SCBU sends me into a panic attack, but I'm working on it!

I would also like to add he was feeding from the breast at 32+2, exactly one week old, despite the SCBU nurses saying he wouldn't till 34+ weeks. Instead he was home weighing 4lb 10oz at 34+4! To calculate age for a premature baby they refer to them with their gestational age until their due date and then it becomes their corrected age. So on Sam's due date he was nine weeks old, but newborn corrected. This applies to developmental abilities, not medical ones such as immunisations which will follow actual age. I came home with a substantial milk stash which I donated to the milk bank to help other babies as had I been unable to express any I would have requested donor breastmilk for Sam. Donating the milk was also a fantastic feeling of helping others and they sent me a lovely certificate.

Fast forward to today and he is thriving – he's on target for his actual age of 20 months old now, busy as anything and a little daredevil. There is light at the end of the tunnel, so hang in there!

Mike

Our premature baby was our third pregnancy after a first missed miscarriage and a following successful pregnancy. My partner and I had a difficult time with both pregnancies that followed the missed miscarriage, including constant anxiety and bleeding throughout the pregnancies.

On the day of the birth my partner complained of abdominal pains, so we went to the antenatal ward in the morning. She was checked over and we were discharged home with no concerns. Roughly an hour or so later the pain had worsened and so we decided to drive back to the antenatal ward. On arriving at the hospital, the pain was too much and my partner was unable to walk through the door. We grabbed a porter and a wheelchair, and she was wheeled up to the ward. My partner was helped onto an examination bed for a check, but in doing so her waters broke and soon the room was full of doctors and nurses while I was ushered out into the waiting room with our two-year-old daughter. There was a lot of commotion, but my focus was on keeping our daughter safe and as calm as possible. After a while I was brought back into the room to my partner, and our newborn was taken off to the neonatal care unit. My wife was taken to surgery to remove the placenta and recover. A few hours later, we could visit him to see how he was doing, but obviously he was still in a care unit so we could only look. He was also soon transferred to another hospital more designed to care for such premature babies.

Over the time of his care in the various units we were allowed various levels of interaction, from only observing him in the neonatal ICU to being able to eventually hold him in the Special Care Baby Unit. Overall, he was in care for just short of four weeks, which required a lot of back-and-forth visits and continuous care for mum and daughter.

How did you feel?

The initial birth was a fast situation, but I spent most of the time in a waiting room with our daughter, answering her questions about the situation and making sure she was okay. There were obviously questions I had but given that everyone was understandably more preoccupied with my partner, asking them anything was the last thing on my mind.

Seeing my partner upset was obviously upsetting, but again it was important to be reassuring and dwelling isn't usually how I deal with the problematic aspects of a situation. I spent my time with my partner and daughter for as long as we could so that we could just process. After this time together my partner remained in the hospital, and my daughter and I returned home.

In the time after the birth, when Sam was in SCBU and NICU, my partner remained as an outpatient and me and my daughter regularly made the daily trip to see both mother and newborn. These trips were a mixture of nerves travelling to the hospital, happy-sadness at seeing our son in the care unit, and guilt when travelling back home at the end of the day.

Once our son had returned home there was a good deal of initial happiness, excited that we could finally return as a family. This was also combined with apprehension in caring for a still very tiny child, and the worry of what the next few years would have in store for us and him. There was also a good deal of concern about my partner's experience of the whole situation and how we could maximise our bonding with our son.

Now that we have had over a year with him, these feelings of worry have quickly dissipated. In fact for me the memory of 'premature baby' times had passed within a few months. He routinely shows us that he is a bright and well-developed little human, showing all the bossiness and humour that his sister displays. I do not see him as being impacted by his prematurity now at all; the vast majority of the impact seems to have been on my partner, with some impact on myself being much further down the scale. These days are filled more with the emotions of a typical parent, exhausted by busy but lovely children.

What made it easier?

For me it was seeing the professionalism of the staff who cared for our son, coupled with their human-touch approach to care. They understood the importance of us seeing our child, even when he was in a vulnerable state. They were also extremely supportive with breastmilk-feeding our son when it was safe to do so, which helped my partner bond, but also allowed me to support her during times when my partner expressed to tube-feed, even if it was helping prep the sterilisation bags and set up the pumping equipment.

It was also helpful to see our son really grow and develop into himself. It took time but seeing him reach various milestones was reassuring. I didn't focus on any missed milestones – dwelling wasn't beneficial – but we did mention them to his healthcare workers. The key thing was to embrace and enjoy the ones reached.

Explaining the situation to our daughter was also a good experience. She has never expressed concern or worry for her brother's wellbeing or his prematurity, but instead has learned the terminology and the importance of the situation. This also helped us to rationalise things by explaining them and talking about it.

Coping, for me, was relatively straightforward once our son returned home. Without dwelling on issues of the situation, it didn't feel as though our son was hindered by his prematurity, but rather that we as parents had to adjust our expectations of what could be done. Our son now had requirements that our daughter didn't need when she was born, and we simply had to work with those in mind.

I felt work was a beneficial way to cope, although it did produce feelings of guilt at being away during these times.

What did you find most difficult?

Honestly the impact on my partner was the most difficult outcome. The feeling of guilt and worry was difficult to alleviate, and the situation had a strong effect on her. The desire to help, comfort and console is ongoing, but the experience is always a deep and personal one. Slowly, over time, we are developing as a family, and these experiences are being softened with happier ones.

Frantically searching for premature baby clothes and other things is also not a fun experience. These experiences can often come at a moment's notice and finding the things you may need at the drop of a hat can be difficult, especially when you have the perfect 'coming home' outfit planned that is in a full-term baby size.

What would you tell other parents in this situation?

For the mother: try not to dwell too much on the why or how. This experience has happened, and the important thing is to savour the present moments going forward. What seems like a defining moment now may not be so impactful later. Look for those little moments of happiness.

For the partner: take time to support the mother and yourself. Talk to others, including your partner, about how you feel. Remember to collect memories of the time: it may seem like you need to focus 100 per cent, but take the time to take a photo or two for reflection later.

for. But this is especially so with premature babies, as it can feel like they are taken away from you and looked after by machines and professionals who all seem to know just what they are doing. It can feel like the professionals are in charge and your baby is being cared for as a patient – not by you as a parent.

It's okay to feel angry and bitter about this. Yes, of course you are grateful for medicine being able to keep your baby alive, but you can still feel displaced or that you have had your baby's early days stolen from you. Jealousy is normal too. Why are they seemingly allowed to do things to your baby when you are not? Why are they 'in charge' rather than you?

It's also okay to tell staff that you want to take a more active role when possible. Ask if you can hold your baby. Remember, you are asking permission from a medical perspective to hold your baby in their current state, rather than permission to hold your baby as their mother. Good professionals will let you do everything you can to help care for your baby. It might not be possible right now, but never feel like you shouldn't ask.

What about feeding your premature baby?

If your baby is premature, especially if they are in neonatal care, you will likely be encouraged to give them your breastmilk if at all possible. If they are very small or sick it might not be possible for you to feed them directly from the breast at first, so instead you will be encouraged to express your milk and it will be given to them via a tube through their nose or stomach or perhaps in a cup or bottle. As they get bigger and stronger you will be able to move towards breastfeeding them. For more information on breastfeeding, expressing and making more milk, see Chapter 9.

Sometimes, if your baby is very small and sick they might need some specialist human milk fortifier added to your milk. Sometimes these are based on human milk and sometimes on cows' milk. Fortifier may be needed because very small babies need a lot more protein, calcium, phosphorous and other vitamins and minerals than there are in breastmilk. These nutrients are particularly important for later bone health.

The decision on this will be made very carefully by your healthcare team, weighing up the benefits and risks of adding fortifier to your milk. There is little evidence that babies over 33 weeks need fortifier, and if your baby weighs over 1,250–1,500g and is getting enough breastmilk to gain weight they may not benefit either. If cows' milk fortifiers are used, the risk of NEC (necrotising enterocolitis, a serious illness affecting the gut – see below) starts to increase, alongside the risk of other gastrointestinal issues and infections, in part because cows' milk fortifier appears to stop some of the immune properties of breastmilk from working.[1]

Breastmilk is especially recommended for sick and premature babies for a number of reasons.

1. It is full of antibodies that help protect your baby against infections

Babies receive some antibodies direct from you through the placenta, but this happens particularly in the last months of pregnancy. If they are born very premature, they will not have received these antibodies. Also, breastmilk has additional antibodies. Colostrum – the very first milk you will produce – is particularly high in these antibodies, so even if you do not plan to breastfeed longer term, giving your baby even just a few days of milk will help pass these antibodies on.[2] Premature babies who receive human milk have lower rates of infections, sepsis and readmission to hospital.[3]

2. It helps to prevent necrotising enterocolitis

Necrotising enterocolitis (NEC) is a very serious illness in which tissues in your baby's intestines become inflamed and start to die, potentially leading to holes developing and the contents of the intestine leaking into the abdomen. This can cause serious, life-threatening infections. It is much more common in premature babies than those who are full-term, particularly those who are born very prematurely at less than 32 weeks or those weighing under 1,500g.

Although researchers are not exactly sure why, babies who receive human milk are a lot less likely to develop NEC. Having only human milk is ideal, although any amount of human milk you can give your baby helps them. For example, one study found that babies who only had formula milk were 6–10 times more likely to develop NEC, but three times more likely if they had breastmilk and formula. It is thought that human milk prevents NEC by reducing the risk of inflammation in the gut, and by helping create a healthy microbiome which appears to help reduce the risk of NEC.[4]

3. Breastmilk is easier to digest than formula milk

Breastmilk is easier for babies to digest than formula milk. One reason for this is that it contains live enzymes that help break it down, which formula milk does not. Babies find formula, which is based on cows' milk, more difficult to digest than human milk. This is important for premature babies or those who are sick, as they need to keep as much energy as possible for growing and fighting off illnesses.

4. It helps with their physical development

A number of studies have shown that premature babies benefit from receiving human milk in terms of their brain development and later measures of intelligence.[5]

What about donor milk?

If you find it too difficult to express enough milk, or are on a medication that is not recommended for breastfeeding, you may be able to access donor milk for your premature baby. In some hospitals this is reserved for babies under 32 weeks old. Donor milk is donated by other women who are breastfeeding. Milk donors are screened to ensure they are healthy, and the milk is pasteurised to make sure it doesn't contain bacteria or viruses such as HIV, hepatitis, or cytomegalovirus. Although this reduces some of the beneficial immune properties in breastmilk, they are still much higher than in formula milk (which contains none). This means that premature babies who receive donor milk are less likely to develop infections, including NEC. They also have better brain and eye development. Donor milk is also easier for them to digest.[6]

If you'd like to read more about donor milk, including experiences of receiving it or going on to be a donor yourself in the future, have a look at the work of the Human Milk Foundation. The foundation works to help families feed their babies with human milk, including helping more families receive milk, raising funds to provide milk and research into the impact and experience of receiving donor milk. They also have information on who can donate milk and how, what happens to it and who receives it – alongside a link to donate money to support their vital work humanmilkfoundation.org.

More information on feeding your premature baby

- My own *The Positive Breastfeeding Book* has lots of background and guidance, including tips on making more milk, tube feeding and transitioning to a bottle.
- Kathryn Stagg IBCLC is a lactation consultant who has particular expertise in feeding twins and premature babies. Her blog has lots of useful information on feeding small and sick babies and transitioning from feeding tube to feeding from the breast kathrynstaggibclc.com.
- La Leche League Great Britain has a great guide to preparing for and caring for your premature baby www.laleche.org.uk/successfully-breastfeeding-premature-baby.

Your premature baby's physical development

Your premature baby's development will be individual to them and their circumstances. Do talk to your health visitor, GP or any specialists involved if you are concerned. Remember, when your baby is born prematurely, they need to do all the growing and developing they would have done in the womb on the outside. This means that compared to a baby born at full term on the same date, they're likely to take longer to reach developmental milestones such as sitting up or walking. And that's fine and to be expected.

Usually any suggested age guides for your baby will be what is known as 'corrected'. To do this, take your baby's age, subtract how many weeks premature they were and then look at the guidelines for that age rather than your baby's actual age. So for a six-month-old baby born two months premature, look at the guidelines for around four months, not six.

Premature babies do tend to catch up and by the time your child is around two years old they will probably be meeting milestones at around the same time as their peers. If they were very premature (weighing less than 1-1.5kg) then they might take a little longer to catch up, perhaps meeting their peers at around three years. Remember these are guidelines, and not meeting them isn't an automatic sign something is wrong. The main thing is that they are developing and moving forward – how quickly they do it is secondary to that. If you have any questions or concerns, just ask. Your professionals are there to reassure you.

Further reading about premature babies
- The BLISS website – for lots of support about caring for your baby. www. bliss.org.uk
- The Tommy's website – particularly the section on growth and development after prematurity. www.tommys.org/pregnancy-information/ pregnancy-complications/premature-birth/taking-your-baby-home/growth-and-development-after-prematurity
- The Baby Buddy App by Best Beginnings also has a video and information on premature babies. www.bestbeginnings.org.uk/small-wonders
- Some good books include *Preemies: The Essential Guide for Parents of Premature Babies* by Dana Wechsler Linden, *Preemie Care: A Guide to Navigating the First Year with Your Premature Baby* by Karen Lasby and Tammy Sherrow and *Hold Your Prem* by Jill and Nils Bergman

My baby has been diagnosed with a health condition

Some babies who are born prematurely or too small will overcome this initial challenge and grow and develop as expected. However, some parents will also be dealing with their baby having an illness or disorder, perhaps one that caused their baby to be born too soon in the first place, or one that developed due to prematurity. This of course is a deeply distressing and difficult time and will be different for every family dependent on their individual baby's needs. Importantly, there is support out there.

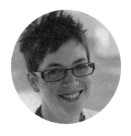

Five common emotions you may feel when your child is diagnosed with an illness

Lyndsey Hookway is a paediatric nurse, specialist community public health nurse, health visitor and IBCLC. Lyndsey has worked in hospitals, neonatal intensive care units, clinics, communities and in families' homes. She has supported families within the NHS, in international private practice, in voluntary outreach, and as part of research projects. She is the founder of the Breastfeeding The Brave project, and the clinical director of the Holistic Sleep Coaching Program. She has experience of her own daughter having leukaemia and the impact that can have on families.

Childhood illness can bring about some pretty intense emotions. Anger. Grief. Shock. Stress. Whether you knew your baby's condition even before they were born, or your baby has become unwell in the early days, weeks or months, you will undoubtedly feel a bewildering array of feelings.

You may wonder 'why my baby', only to then quickly feel guilty because you wouldn't wish this on anyone. You may wish you could take your child's illness upon yourself, to spare them the treatment or problems they will face. You may be angry at those around you with healthy children, despising those who complain about seemingly trivial problems when you have a bigger mountain to climb. All of these feelings and more are completely normal. You are not strange, and you are not alone.

We need to learn how to thrive through illness. Because it deviates from the normal course of childhood, thriving through adversity requires adaptations. It may initially provoke a 'rabbit-in-headlights' response as we realise that aspects of family life we had planned may now need altering.

Of course, not everyone feels all these feelings, and different illnesses and conditions may bring about different responses. Having a sudden admission to hospital in the middle of the night is very different from finding out at your 20-week scan that your baby has a congenital condition. And a long-term illness that requires treatment for many months or years is very different from a condition that can be cured quickly, albeit with intensive treatment.

Your baby is unique, and so is your experience of illness. However, many of the feelings that can crop up are shared by parents experiencing a variety of health-related dramas for their little ones, including grief and shock, anxiety and stress, anger and frustration, exhaustion and overwhelm and also making sense of the situation and adjusting to a new normal.

1. Grief and shock

You may have had many aspirations for your baby. Ultimately though, what most parents want for their child is for them to be healthy and safe. An illness, whether brief or longer lasting, or a disability or other condition fundamentally challenges that most basic and primal desire for a healthy child. Illness is never something any parent plans or wants for their little one. Accepting the reality of illness can cause feelings of shock. You may also grieve what 'might have been'.

How to cope

You may have a tried and tested way of coping with difficult times. Perhaps you will utilise your 'go-to' strategy in this situation as well. Here's how some people respond to grief and shock:

- Information finding. Although there is a danger of over-googling something and ending up more stressed than you started, to a certain extent knowledge is power. Being informed about your baby's condition and knowing what to expect in the next few days can be a constructive way of coping. I strongly suggest you request a meeting with your baby's doctor, who will be intimately acquainted with the details of your child's condition and can advise you on an individual basis. The internet can be a scary place, and other people's experiences may not be relevant to yours.
- Journaling. It can be very cathartic to write and diarise your experiences. This can also be a way of getting your thoughts out of your head and stop your brain from buzzing and whirring in the small hours.
- Try to eat snacks. During times of acute stress, sometimes you lose your appetite completely. Rather than feeling daunted at the idea of a large meal, try to keep a steady flow of healthy snacks going. This is something really practical that others can do to help you as well. You will probably have lots of nebulous offers of help, and this is a very specific task that you can delegate.
- Be prepared. When your baby is diagnosed with an illness, it helps to have an emergency bag ready. Perhaps leave it in your car if you have one, or by the front door, ready to grab as you go. Include changes of clothes for you both, non-perishable snacks, phone charger and a book.

2. Anxiety and stress

When a baby is diagnosed with a health problem it is natural for parents to feel anxious and stressed about it. On a scientific level, you have an automatic stress response, over which you have little control. This includes the physical reaction to stress – such as sweaty palms, racing heart, nausea, loss of appetite, and so on. It also encompasses some of the automatic emotional processes, such as panic, irrational thoughts, and behaving as if on 'auto-pilot'. You may find that you do procedural tasks without even realising what you've done. You may pace the floor or tap your foot.

How to cope

You can't always control the automatic responses of your stressed brain. But you can develop intentional coping responses and strategies.

- Some people choose to distract themselves when they feel stressed or anxious – sometimes keeping your hands busy is enough, such as with knitting, or colouring in.
- Sometimes you may need to direct your brain away from anxious thoughts, with activities such as jigsaws, crosswords, or sudoku.
- You may feel like your brain isn't up to its usual speed, so a book you have read many times, or a novel that you can dip in and out of, might help.
- Practise mindfulness, guided relaxations, meditation or yoga.
- Talk to friends and family.
- Get support from a professional. There are people who can help you to move through the heavy negative feelings of anxiety and stress. Ask your doctor to refer you, or find a local psychotherapist or counsellor.

3. Anger and frustration

It might sound strange to talk about feeling angry or frustrated, and yet this is a common response to a diagnosis of illness or a chronic condition. You may feel angry at a higher power, the medical professionals, yourself, or even your baby. It's very common to feel like you want to blame someone, even when rationally nobody is to blame. You may also feel out of control and frustrated by some of the implications of having and caring for a sick child. While your prime concern is likely to be your child, it's also normal and common to feel frustrated about the impact of your child's illness on you, your career, your home and family life and your experience of parenting.

How to cope

Here are some tips to get on top of the negative feelings:

- Try some exercise if you can. Even if you are in hospital with your little one, take the stairs instead of the lift. Go for a walk – hospitals are big places, so it's pretty easy to get your step count up as long as you are able to leave the ward for a while. You might even be able to take your baby out for a walk with you sometimes.
- Try to shift your anger away from people. Write a letter to your child's illness instead of feeling the need to play the blame game.
- Let go of things that are outside your control and focus on things you can control.
- Talk to a friend who is a good listener. Sometimes it helps to rant, cry, shout or offload on someone who knows you well and can listen non-judgementally.

4. Exhaustion and overwhelm

The experience of having a baby with an illness or condition can be crushingly exhausting. Not only is the stress and worry of this time mentally exhausting, but you might also struggle with your own sleep. It can be hard to switch off, and you might still feel tired when you wake up. Stress can make it harder to fall asleep, stay asleep, and achieve good quality, restful sleep. On top of this, there may be other aspects of caring for a little one that are physically demanding and overwhelming as well.

How to cope

Here are some ideas for looking after yourself:

- Try to rest whenever you can. Just lying down and reading a book can help to recharge your batteries. Instead of focusing on times when sleep doesn't come easily, focus on resting your body and mind.
- Accept offers of help. People will be keen to help, so don't feel self-conscious about accepting. Have a list of what people can do to help handy, and get a close friend to send it to people on your behalf. Others can also coordinate a support response, to save you endless organising and corresponding when you may not feel like it. Delegate caring for your home, pets, and any other children. Ask for help with grocery shopping and bringing in meals and snacks for you.
- If possible, ask someone to come and sit with your little one for an hour while you leave the ward, take a shower, or have some time at home.
- Develop some soothing routines for yourself. Hospital routines can be quite disruptive to sleep, so find out what care your baby will have and plan your routines around when you are likely to be disturbed.

5. Making sense of it all

How do we make sense of and come to terms with something that doesn't make sense? Well, in one respect, we can't. It's never okay that a little one becomes unwell – it feels particularly unfair that a baby can become sick. Many people feel the need to mark and validate their experience in some way, or somehow adjust to a 'new normal'.

How to cope

You may find some of the following suggestions helpful if your child has a more long-term health condition.

- Depending on your baby's condition, they may be eligible for the Beads of Courage programme. This is a lovely charity that provides a decorative bead to mark certain procedures your baby has borne with bravery. Beads of Courage support children with chronic serious illness, premature babies and siblings. See **www.beadsofcourage.org**

- You may want to fundraise for a particular relevant charity that has supported you and your baby, whether that is the in-hospital charity, a hospital accommodation charity, or a condition-specific charity. This can help to give back, and also provide something meaningful from a challenging experience. Some people run marathons, others brave the shave, still others organise black-tie gala dinners, and some decide to host a nearly new sale with proceeds going to charity.

- You might want to mark your baby's illness in a tangible and positive way – such as making a photobook, planting a beautiful tree, or writing a poem.

- You might want to join a support group for other parents whose children are coping with the same condition. There is nothing like being able to talk to other people who understand better than anyone what it is like to walk in your shoes.

Childhood illness is many things, but I think above everything else it wants to be a thief. It tries to steal joy, fun, family time, togetherness, carefree days, normality, socialising, school days, and laughter. However, if you can learn to develop coping mechanisms, and accept some adaptations, you can stop the thief in its tracks. I don't mean you can stop the course of the illness. I don't mean that it will be easy. But over the years I've learnt that you can develop character, resilience and grace that you didn't know you were capable of. You'll discover that friends and family who matter are the ones who show up. You'll learn that bravery isn't the absence of fear, but the quiet, steadfast perseverance in spite of it. You'll learn that you can admire and respect a tiny human for coping with something that even an adult shouldn't have to cope with. You'll learn that as a parent, you can't always make everything okay, but you can make things better simply by being there.

Chapter seven

When your baby is developing differently

→ This chapter considers the different emotions and thoughts you might be having, what you might be thinking and where to find support when your baby is developing differently to other babies. They might, for example, have Down's syndrome, a brain injury or developmental delay. There are many different conditions your child might have been diagnosed with, and each will have their own specific symptoms and pathways of care. I won't detail each here from a medical perspective, but rather consider something that most likely underlies all parents' experiences – how you feel and where to get support.

Although the specifics of care for your baby will differ based on their needs, it is likely that you share a number of experiences, emotions and fears with other parents whose baby is also developing differently. As is common on becoming a new parent anyway, it's likely these emotions and worries are varied and polarised, exacerbated as the future you may have imagined changes around you. But as Anita, mother to a daughter with Down's syndrome, explains in this chapter, 'different' or 'changed' doesn't mean less or worse... it just means, well... different.

Maybe you found out that your baby was developing differently during pregnancy. Maybe it came as a shock after birth. Or maybe it has been something

> **" 'Different' or 'changed' doesn't mean less or worse... it just means, well... different. "**

that you have seen developing slowly as they are growing older. Every baby will be different, even those with the same condition. But seeking out more information, emotional support and solidarity with other parents in similar situations can be a way of riding the rollercoaster and adapting to that change.

Remember that your child is not simply their diagnosis. They are a baby with their own personality and future, who happens to be affected physically, cognitively or emotionally by differences in the way they are developing. They are a child with autism or Down's syndrome – not 'autistic' or 'a Down's syndrome child'. They are more than a label. And you might hear many labels that you come to wholeheartedly disagree with. Your child does not have a 'defect' or 'disorder', which you might hear tossed around as 'medical' terms. You will know they are much more than this. I know it stings to hear such words, and that it provokes emotions you are trying so hard to control.

This is why support from organisations and other parents who know what you are experiencing is so important. At the end of this chapter there is a list of organisations and sources of support that can help. I bet you there is also a Facebook group, no matter how rare your baby's condition may be. A huge upside of social media has been to bring people together from around the world to share and support each other. It can be so reassuring to read stories from people further along on the journey than you, to see what the future might look like and learn about positive things you can do, especially if you are feeling terrified right now. Let people support you and care for you and one day in the future you might be that person comforting and reassuring another new parent in the group.

The early days and weeks with your baby may have been even more of a whirlwind than you expected. Tests and conversations and having to adapt your plans. Therefore, what I have already said in previous chapters gets emphasised a million times more. You matter too. Looking after yourself is so important. Proactively think about who can help you and how, so you get chance to rest: both to physically recover from birth, but also to process and reflect on what has happened. Time together with your partner (if you have one) is probably even more important than ever so you can just be together and support each other. Surround yourself with care and support as much as possible, in a way that feels right for you.

Again, as with any parenting experience, different people will have different emotions and fears. There is absolutely no one way to react. You might feel heartbroken. You might not feel as fazed as you expected. You might be confused, feel shocked or be in a state of disbelief. You might spend every night reading as much as possible, or try to avoid any information at all. You might ring everyone you know or you might feel like hiding away. You may want to celebrate and share, or you may need time to yourselves as a family. Never feel like there is one right way to react, or that you are a 'bad parent' for not feeling certain things. Give yourself time, care, space and permission to just be and feel whatever you want.

Some people find the piece of writing 'Welcome to Holland' by Emily Perl Kingsley[1] a really helpful piece to think about and reflect on. I know, however, that others don't like it, or feel conflicted. When reading about it, I found a great blog piece by Kristen Groseclose called 'The Trouble with Welcome to Holland'[2] that I thought expressed it better than I could. Essentially, some parents feel that it diminishes their experiences, and underestimates, or ignores, grief. Others find it intensely useful. Some people feel all of those things consecutively or simultaneously. As I keep emphasising, how you feel about it is very much up to you.

At the end of the day everyone's baby and experience as a family is different. On the next page Anita tells us about her life with her daughter Magdalena, who has Down's syndrome.

Further support

Cerebra: Cerebra.org.uk Tel: 01267 244 200
A charity dedicated to helping families with children with brain conditions discover a better life together.

Contact: Contact.org.uk Free helpline: 0808 808 3555. This organisation works with families to support all aspects of life parenting a child with a disability. It provides a national advice information and support service.

The National Portage Association: www.portage.org.uk/about/what-portage
Tel: 0121 244 1807 info@portage.org.uk

Family Fund: Familyfund.org.uk Grants to improve quality of life and ease the financial pressures of raising a child with a disability.

Scope: Scope.org.uk Helpline: 0800 800 3333. A disability equality charity providing practical and emotional support as well as campaigning for a fairer society. They also have an online community.

PADS (Positive about Down syndrome): www.positiveaboutdownsyndrome. co.uk PADS is run by parents for parents and parents-to-be. The Facebook page shares everyday stories of people with Down syndrome. They run a welcoming closed Facebook group for new parents too. They also link to a network of support groups around the UK that they can put families in touch with.

Future of Downs: www.futureofdowns.com Support, chat and information for parents of children with Down's syndrome. They run a large, active Facebook group specifically for parents.

Down's Syndrome Association: www.downs-syndrome.org.uk Helpline: 0333 121 2300. The national organisation with lots of resources and information here.

Autism: autism.org.uk Helpline 0808 800 4104

Support organisation for Trisomy 13 and Trisomy 18 and related conditions: www.soft.org.uk

Financial support available as listed on the government website: www.gov.uk/browse/benefits/disability

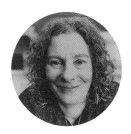

Five things to think about when your baby is developing differently

Anita is mother to Magdalena, who has Down's syndrome, and is author of a forthcoming book called *Magdalena's Milk* about breastfeeding and Down's syndrome. You can find out more by emailing magdalenasmilk@gmail.com

Hello and congratulations on your baby! I'm mother to three daughters, aged 25, 18 and 14. My youngest was diagnosed with Down's syndrome a week after she was born. A few years after that, she had an additional diagnosis of visual impairment and then some years after that, autism.

But that doesn't describe my daughter at all! And those words are no longer heavily loaded; they are as light to me as 'leaf', 'sky', 'blossom'. My daughter is Magdalena; she is graceful, gentle, sensitive and strong-willed. Fascinated by how things work, she retains focus in what interests her and repeats something to know it intimately. She is intrigued by the natural world and has an extensive knowledge of insects and animals. She is enthralled by Greek myths, which she has learnt off by heart through asking her dad to tell her the stories repeatedly until she knows them herself. She is excited by the sea and will plunge in no matter the weather. She loves to spin, like a whirling dervish; feeling the wind in her hair while she sings along with heartfelt emotion to her favourite songs. Magdalena and her big sisters got up to the usual sibling fun and mischief when they were little and Magdalena starred in an award-winning film series that her sister made about the things they got up to together. Family life is both ordinary and beautiful, and ever-changing.

I'm remembering the many emotions, which swelled up amidst the intense physical work of keeping my daughter alive during her first year. And I'm thinking it's likely that you've not had a moment for yourself yet; let alone time for friendships that you'd normally turn to for support. You are likely coping with de-coding medical terminology, possibly feeling anxious about the future and you may be grieving the loss of how you expected your life with your new baby to be. It is very likely that your head feels foggy from trying to make sense of what it all means... for your baby, you, your family. These feelings are normal, and if I could I'd want to just give you a hug right now, admire your beautiful baby, make you a cup of tea, cook you some comforting soup and let you know that this rollercoaster of emotions will pass, and that there are some practical tips which can help during the first year of parenting your beautiful baby who needs that bit of extra care.

1. Include your child in all of your family life

Everything may be different to how you imagined. But 'different' isn't 'less' – many would say that life becomes richer as we learn to live more fully in the present. Providing a nurturing environment will nourish your child's physical, mental, and emotional development. You are planting the garden in which they will find their interests, and in which their curiosity will develop. Everything that a child is or isn't exposed to can have an effect on development. If we include our babies in everything our family loves to do, then there's a good chance that they will grow up enjoying those things too, or at least accepting that this is part of their normal family life! So don't listen to the naysayers, include your child in your usual family life. Find people who empower you on your journey, who celebrate and enjoy your child for who they truly are. Your child is unique, and your relationship and particular life circumstances are unique.

Ignite your imagination. If your child's interests (or yours!) lead you towards an activity which appears impossible for your child to access because it is designed for typically developing children, don't give up, explore it further! Humans are gloriously inventive and forever designing adaptations and technological gadgets that make a world of inclusion and active participation increasingly possible. Also, try out new things... and be willing to be surprised. For example, my daughter loves playing with balls: kicking them, catching them, throwing them. With her sight impairment and low muscle tone we certainly didn't expect this to be something that she would enjoy, but she does.

2. Reach out to friends and groups in your own way

Parent and baby groups can be great, but they can also be an ordeal that zaps the limited energy you have. Especially when the groups revolve around mainstream conversation about typically developing babies. It takes energy to educate people about your need to be included in the conversations by them not assuming that all parenting experiences are the same. Whereas they may be complaining about sleepless nights, for example, your greatest wish may be that your baby would wake by themselves to feed. A room full of tired parents in an echoing community hall is a challenging place to have sensitive conversations and if you try and people don't get it, that can hurt.

So, if a baby and parent group isn't nourishing you, then don't go. Look for different groups to try; maybe a baby massage group, a parent and baby yoga group, or a sing-along-with baby group. Look for just one person in each group that you feel you may be able to connect with. Get a phone number, try and connect outside of the group. If after three sessions you aren't feeling any connection or love from the group, don't continue. You don't have to put yourself in situations where you feel drained, upset, unacknowledged or invisible. Walk away and say no when you need to: now is not a time for duty or obligation.

It's okay to do less generally, do life slower; at a pace that is good for you. It's okay to stay home. Your baby needs you right now and you need your baby. You'll feel better for taking this time to slow down to align with your baby's pace. Give yourself permission to cuddle and be with your gorgeous little one. They need you. Breathe together, holding your baby skin-to-skin. It will be good for both of you.

You can try inviting one friend at a time to come and visit you, and ask them to bring a dish of food. This will give you both space to be connected, and have conversations together, while fitting around what you and your baby need and saving the energy it costs you to go outside of your home.

3. Dealing with appointments

When your baby is developing differently many different specialists become involved in their welfare. Much of this support will be welcomed and reassuring, with access to services that will be valuable now and through the years. But it can feel overwhelming.

A specialist's job is to support our babies' health and development. To do this they need to listen and work together with us. We can ensure they do this through asking questions and for clarification when we need it. We can request second opinions where necessary, and ask that medical terms are explained to us in language that we understand. It is important that our voices are listened to and heard. We are the experts in our children. We are also the only ones who have been to every appointment and heard every specialist's opinion, which gives us unique insights that are vital to the decision-making around our children. If you have a hunch or instinct, follow it.

This takes a lot of extra work and the weight of responsibility can feel immense. It's natural to worry that we aren't doing enough, but you probably are doing more than enough. Your baby has the same needs as every other baby: to be loved, fed and cared for. Gathering information when faced with a new situation is what we do; we want to learn how to best meet our babies' needs and for them to fulfil their potential. To prevent burnout and retain balance it can help to write down questions as they arise, then put a daily time limit on your information-gathering. Choose trusted sources of information to find answers to your questions – start with taking a look through the links that I've recommended. Equally, if the thought of reading more 'stuff' brings you down or fills you with dread – don't do it! It's not necessary: you are all your baby needs right now and they won't be getting 'you' while you're online or exhausted from doing research in the middle of the night!

You can take a friend (without a baby) with you to appointments. This can be so supportive in helping you remember key points, and having someone to discuss them with afterwards. Also why not make the day into something enjoyable? You can chat while in the waiting room, plus they get an insight into your world without you having to try and explain the peculiar world of hospitals, appointments, paperwork and procedures. Especially when it feels like you are being robbed of time to be with your friends, just chatting on the journey to and from appointments can be a way of staying connected.

4. Remember your baby is an individual

The first year of life is riddled with babies' 'first' everything, with a lot of box-ticking, growth checks and milestones. Our society is obsessed with measuring and quantifying to mark progress and signal success. This implies a forward linear trajectory, which is not applicable to the reality of life. Humans never stop learning and we learn in different ways at different times – these boxes don't predict the future. Plus the really important bits about someone's life are left out... because they can't be measured, like the love and the friends, and the fun and laughter of life.

When our babies (who are developing in their own way, in their own time) don't meet the typical tick-box milestones at the same time as their typical peers they get more closely monitored with extra appointments and home visits from a whole range of people. This can be reassuring, but it can also feel like we don't have the same rights to a private life as other families. We may find ourselves craving the 'normality' of life with a typically developing baby, where our weeks aren't punctuated by an array of people 'concerned' about our babies – often reinforcing all the things that our babies 'aren't' doing. Of course it's not always like this, and for many people the extra care and attention is helpful, appreciated and welcomed. And indeed some families have to fight to access the services and support that their baby needs.

Remember that you can make decisions about which appointments are essential and which ones aren't. It may be that you can space them out better, or have several in one day. Check that your baby has the charts and developmental progress inserts suitable for them. For example, there are special charts for growth and development for conditions such as Down's syndrome, just as there are different charts for formula- and breastmilk-fed babies.

5. Never be afraid to ask for help

You deserve to be supported during the intensity of all that needs juggling during the first year. But, how do we get the support that we actually need, especially if it feels impossible to ask for any help at all? First, know that when we give others the opportunity to help us we are actually giving them a gift. We are inviting that person to become an important part of our life and to be appreciated for their contribution. Next, know that by looking after ourselves, we are being responsible; we are preventing ill-health, exhaustion and burnout. You deserve this, and so does your family and community. It won't be forever, but it's what's needed right now.

I call this 'Intentional Support'. Intentional means that you have stated with clear conscious intent what you need to make life manageable, and distributed these requests between many people over a rota with a spacious timescale, one that repeats fortnightly or monthly for example. Requests are matched with people who choose what they want to give from the things that are needed and they choose the time frequency that suits their capacity. It is enjoyable for everyone.

People can give the support that is needed, at the time that it's needed. It means that you don't end up with three cooked meals on your doorstep on the day that you've made an almighty effort to cook a proper meal yourself. It means that you won't end up with so many flowers that you are down on your knees rummaging in cupboards for jam jars and buckets to put them in, when all you really want is a bowl of homemade soup and someone to hold your baby so that you can have a bath.

Seek out support from a range of places. This shares out responsibility and work, enabling people to take a break on a week that's difficult for them, knowing there are others to cover them. Be specific about what is needed. This is honest and respectful to everyone. People often want to be involved and help out, but fear can stop them offering if they think that they will be solely relied upon. Also, tell them that it's okay if they say no. And that it can just be a 'no, not right now, please ask me again in a few weeks' time'; it doesn't need to be a 'no, never', nor will you be shut out of each other's lives if they say no. This takes the emotional charge away from asking and being hurt by negative responses. This is also a good moment to be truthful about your responsibilities right now and for friends to understand that you won't be available to them in the same way you were before and for them to not take this personally and to be more proactive about checking in with you, even if you haven't replied to their last five messages.

Also, find out what support exists locally through libraries, local council websites and local social media hubs. Ask your health visitor and ask national organisations about local groups in your area. Local parent-led support groups are the places to go to for local knowledge and to get support for the whole family and to grow life-long friendships. There is nothing that replaces being with other humans in a safe, non-judgemental, caring group with parents who just 'get it'. These are places of joy where you can celebrate your children together and support each other through the highs and lows of parenting. Online support groups are great for connecting with other's lived experiences too.

Chapter eight

Feeding your baby – making a decision

→ How we feed our babies is a big decision, and one that can be affected by many factors. For many families it's not just about what milk to choose, but how feeding fits with your family and caring for your baby. Getting as much information and support as you can is therefore really important.

If you are pregnant and reading this and haven't made the decision yet on how to feed your baby you might like to think about the options available to you:

- **Just give your baby breastmilk** (known as exclusive breastfeeding). It is possible to express breastmilk and give it to your baby in a bottle occasionally, or sometimes women do this for all feeds for various reasons.
- **Give your baby both breast and formula milk** (often known as mixed or combination feeding). This is possible, but is often easier after the first six weeks once you've established a good breastmilk supply. If you wanted to breastfeed but were unable to do so, giving breastmilk alongside formula still helps your baby get some of the protective immune properties of breastmilk.
- **Just give your baby formula milk**. They will need first stage infant formula until they are 12 months old when they can move on to cows' milk.

"Just think about the days and weeks ahead – the future will sort itself out."

Deciding how you are going to feed your baby is not always straightforward. You might decide that you want to breastfeed your baby, but encounter challenges and then decide that the best thing for your family would be to move to formula milk, even if personally you really wish you were still breastfeeding. Alternatively, you might decide to introduce formula or expressed milk to your baby alongside breastfeeding, but they refuse flat out to take a bottle or you decide you want to breastfeed for much longer. Staying flexible and knowing that in most circumstances you can make a decision, and then make another decision later, can be helpful.

Feeding really is a very individual decision (or series of decisions) and you don't actually have to think about it in the long term right now. Just think about the days and weeks ahead – the future will sort itself out. Saying that, you might have your partner, family and friends all telling you what they think you should do or what they want to happen. Again, take your time, get informed and do what's best for you and your family, not what anyone else thinks you should do.

If you've decided to formula feed then you may or may not want to read the next section. If you're already formula-feeding your baby, particularly if you have had a difficult experience trying to breastfeed, then I fully understand how difficult reading about breastfeeding can be (or you might just not want to). So you can skip to Chapter 10 now – although if you are struggling to come to terms with a difficult breastfeeding experience I would recommend reading my short book *Why Breastfeeding Grief and Trauma Matters*. Based on research with over 2,000 women who couldn't breastfeed for as long as they wanted to, it explores difficult emotions and where you can get more support if you need it.

If your baby isn't here yet, or you want to read more about the reasons you might like to consider breastfeeding, read on...

Why might you want to breastfeed or give your baby breastmilk?

There are many reasons you might like to breastfeed your baby. Lots of these are to do with health.[1] In particular breastmilk contains lots of immune properties that help protect your baby against infections. Babies who are breastfed are less likely to get gastrointestinal, respiratory or ear infections in particular. The very first breastmilk you produce – known as colostrum – is particularly high in these immune properties. It passes immune protection to your baby from you. Without this, babies would have to develop this immune response themselves, so colostrum is often viewed not just in terms of milk, but as a vaccination of sorts for your baby. For this reason, some women give their baby breastmilk for the first few days, even if they don't plan to breastfeed longer term.

There are also lots of other properties found in breastmilk that help your baby's health and development in different ways. For example, breastmilk contains something called lactoferrin that helps with iron absorption, long-chain polyunsaturated fatty acids support your baby's brain and eye development, and melatonin in your milk helps your baby sleep at night.

Breastmilk is also really easy for your baby to digest, which has the added bonus of making their nappies less smelly! Because breastmilk is designed specifically for baby humans, it contains just the right amounts of things like protein. Infant formula milk is based on cows' milk, so although they modify it to be suitable for babies (such as adding vitamins and minerals) it is more difficult for them to digest.

There is also some evidence that babies who are breastfed are less likely to be overweight when they are older. This doesn't mean that all babies who are formula fed will be overweight, just that there is a higher chance. One reason for this is that it's quicker to get milk out of a bottle than it is a breast, so babies drink formula more quickly and in larger amounts. It's also easier to persuade them to finish a bottle as you can see how much is left, rather than letting them decide how much they want. The good news here is that it is possible to bottle-feed a baby carefully so you let them be more in control of the feed and that is really important – more on that in the bottle-feeding section.[2]

Finally, breastfeeding can also help your health. There is evidence that women who breastfeed, and the longer they breastfeed for, have lower levels of reproductive cancers such as breast and ovarian cancer, heart disease and diabetes. It also helps some women lose weight – but sadly this doesn't work if you eat cake each time you feed the baby.[3]

But what else? All of this health stuff is great. After all, no one wants a poorly baby. But this book is about you and supporting you in making decisions, so let's look at some more reasons relevant to you. Although many women say breastfeeding can be tricky to get the hang of in the early days, once you have got into the swing of things and are producing more milk and getting to know your baby, most then say it gets much easier – as long as you are well supported with any challenges that might arise. Therefore breastfeeding has other benefits that are more personal, such as:

- **Breastfeeding can be more convenient.** No preparing, cleaning and sterilising bottles. No having to make bottles up in advance or warm the milk up. Really easy at night. You can't leave your breasts at home accidentally. And it can be a brilliant excuse to take yourself off somewhere quiet if you have annoying house guests.

- **Breastfeeding can make mothering easier.** Breastfeeding can also be a great way of soothing any other issues your baby has. Crying? Feeding will solve that. Can't sleep? Feed. Unsettled after injections? I know what will work. And so on.
- **Breastfeeding can be really empowering and healing.** Think about it. You're keeping a baby alive with your breasts. You're in charge. No one is selling you something. Just you, feeding your baby and making them grow. This is a great feeling at the best of times, but if your baby has been in special care or you've had a difficult birth, or maybe a difficult relationship with your body in the past (such as an eating disorder or you've been abused), breastfeeding can feel like a way of reclaiming the power your body has.
- **Breastfeeding can help you feel calmer.** When you breastfeed your baby you release the hormone oxytocin. Oxytocin, often known as the hormone of love, makes you feel more relaxed, lowers your blood pressure and helps reduce anxiety.
- **Breastfeeding can help you get more sleep.** No, seriously, it can! It might not feel like it, but breastfeeding helps both you and your baby to fall asleep more quickly after a feed. Your breastmilk contains melatonin, the hormone that helps sleep. Breastfeeding also releases the hormone prolactin in you, which has been linked to helping you sleep better.[4]
- **Breastfeeding can help you fight stress.** When our bodies are under stress (and that can include exhaustion and feeling like everything is too much) we release a series of hormones to try to counteract whatever is stressing us. This can cause an inflammatory response in our bodies which can do harm in the long term. Breastfeeding appears to help dampen down this inflammation.[5]

Will I be able to breastfeed my baby?

The majority of women should be able to breastfeed their baby if they want to. That doesn't mean that all women will be able to, and a small percentage adds up to a large number of women over a big population.[6] You have probably heard lots of stories about women having breastfeeding difficulties and having to stop before they are ready. This is a really serious problem. In the UK, for example, over 80 per cent of women want to breastfeed, but less than half are doing so by six weeks. Most of the women who stopped feeding during this time weren't happy to do so but felt they had to because they were having too many difficulties.[7]

It's really important that we look at these experiences closely, especially if you're making a decision whether to breastfeed or not and are worried. There is a difference between having a physical reason why you would not be able to breastfeed or make enough milk and having bad experiences that mean you end up in pain or not making enough milk when with the right support you might have been able to breastfeed for longer. Unfortunately, in the UK we have many, many women in the latter group. They end up having difficult experiences because they weren't able to get the right professional support. Maybe they received poor information, or others put pressure on them to stop feeding. If you want to read more about all these influences I recommend several books:

- *Breastfeeding Uncovered: Who really decides how we feed our babies* - Amy Brown
- *The Big Letdown: How medicine, big business and feminism undermine breastfeeding* - Kimberly Seals Allers
- *The Politics of Breastfeeding: When breasts are bad for business* - Gabrielle Palmer
- *Unlatched: The evolution of breastfeeding and the making of a controversy* - Jennifer Grayson

These challenges are why it's really important if you're breastfeeding to know where to get support, understand normal breastfeeding behaviour and know when to spot a problem. The breastfeeding chapter that follows will help you with this.

There are some fairly rare circumstances in which you might not be able to breastfeed. These include:

1. If your baby has a rare illness known as galactosemia

Galactosemia is a metabolic disorder that means an individual doesn't make enough of the enzyme that is needed to break down a sugar (galactose) that is found in milk into a usable form. This means the sugar builds up and can cause damage to the brain, liver and kidneys. Babies who have galactosemia will need special formula, although some babies have a version known as Duarte glacatosemia, which occurs when they produce some enzymes and can have a couple or more breastfeeds a day.

2. If you have certain health conditions

It is rare that a health condition will stop you breastfeeding, but there are some cases where this is true. For example, your baby should not have your breastmilk if you have been diagnosed with human T-cell lymphotropic virus, untreated brucellosis, or Ebola.

If you have HIV you should talk to your health professional, as the British HIV Association and American Academy of Pediatrics state that mothers should be supported to breastfeed as long as they are taking antiretroviral therapy (and have a low viral load) and do so exclusively, as mixed feeding

> **"Many mothers worry about medications, but the majority are safe to take when breastfeeding."**

increases the risk of transmission. In these cases the risk is almost negligible until solid foods are introduced. At this point, the risk increases slightly but is still low. There is around a 2 per cent transmission rate if breastfeeding past a year. However, if you experience complications such as your baby having sores in their mouth from thrush, cracked nipples, mastitis or breast inflammation you should talk to your health professional as these increase the risk. Have a look at the La Leche League leaflet here for more information **www.laleche.org. uk/breastfeeding-hiv**.

For some illnesses, there is little risk of your baby getting sick from your milk, but they might catch the illness from you. Therefore it is recommended that you give your baby expressed breastmilk if you have active tuberculosis, herpes lesions on your breast, or chickenpox.

Many mothers worry about medications, but the majority are safe to take when breastfeeding (or there is a safe alternative), as either they do not pass into your breastmilk or they pass in such small amounts that they will not affect your baby. Medications that are contraindicated when breastfeeding include lithium, Methotrexate for arthritis and chemotherapy or radiation.

If you're unsure whether you can breastfeed and take a medication the Breastfeeding Network Drugs in Breastmilk service has a range of factsheets on the safety of different medications. You can also contact a pharmacist with specific queries **www.breastfeedingnetwork.org.uk/drugs-factsheets/**.

3. If you have a health condition that affects your milk supply

There are some conditions that might affect your ability to make a full milk supply for your baby. It is important to note that it is fairly rare to make no milk at all, but you might find that you need to give formula milk as well. In these cases always seek support from an expert in breastfeeding to help you make as much milk as possible. These include:

Hypoplastic breasts

Hypoplastic breasts or 'insufficient glandular tissue' means that the tissue in your breast that supports milk production didn't grow enough, or at all. If you spot any of these signs in yourself you might have issues with your glandular tissue.

- Widely spaced breasts (more than 1.5 inches apart)
- 'Tubular' looking breasts, e.g. long and thin
- Your breasts didn't increase in size during pregnancy or after the birth
- One breast is quite a bit bigger than the other

Many women with hypoplastic breasts produce some milk but may need to supplement with formula.

Hypothyroidism
If you have a thyroid disorder that is well managed then this shouldn't have an impact on your ability to make enough milk. However, if you find yourself struggling to make enough milk you might need an increase in your thyroxine medication.

Diabetes
If your diabetes is well controlled then this shouldn't have an impact on your milk supply. The problem comes when your insulin levels are not well controlled, or you don't realise you have diabetes. Insulin plays a role in milk production and if your levels are too low, your milk might take longer to come in.

Polycystic ovary syndrome
Different women have different experiences depending on their hormone levels. Some will be fine, some might produce too much and some too little milk. Speak to your health professional if you are having difficulties, but be reassured that if you are taking Metformin it is fine to continue to breastfeed.

4. If you have had breast surgery (maybe)
This all depends on the type of surgery. If you had a reduction with glandular tissues and ducts removed there are no hard and fast rules, but if you had lots removed you might struggle to make a full supply. If your nipple and areola were fully severed to reposition the nipple you may struggle as the blood supply and ducts will have been affected. However, over time milk ducts can actually start to regenerate and reconnect, particularly during pregnancy! Nerves can also begin to heal over time.

If you have had breast implants you are more likely to be able to breastfeed. However, this depends in part on why you had the implants. If you had signs of hypoplastic breasts (e.g. lack of fullness, smaller, uneven, or underdeveloped breasts), then implants will not solve the issue. Don't worry about the content of the implant leaking into the milk though – it can't.

So you can probably breastfeed if you want to. Even with some of the conditions listed there is a good chance that you will produce at least some milk, especially if you can get the right support. The key thing is making sure you get the right information and support. The next few sections cover this and also point you in the direction of more detailed information.

Chapter nine

Breastfeeding your baby

→ This chapter covers all the key things you need to know to get breastfeeding off to a good start. As this is just one part of your first year, it's not possible to go into all the detail you might need, especially in trickier situations. So if you are breastfeeding and want to know more I recommend:

- *The Positive Breastfeeding Book* - Amy Brown
- *You've Got It in You: A Positive Guide to Breastfeeding* - Emma Pickett
- *The Womanly Art of Breastfeeding* - La Leche League

You may also find the following websites useful:

- Dr Jack Newman **ibconline.ca**
- KellyMom **kellymom.com**
- Global Health Media **globalhealthmedia.org/videos/breastfeeding**
- Biological Nurturing **www.biologicalnurturing.com**
- Unicef UK Baby Friendly Initiative **www.unicef.org.uk/babyfriendly**

Who is there to support you if you are breastfeeding?

One of the most important things you can do to help breastfeeding to get off to a good start is to get the right support – whether that's practical support on how to latch your baby on, the answer to a query about how often they are feeding, or just wanting someone who understands to reassure you. Your midwife or health visitor is there to support you, but if you have lots of questions or specific complications and need support right now, or want some moral support from another mum, you can get in touch with one (or more!) of the following:

Lactation consultants (full name International Board Certified Lactation Consultant – or IBCLC). They will have trained for many years to become qualified, spending over 1,000 hours helping breastfeeding mothers after they have qualified as a breastfeeding counsellor or health professional and taking at least 90 hours of breastfeeding education... before sitting an exam. Some work in hospitals and some work privately. They are great for any level of support but are particularly useful if you have a complicated issue. You may be able to access them in person, by video chat or over the phone. The Lactation Consultants of Great Britain website has a full list of qualified IBCLCs www. lcgb.org/find-an-ibclc.

Breastfeeding counsellors are accredited by a major breastfeeding organisation – in the UK that's either the Association of Breastfeeding Mothers, or the National Childbirth Trust. The Breastfeeding Network also train Breastfeeding Supporters and La Leche League Great Britain train Leaders. All these people have the training to answer common breastfeeding questions and can support you to find more specialist help if necessary. If you contact any of the breastfeeding charity helplines you can speak to one of these lovely people for free. The numbers for the main charities are:

- National Breastfeeding Helpline: 0300 100 0212 www. nationalbreastfeedinghelpline.org.uk
- Association of Breastfeeding Mothers: 0300 330 5453 abm.me.uk
- La Leche League: 0345 120 2918 www.laleche.org.uk
- National Childbirth Trust (NCT): 0300 330 0700 www.nct.org.uk
- The Breastfeeding Network supporter line in Bengali and Sylheti: 0300 456 2421

Peer supporters (or mother supporters, breastfeeding buddies, or peer counsellors) are typically mums who have breastfed their own babies and undertaken some training in order to be able to support others to breastfeed. Peer supporters are there for general information, tips and moral support, but cannot diagnose problems or reassure you about health issues such as weight gain. For that you need to speak to a health professional or breastfeeding counsellor or IBCLC.

You might find peer supporters holding their own breastfeeding drop-in groups (often supported by a breastfeeding counsellor or midwife) either at a children's centre, hospital or any location they can find. Church halls, community centres and libraries are popular. Ask your midwife or health visitor for details of your local one. They may also have an online Facebook group, which is really handy for getting to know people if you don't feel up to getting out of the house, or simply need someone to chat to at 3am. If you're reading this while still pregnant – pop along to get to know people and actually see breastfeeding happening. They welcome new blood, sorry, I mean mothers, with open arms and cake.

Finally, be wary of information provided by anyone who is advertising a paid-for breastfeeding support service but cannot show you their qualifications.

How long should I breastfeed for?

I don't know. How long do you want to breastfeed for? Seriously – this part is absolutely up to you. Maybe you want to do three feeds, three weeks or three years. I'd probably advise stopping before they go off to university or get married. But jokes aside, this really is a personal decision that you need to make within the context of your own family life. Although actually you don't really need to make a decision at all, other than to perhaps carry on for today, or this week.

Based on research the World Health Organization recommends six months of exclusive breastfeeding – that's just breastmilk, vitamin drops and any medication needed – followed by introducing solids and continuing to breastfeed alongside for as long as you want. That's because the research showed that giving just breastmilk for six months offered babies the best protection against infections while not compromising growth. If you were a gambling person you might say that it offered babies the best odds, or roll of the dice.

But it's not a case of either breastfeeding exclusively for six months or don't bother. The longer you breastfeed, the longer your baby has the protection of breastmilk. The more breastmilk they get, the better. So that generally means that breastfeeding for three weeks offers more protection than not breastfeeding at all. And breastfeeding alongside formula offers more protection than not giving any breastmilk. We simply don't have enough data to be able to accurately state that 'breastfeeding for six weeks means your baby has X percentage likelihood of getting sick compared to Y percentage for 12 weeks'. And if we did, that would only apply across a population of all babies – it wouldn't give an exact figure for *your* baby getting sick or not. Health is affected by so many factors – your genes, where you live, what's going on around you and a bit of luck thrown in.

So you need to make the decision that's right for you, taking into account what you want, other factors in your life like work or other responsibilities and your own health and wellbeing. Ideally of course none of these things would matter – women would be supported to breastfeed for as long as they wanted through well-paid maternity leave, help and support on tap and someone to do all your cleaning and give you regular massages. But we know in reality that decisions are more complicated than that.

You might want to think about how long you will breastfeed for in small chunks. Sometimes holding a tiny baby and thinking you have to keep feeding them for the next six months is overwhelming, especially if you are finding things difficult. Set yourself a manageable goal of the end of the week, or the end of the day or even just the next feed and tell yourself you'll re-evaluate then. You might just find you end up breastfeeding longer than you planned.

At the other end of the scale, thinking about continuing to breastfeed an older baby or child, again this is absolutely up to you. Breastmilk is 'species-specific' milk – it's designed for baby humans. There is no upper age limit for it, and it continues to not only be a nutritious food for your child, but also to provide them with all those immune-boosting properties. It does not make them overly dependent on you (whatever misinformed people might tell you) – research actually suggests it helps promote confident pre-schoolers. And while it might seem strange to think about breastfeeding an older child when you are pregnant, or have a tiny newborn, it can seem less strange as they grow because feeding an older child is very different from feeding a very young baby.

How do I hold my baby to feed them?

There are lots of different positions in which you can hold your baby to feed them. The key is to get them into a position that is comfortable for you and that gets your nipple and the baby's mouth to align in the right way. You might like to try different options to see which one you feel most comfortable with. These things are really best learnt by looking at a video or diagram, or another breastfeeding mother. La Leche League has lots of different pictures of how to position your baby at **www.llli.org/faq/positioning.html** and Dr Jack Newman has some great videos here: **breastfeeding.support/breastfeeding-videos**. The Global Health Media videos are also definitely worth a watch for lots of different aspects of breastfeeding: **globalhealthmedia.org/videos/breastfeeding**.

Here are some different positions you might like to try:

- **Cradle hold** – this is the traditional breastfeeding pose you usually see in pictures, although actually not everyone finds it particularly easy or comfortable. You hold your baby across your body, with them latched on one side and their feet on the other. Their head will rest on your forearm, with their whole body and tummy against you.

- **Laid back** – this is often very comfortable once you get the hang of it. Here you sit in a reclined position, aiming for your sacrum (the hard part at the back of your pelvis) to be supporting your lower weight. You can use lots of pillows to make yourself comfy. Place your baby on their tummy, lying along your body, with their head near your breasts. It's easier to angle them so they're facing your nipple. Make sure their feet are away from any wound if you have had a caesarean section. Make sure they are secure, but give them room to move themselves into position – which they will do using their hands and feet to get to your nipple. They will know what direction to go from smell and will automatically open their mouth wide as they come up to your nipple. Dr Suzanne Colson, author of *Biological Nurturing*, has a great video showing this in more detail **www.biologicalnurturing.com/video/bn3clip.html**.

- **Rugby ball hold** – this is when you position your baby along the side of your body so their feet are behind you, and their head round at your breast. It's useful for feeding twins at the same time, or if you have had a caesarean section.

- **Lying down** – this can be great to let you get some rest, or if you are in pain sitting up. It is also useful if your milk flow is very fast as your baby can let a little trickle out. Putting a towel or muslin underneath you can save your bed from getting damp.

- **Toddler style** – this is when older, mobile children launch at you from any angle. The weirder the position, the better!

How do I latch my baby on?

Again, this is best viewed rather than explained, given how easily we can watch videos on smartphones and other devices these days. If you're pregnant, watch them now rather than waiting until you have a wriggly baby to try and hold too. Dr Jack Newman's page and the Global Breastfeeding Media videos are great tools. Unicef Baby Friendly also has a good factsheet here: **www.unicef.org.uk/babyfriendly/wp-content/uploads/sites/2/2010/11/Off_to_the_Best_Start_Leaflet_4_Pages-2017_.pdf**.

> **"You will likely hear that breastfeeding is meant to hurt at the start. It really isn't. It might feel like a very new and quite powerful sensation, but pain is not 'normal'."**

Getting a good latch is probably one of the most important parts of breastfeeding. Some seemingly tiny changes can make a huge difference. A bad latch will at best hurt and at worst shred your nipples to pieces – and also mean your baby doesn't get as much milk. So take time to get it right, and if you are in any pain at all please, please, please seek support. You will likely hear that breastfeeding is meant to hurt at the start. It really isn't. It might feel like a very new and quite powerful sensation at first, but pain is not 'normal' or to be put up with. So if it hurts, ask your midwife to look. And again and again and again if it still hurts. If it still hurts, seek more support from a breastfeeding counsellor or IBCLC.

The key to a good latch is getting your nipple deep into your baby's mouth. Many people think babies drink from a nipple like you would suck from a straw. However, when a baby latches on effectively they will take a big mouthful of your nipple and the surrounding darker skin (your areola) and draw your nipple right back into their mouth (don't worry, it's designed to stretch!), massaging the underside of your areola with their tongue as they feed. Milk goes to the back of their mouth rather than the front – so aim your nipple towards the back and roof of their mouth.

Here are some simple instructions to help (and watch the videos too):

1. Hold your baby with your nipple level with their nose

2. Brush your nipple against their top lip to encourage them to open their mouth wide

3. Hold their head so it is tilted back slightly, so that the first connection they make with your breast is their chin – this will allow them to take a big mouthful

4. Let them latch on – aiming to see more areola (the darker skin around your nipple) above their mouth than below

5. You should aim your nipple towards the back and roof of their mouth

6. Their bottom lip should be flanged outwards, not tucked in

7. Support their neck but don't hold the back of their head – this allows them freedom to find the nipple and be comfortable (and also lets them breathe)

Remember, a good latch will not hurt. If it hurts at all, or when you reclaim your nipple it is at all misshapen, get help.

How often should I breastfeed my baby?

Lots! And then lots more! Breastfed babies do feed really frequently. There are a number of reasons for this. Firstly, breastmilk is really easily digested. Most babies will digest a feed within 2-3 hours. Breastfed babies also tend to take just as much as they need at each feed rather than overfilling themselves. This means that they tend to have more smaller feeds.

Frequent breastfeeding helps stimulate a better milk supply. Simply put, the more you feed, the more milk you make and vice versa. Your baby is programmed to want to make sure there is as much milk as they need, so they are designed to feed often. They also know (well, subconsciously I presume, rather than having calculated thoughts) that they need more milk during a growth spurt so will feed lots and lots around these times – think of it as them putting a big order in.

They may also not feed in any particular pattern. Some days they might feed roughly every two hours, while other days they will feed at 2pm, 3.15pm, 4pm, 7pm and so on. Many babies have a period in the evening when they seem to be a bit unsettled and may feed very often, on and off ... on and off... on and off... napping in between over a period of a few hours. This is known as cluster feeding and is thought to help stimulate your milk supply.

Also, if it's hot they may feed more. Breastmilk is over 80 per cent water, so just keep feeding rather than offering water. In hot weather your milk will adapt to having an even higher water content to keep your baby hydrated. Magic!

It's important to remember that all babies are different. Some babies will feed less often. Others will feed more frequently. The main thing is to follow your baby's lead and let them feed whenever they want. This is known as 'responsive feeding'. When babies are fed this way it is more likely you'll have a better milk supply, fewer problems, your baby will gain more weight and you'll feed for longer. Complications can arise if you try to restrict feeds. Remember, the more you feed, the more milk you make – but also vice versa.

How do I know my baby wants to feed?

Spotting the early signs your baby wants a feed – known as feeding cues – is an important part of responsive feeding, because it helps you recognise when they are asking for a feed rather than having to calm them down because they've got upset because they are really quite hungry now. Cues include:

- **Early cues:** opening their mouth, turning their head about to try and find a nipple, licking their lips and making sucking sounds.
- **Further cues:** putting their hands in their mouth,* starting to wriggle, and getting louder.
- **Late cues:** crying, fussing and really squirming.

A note on hand sucking - once babies are a bit older and have discovered their hands at around 2-3 months, they may spend a lot of time sucking on them. If they are teething they also love a bit of munching on their fingers. So it's best not to take this sign alone as a need for more milk.

How do I know my baby is getting enough milk?

It's really common to worry that if your baby is feeding and feeding and feeding it's a sign something is wrong. Here are some things you can check:

- Your baby is feeding at least 8-12 times in 24 hours. There is no set length of time your baby should feed for, but if they are feeding for less than five minutes at a time, or for more than 45 minutes, it's best to check with a professional that everything is okay. Some babies just eat quickly or slowly, but it might be a sign they are not getting enough.
- Check whether they are swallowing. Can you hear them swallowing during a feed? At the start of a feed your baby will usually make a series of quick sucks, followed by a more rhythmic suck-pause-suck pattern. Your baby swallows during the pause. Look at your baby's jaw and chin - their jaw moves downwards as they suck and you might see their ears wiggle. Their cheeks should stay full, not be hollow as if they were sucking on a straw.
- Check what is coming out. Remember, your baby's wet nappies should gradually increase over the first week, with six or more each day by the end of the week. Bowel movements should get looser and yellower with at least two dirty nappies per day by day three. Check out the box on page 86 for a reminder. Once breastfeeding is established, by around six weeks, some babies can go longer in between dirty nappies. Before this a lack of dirty nappies might be a sign something is wrong.
- Check your baby looks hydrated - they should have firm skin. Their eyes and the soft spot on their head (the fontanelle) should not be sunken.
- Is your baby alert and active between feeds? If they are a newborn they are not going to be dancing the conga round the living room, but there should be a distinction between asleep and awake, even if that's just staring at you for a bit.
- Check your baby's weight gain - your baby will gain around 4-7 ounces per week once they are about four days old, and will continue to grow in length.

Once they have had enough milk, most babies will start to suck more slowly. Some women notice that they may make fluttery movements with their tongue/jaw. They may gradually become floppier, especially if they are going off to sleep (which many young babies do after a feed). They may even feel heavier to you. You may notice their hands become more relaxed – going from a clenched fist to being more open, although this doesn't always happen. Many babies then let go of the nipple (sometimes spitting it out) and make a 'milk drunk' face – their eyes will roll back in their head and milk may trickle out of their mouth. Older babies may not fall asleep at the end of a feed, instead preferring a good nosey at what's going on in the room.

Can I really make enough milk for my big baby?

Yes, most likely, especially if you feed them responsively. The more you feed, the more milk you make, and many women successfully breastfeed twins and triplets or tandem-feed a newborn and an older baby. You will gradually make more and more milk as your baby grows, from just millilitres in the first days through to around 675ml per day by two weeks, 750ml by a month and around 900ml from six weeks onwards. Although there will be small variations in how much milk babies take, babies from six weeks to six months old take in on average around 900ml a day.

How much milk you produce isn't related to breast size, although women do seem to have slightly different storage capacities, with some storing a bit more and some a bit less. If you have a smaller capacity your baby might feed a little more often, but milk is being continually produced, even during a feed. Your breasts don't fill up and get drained completely at a feed.

Can I feed them too much?

No. Breastfed babies are pretty much in control of how much they feed. They have to actively latch on to your breast to get the milk out, so it's not possible for milk to continue pouring out if they stop. Also, as you don't know how much they are feeding you have to put your trust in them to take as much as they need, rather than seeing how much is in a bottle and encouraging them to finish it. Breastmilk also contains some bioactive properties that help regulate appetite, including ghrelin and leptin, which help signal to babies when they are hungry and when they are full.

Remember that breastfeeding isn't just about milk. It's also about comfort and security for your baby. They get a lot of comfort from suckling and being close to you. Sometimes it is clear that they are not particularly hungry but just want a quick feed while they doze off to sleep, protesting if you try to reclaim your nipple or move. This is normal. In many cultures babies are carried most of the time in a sling and will have very short feeds, being comforted by being held close. In my own research when we asked mothers whether their baby seemed to feed 'differently' when feeding for comfort they often said yes – feeds were shorter and the suck less strong.

However, unfortunately people will often tell you that your baby is feeding too often. We seem to have a bit of an obsession with this as a culture. Breastfed babies do feed on average more often than formula-fed babies, but they take shorter and smaller feeds. They are also less likely on average to over-feed or become overweight – in part because they are more in control of their milk intake.

Breastfeeding isn't just about food, it's also drink and comfort for your baby. Think about how often you have something to eat or drink during the day. Do you have a set amount every few hours, or is it more irregular? Might you enjoy having a hot drink or favourite snack for reasons other than just being thirsty? I find the worst offenders for criticising how often babies feed tend to be those who barely miss a beat between cups of tea for themselves.

What if my baby isn't getting enough milk?

It is really important to keep an eye on the signs your baby is getting enough milk and their growth, particularly in the early days. Although most women, given the right support and time, should be able to make enough milk for their baby, others will struggle. This might include:

- If you have one of the health conditions listed on page 129.
- If you have had a particularly difficult birth. Interventions during birth such as a caesarean section, lots of pain medication or a post-partum haemorrhage may mean that your milk is slightly delayed in coming in, meaning your baby might lose more weight in the early days.
- If your baby isn't effectively latched on to the breast or doesn't take full feeds – perhaps because they are very small and get tired easily.
- If you are trying to feed your baby to a routine, delaying the time between feeds or giving your baby a dummy to suck on, then they might not be stimulating your breasts to make enough milk.
- Some medications, including those that are oestrogen-based (such as the combined pill), or cold medications that contain pseudoephedrine, can decrease your milk supply.

Your health professional should be monitoring your baby's weight and growth and checking to make sure that breastfeeding is working effectively. If you notice that your baby is showing signs of not getting enough milk it is important to act quickly. If you want to continue breastfeeding the first port of call should be your health professional to support you to make more milk.

Troubleshooting

There are a number of challenges you might experience when breastfeeding. Knowing what the signs are, being able to spot them and seeking help from a health professional or trained breastfeeding expert are key steps to making sure they don't get any more serious. Some of the most common problems are discussed below. For information on seeking support if you have been prescribed a medication look back to Chapter 8. However, other complications can arise and for those I would recommend that you either

- Seek support from a health professional or breastfeeding counsellor
- Have a look at the leaflets available on the Breastfeeding Network website
- Read a more detailed book, such as my own *The Positive Breastfeeding Book,* or *The Womanly Art of Breastfeeding.*

1. Engorgement

Engorgement is common in the early days as your milk starts to come in. Your breasts will likely feel very swollen, hard and warm and you'll feel very uncomfortable, if not somewhat impressed by what your body can do! Engorgement is pretty much a catch-22, as the main way to get rid of it is to feed your baby, but it can stretch your areola and nipples so much and make your breasts so large that your poor baby can't latch on. Argh.

Don't panic though – it will pass, I promise! If this has happened when your baby is newborn keep trying to feed as much as possible. It can help to try and express a little before each feed so things deflate a bit and your baby can get a look-in. To make this easier try having a warm shower, or putting a warm compress on your breasts and massaging them gently. Very gently. Some women then find that using a cold compress – either a special one you can buy or simply a pack of frozen peas – can help ease the swelling. Never put ice directly on your skin – try a muslin cloth or towel in between. Some people might recommend you put chilled cabbage in your bra – whole leaves, not shredded – but be cautious, as there is some evidence they could reduce milk supply.

If your baby is older you might find you get engorged the first time they sleep through (yes, they will one day!) or when you go back to work or are separated from your baby for whatever reason. It can be worth expressing a little to ease the pain, even if you don't plan to save the milk.

> **"The key is spotting when something is wrong and getting support from a health professional or breastfeeding specialist."**

2. Pain and cracked nipples

Pain is a very common reason for stopping breastfeeding, but it should not be considered 'normal'. With the right support many women find that their pain eases and they can continue breastfeeding. The key is spotting when something is wrong and getting support from a health professional or breastfeeding specialist if it happens to you. Although many women will say things can feel a bit uncomfortable at the start, if you are experiencing pain and it isn't easing please do get help.

One of the most common reasons for nipple pain is a baby who isn't latched on to the breast correctly. They might not be latched on deeply enough and be putting pressure in the wrong place, or the latch may be squashing your nipple against the roof of their mouth or rubbing on their tongue. Babies who are not latched on correctly will also suck harder, because they're not getting as much milk out. Some babies tuck their chin in, or have a recessive chin, meaning they struggle to latch on deeply. A very shallow latch might also leave your nipples looking like a 'lipstick' from compressing your nipple.

The good news is that most mothers find that if they get help with positioning and attachment their pain will go away, although for a very small minority of mothers it still seems to hurt even when everything is fine. Getting help with your positioning is important not just to make the pain go away, but to also make sure your baby is getting enough milk. An effective latch means they get more milk more easily – also reducing the amount of time they spend feeding.

If your nipples have been damaged the very first step is to make sure you get some help to work out how things can be better. In the meantime, try watching those latch videos again, experimenting with the position and the way you hold your baby. You might find that small adjustments make a huge difference. Some women find that holding their baby in the rugby ball hold or laid-back position is less likely to cause pain and damage.

To help your nipples heal, after a feed express a few drops of milk and rub gently around your nipples - breastmilk has antibacterial properties so can help prevent infection. Moist wound healing (healing without a dry scab forming) has been shown to help - but you don't have to buy expensive creams. If you have deeper wounds, Vaseline, hydrogel dressings or lanolin creams can help.

Remember to keep damaged nipples clean. The current advice is to simply use soap and water to wash them. If you have damage and are a bit sticky, you could also use a saline soak - as is often recommended to help heal piercings.

If you are in too much pain to feed directly, it's important to try and keep expressing milk from that side as otherwise your supply may drop. Hand expression might be gentler. Even if you have decided to stop feeding, it's important that you continue to express rather than just stop cold turkey or you will likely get very engorged on top of everything else (see the guidance on stopping breastfeeding on p 151).

If you are worried about any damage or things really do not look right, do seek advice from a health professional.

3. Thrush

Thrush is a fungal infection that can infect warm moist places like your nipples or your baby's mouth. It particularly likes cracked or damaged nipples. Basically, it's a bit evil. Signs of thrush include:

- Itching nipples
- Painful nipples – often a burning pain
- The skin on your nipples may look shiny or flaky
- Stabbing pains behind your nipples

Pain is often worse during feeds and for up to an hour afterwards, but can persist in between. It can occur on one side, but often affects both as your baby will transfer it during feeds. It often occurs after antibiotics.

Signs your baby might have thrush:

- White patches in their mouth that look like milk but do not come away if gently cleaned, or do but leave red patches that look sore or may bleed
- A white film on their lips
- Becoming fussy during feeds
- Some babies can get a nappy rash that doesn't seem to clear up

If you have thrush do talk to your health professional as soon as possible. They may take swabs of your nipples and baby's mouth. Medications they can prescribe include:

- The topical treatment of miconazole cream (Daktarin) for your nipples and a gel treatment including miconazole for your baby's mouth. Treating you both is best as obviously just treating one could mean you keep transferring the infection back and forth. The treatment should work in a few days.
- If this doesn't work, and particularly if you are experiencing deeper breast pain, your GP may prescribe you oral fluconazole. Treatment usually lasts around 10 days or more.

Meanwhile you should try to kill the infection and stop the spread by regularly hot washing everything that comes into contact with your nipples, as well as:

- Washing your hands after touching your nipples and using a separate towel from the rest of the family to dry them
- Trying to avoid using breast pads, or using disposable ones and changing them very regularly
- Wearing a clean bra every day
- Thinking about anything else that comes into contact with your nipples – clothes, cloths, bibs, slings and so on
- Regularly clean any dummies, teats or toys if your baby can get them in their mouth
- If possible don't express milk for use later as freezing will not kill the infection

You might also like to consider changing your diet to see if that helps – cutting down on refined carbs and sugar can help some women, alongside trying to avoid foods heavy in yeast such as alcohol, bread and mushrooms. Supplements such as lactobacillus acidophilus, triple-strength garlic tablets, grapefruit seed extract, or vitamin B supplements may also work.

4. Blocked ducts and mastitis

Sometimes milk can get stuck in your breast, literally plugging or blocking one of the ducts. You might feel a lump, see a red patch, your breast might feel hot or sore and it might feel painful to feed on that side.

It is important to try and get rid of the blockage, not just to get the milk flowing again and the pain to go away, but also because a blocked duct can become inflamed leading to mastitis. This can happen quite quickly, so as soon as you notice a blocked duct take steps to remove it. Mastitis feels very similar but with worse symptoms. You might see red lines streaking out from the infected area and you may feel as if you have flu – achy, exhausted and hot or shivery.

Blocked ducts and mastitis often occur in the early weeks as you are getting used to making more milk, or they can be a consequence of a baby not removing milk effectively as their latch is too shallow. Mastitis is also more common if you have damaged nipples, as bacteria have an entry point. But blocked ducts can also occur if you get engorged when going back to work or your baby changes their feeding pattern. You might also get a blocked duct from things pushing on your breast such as a bra, bag strap or even seatbelt.

Instinct – and sometimes bad medical advice – may suggest you stop feeding, but that is actually the worst thing you can do. The key is to try and remove the blockage by draining the breast. Feeding as frequently as possible helps with this. It is fine to take painkillers such as ibuprofen or paracetamol (if these are usually fine for you to take). Ibuprofen in particular can help with inflammation and swelling.

The next thing is to try and encourage that blockage to come away. Massage helps. Massage gently around the lump, stroking towards your nipple. Try not to pull on the skin. A good idea is to do this in the shower – the heat of the shower helps and you can use conditioner to help with the massage. If you can't get to the shower, try a heat pack. You can also use an electric toothbrush or anything else you might have that vibrates to help ease it. Drink lots of water too.

If you are not feeling better after 24 hours, both breasts are infected, you see pus or you feel really unwell, go to your GP. They can prescribe you antibiotics.

5. Tongue-tie

Tongue-tie occurs when a baby's frenulum (the membrane underneath their tongue connecting it to the bottom of their mouth) is too short, meaning they cannot latch on to the breast effectively. Having a very thick or tight frenulum means your baby cannot move their tongue either out or up enough to be able to latch on or remove milk. Ideally all babies should be checked for tongue-tie, but if they haven't been and you are struggling to latch your baby on, do seek help. A tongue-tie does not necessarily mean your baby won't be able to latch effectively, but it does certainly place them at higher risk. Always remember it's okay to get a second opinion from an infant feeding co-ordinator, breastfeeding counsellor or IBCLC if you are told there is no issue with your baby's tongue but they are still having problems.

Signs of tongue tie include:

- A shallow latch
- Painful nipples even if your latch looks fine
- Very gassy baby from swallowing air
- Low milk supply
- Slow weight gain
- Very frequent feeds (as your baby isn't getting enough)
- A head-banging baby – not to music, but them popping on and off the breast repeatedly, sliding off once they try to latch on
- Very short or very long feeds
- Your nipple comes out looking flattened or lipstick-shaped

If you are having these symptoms the first step is to make sure it is not down to positioning and latch. If these things all seem okay, yet you still have these difficulties, it may be possible to have your baby's frenulum 'snipped' (divided). This can really help some babies with breastfeeding, but it's important not to do it unless it is necessary, as in some cases it can lead to pain and infection. Unfortunately it does not seem to help all babies, but NICE guidelines suggest it should be offered if it could help breastfeeding. Your health professional may refer you for this or you might want to seek support more quickly yourself by paying privately. It is really important that a trained specialist does this. You can find a list of accredited practitioners on the Association of Tongue-tie Practitioners website **www.tongue-tie.org.uk**.

A tongue-tie division involves swaddling your baby and cutting the tie with special (sterile) scissors. There will be a small wound (which may turn white as it heals) with a small amount of blood, but the inside of the mouth heals so quickly that it shouldn't cause any lasting issues. Your baby may not need an anaesthetic depending on their age and development. Each area has different guidance. Some will cut without it if your baby is less than eight months old. Others will want to use anaesthetic if your baby has any teeth. Some babies sleep through the whole thing and most only cry for about 15 seconds. Many are angrier about being wrapped up. You will be encouraged to feed your baby as soon as possible afterwards.

Ideas for partners or others to help you if you're breastfeeding

If you're looking for ways to help a breastfeeding mother, there are many things that you can do to support her, both in continued feeding and getting a break. A common suggestion is often to offer to give a bottle, either of formula or expressed milk. You can understand why – it seems at first like an obvious solution, and other people may want to join in with feeding the baby. However, while it can work for some families, it's important to make the decision, taking into account all the information. If you're thinking of giving a bottle of formula, here are some things to consider:

- The time involved with the additional preparation, including making sure bottles are made correctly and safely. Will it actually save time overall?
- The impact on milk supply. Some women will find that if they start to replace feeds with formula milk then their milk supply will drop, as the body thinks less milk is needed.
- A small risk of increased chance of illness. On an individual level this risk is likely to be small, but we know that in general babies who have formula milk are at increased risk of becoming ill, particularly with infections. On an individual level this risk is small and plenty of babies are just fine. But it is something you might want to weigh up against the benefits you see of giving a bottle.
- Whether the mum is happy. Some women don't want their baby to have formula, for many reasons. Whatever her reason, support her.

Another option is to give a bottle of expressed milk. For this, it's best to wait until around six weeks after the birth for a few reasons. First, she will still be getting to grips with breastfeeding and adding in expressing milk might feel like one step too far (remember this is about supporting her). Also, in the early weeks, her body is trying to establish just how much milk she needs to make, so she has enough but isn't left with engorged and painful breasts. Adding in expressing milk for the occasional bottle might confuse her body (this is a bit different if she is returning to work and regularly giving expressed milk). Basically, it's easier to wait a bit. Again, if you are going to try this there are a few things to consider, as giving expressed milk doesn't work for everyone.

- Whether the mother would actually find this useful. Some might jump at the chance, while others will have a long list of other things they would really prefer that you did, like the washing up.
- How difficult she finds expressing. Some women can express loads of milk really easily, while others will struggle for every last ounce. Some find it pain-free, others can find it painful.
- Consider if you're actually helping. This leads back to the previous point. Some women find expressing easy and will happily do it to get some time to themselves. Some can catch loads of milk while feeding the baby on the other side. Others find it a complete faff – find the pump, find a bottle, express the milk and so on and so on... for these women, especially if they find breastfeeding quite easy, giving bottles of expressed milk is more hassle than it's worth.
- Whether your baby is happy to have a bottle. Hearing your baby fuss and protest against having a bottle, when you know you have a pair of willing and waiting boobs right there, does not fit with anyone's definition of relaxing.

All in all it's a very personal decision. Consider whether this is more about helping the mother out, or because you want to feed the baby too. There's nothing wrong in admitting that it might be the latter, and of course the mother may be happy to put in the effort to let you do that. But work out how you are going to balance out that effort so it's not just her doing extra work. Also, if you want to feed, do it at a time that helps her out – maybe a last feed before bed so she can get a bit more sleep, or at a time when she can do something she wants (even if that's just staring into space with a hot cup of tea).

Other ways to help that don't involve a bottle

There are lots of ways to support a breastfeeding mother that don't involve giving a bottle. Some of these will apply more to partners than friends or family (mainly because of things like cuddling up to her in bed at night), while others are fair game for everyone. I'm aware that wording these things in this way somehow implies that we've gone back to the 1950s and the mother is doing all the housework. Of course, I do not mean it this way. I mean either doing more than your fair share (if you live with her), or doing things for her (if you don't live with her) – but that's impossible to keep writing over and over. In no way should a new mother on maternity leave have all the housework on her shoulders, but it can feel incredibly stressful to be at home if the house is a tip and she can't do something about it because the baby can't be put down.

1. Help around the house (although of course it's not 'helping' if you live there too).
Sometimes when breastfeeding it feels like all you ever do is feed the baby, or they are asleep on you. If at any point the baby happily goes down to sleep, the last thing she's going to want to do is housework. Seriously, although tiny baby clothes are really cute, if you want to give a new mum a present, get her (or indeed you both, if you're her partner) a cleaner or ironing service or come do it yourself.

2. Feed her
You could see this as indirectly feeding the baby, but caring for the mother is one of the best ways to care for a baby. This might include preparing and/ or cooking dinner (so it could be delivered and they can put it in the oven later), leaving her healthy snacks in reach and in small pieces in the fridge and bringing her something to drink when she inevitably sits down to feed the baby and is suddenly thirsty.

3. Sit with her during feeds
When the baby is having a growth spurt and she feels all she ever does is feed, sit with her. Cuddle up with her on the sofa, pop round for a chat, video call her... whatever. Just make sure she doesn't feel that she is alone. Just because you can't use your boobs to feed the baby, doesn't mean you suddenly have time for long hobbies outside the house.

4. Take charge of other things
Okay, so you can't feed the baby, but you can settle them after a feed. You can put them in a sling and soothe them. You can take them out for a walk (if the mother is happy with them being away from her). You can be chief bath-giver, nappy-changer, book-reader or tummy-time facilitator. If you want to help at night, you could be in charge of bringing the baby to her (if she's not co-sleeping, or maybe if she's in pain after a tricky birth) and settling them after.

5. Be her advocate
If she's having difficulties, find out who she can contact. If someone is giving incorrect advice or criticising her, stand up for her. If she has a question, do some research too.

6. Be proud of her and tell her often
As simple as that. Tell her she's doing a great job.

What about stopping breastfeeding?

Stopping breastfeeding can mean different things to different people. Some will be very ready to stop and be happy and proud of the time they have spent breastfeeding, while others will feel that there is no real choice, feel forced into stopping before they are ready and be very much grieving that experience. Then of course there is a whole spectrum in between.

So when you think about stopping breastfeeding, it's important to look after yourself physically and emotionally. It's also really important, if you are unhappy about stopping breastfeeding, to think about whether there is anything else that could change to mean that you might be able to continue.

If you do want to carry on but feel you have to stop please do reach out to a breastfeeding supporter or IBCLC if you haven't already and see if there is any way around the difficulties you are having. It might be as simple as a small change, finding you more support or working out a way for you to partially breastfeed alongside formula. So do ask before you stop.

Practical tips for stopping breastfeeding

The most important thing to do when stopping breastfeeding is to cut down as slowly as possible. This might mean deciding you will stop feeding soon and slowly reducing the number of feeds your baby or child has. It might mean continuing to express even though you are not directly feeding your child and either giving them the milk or discarding it if you have stopped for medical reasons.

Going slowly helps your body realise it's time to start making less milk. As a general rule, drop/replace one feed and see how you feel for 2-3 days, before dropping another one. It might be that you can go more quickly - some women find they adapt easily and others will find they get engorged very quickly. It's also likely to depend on how much you were breastfeeding. If you were exclusively breastfeeding, you will probably need to go more slowly than if you were just giving one or two feeds a day. Keep an eye on yourself and take your time.

If your baby is under one year old they will need first stage formula milk (see Chapter 10 for more details) but if they are older they can move on to cows' milk. It might help if someone else can try to give those feeds. If you have a partner talk to them about how they can support you. If your baby is over six months old you can try moving to a cup rather than a bottle.

If you are stopping feeding an older child, remember that breastfeeding is not just about milk to them. It's also about connection and security and calmness, so make sure you find other ways to replace those things. The initially logical solution of offering milk in a cup to replace the feed often doesn't work because it's not really about the milk. Trying to get someone else involved as a distraction won't work either like it might for a young baby.

151

" Stay with them. The breast may have gone but you have not. "

Think about the times when your child feeds and how you might do something different but equally connecting instead. Do you feed at bedtime? On coming home from nursery? First thing in the morning? Learning to spot the signs your child is about to ask for a feed, or knowing when they are likely to do so and distracting them with something fun and exciting can really help. In this way they don't need to be rejected - they've still got you. Try going out of the house just before the usual feed time.

You might have used breastfeeding to help an older child get to sleep. One way to help them transition to falling asleep in another way is to start off with your usual routine of feeding them but gradually finish the feed after a shorter and shorter time so they don't fall deeply asleep while still feeding. The first time you might feed until they are drowsy and then gradually shorten this. Stay with them. The breast may have gone but you have not.

Another idea is to use tokens or other limits with your child. This works for some better than others. Basically, they get given a set amount of tokens and they can exchange them for feeds, with you gradually cutting them down. Finally, some might be more bribable than others. Try a special toy or big treat to celebrate them being a big kid now.

Ideas for being kind to *yourself*

However ready you are to stop breastfeeding, it can bring all types of emotions. You might be nonchalant, jubilant or heartbroken. Or all at once or in quick succession. Many women find they feel a bit down or tired after stopping, probably due to the change in hormones, but also it feeling like the end of an era or the passing of time - even if you were ready. The important thing is to think about how you feel and give yourself chance and permission to feel that way. It's okay to be sad or angry, especially if you weren't ready to stop feeding just yet.

Don't be afraid to talk about these emotions - to family, friends or professionals. You absolutely can talk to a breastfeeding counsellor or IBCLC about this - many have had the experience of not being able to breastfeed for as long as they wanted. You might also talk to a doula or counsellor. Doulas are trained in being emotionally supportive and are great at debriefing those for whom things haven't gone right - and that doesn't just include birth. A professional counsellor would be another good option, and you can look for one who specialises in perinatal support. Who might you feel most comfortable with? The important thing is to talk and not bottle it up and think it isn't important enough.

If you have stopped breastfeeding before you were ready it's really common to end up blaming yourself. Stop. This is not your fault. You are doing the very best for your baby in the circumstances. It is highly likely circumstances have conspired against you – fuelled by a society that doesn't really value or support breastfeeding enough. Far too many women struggle to breastfeed because they couldn't get the support they needed – not because they didn't try hard enough.

Remind yourself that you are caring for your baby and meeting their needs. If you didn't love and care for your baby, you certainly wouldn't be worrying or feeling upset about not breastfeeding them. Remember that nothing in life is certain and nothing we do for our health is as simple as either we're healthy, or we're not. Very few people ever get to make every decision just the way they like for their baby and most of us still thrive.

For more reading on working through your emotions when stopping breast-feeding before you are ready you might like to look at the following articles:

- Why breastfeeding grief and trauma matter welldoing.org/article/why-breastfeeding-grief-trauma-matter
- Mourning the end of the breastfeeding relationship thenaturalparentmagazine.com/mourning-end-breastfeeding-relationship/
- Breastfeeding trauma – a mother's story www.mothers-spirit.co.uk/post/breastfeeding-trauma-a-mothers-story

You may also find this podcast by Becki Scott for Doula UK useful anchor.fm/doulauk/episodes/Episode-15-Becki---Understanding-Breastfeeding-Grief-and-Trauma-edt6mg

My short book *Why Breastfeeding Grief and Trauma Matter* explores the experiences of over 2,000 women who couldn't breastfeed for as long as they wanted to.

Chapter ten

Giving your baby formula

→ If you have decided to formula feed your baby, either exclusively or alongside breastfeeding, there are a number of things to think about to have the best possible experience for you and your baby.

Making sure you have the right equipment

If you are going to give a bottle of formula you need both bottles and equipment to keep them clean. This includes:

Bottles, teats and bottle covers
You might like to try out different bottles and teats for your baby, although there is no real evidence that any bottle is better than another. Some claim to be closer to the breast for those combining breast and bottle-feeding, or moving over from breastfeeding, but again there is no consistent independent (i.e. not from the manufacturer who stands to profit) evidence for this. With breastfed babies you might need to try a few before they settle for one. If your baby is older than six months and they are refusing every teat you try, you might like to think about using a cup instead.

In terms of teats, newborn babies are best suited to slow flow teats, whereas older babies might prefer a medium or variable flow. Others will be happier on a slow flow. If you are breastfeeding as well some parents find it better to stick to the slow flow as it means that sucking from a bottle isn't much easier than the effort a baby puts in to breastfeed, meaning they are less likely to reject the breast as 'too slow'. Never be tempted to add more holes to a teat so the milk comes out faster – it damages the teat and could overwhelm your baby.

You can buy bottles that claim to reduce colic symptoms by having tubes or air vents in them. There is no clear evidence that these work and they can be more difficult to clean. However, some parents do find they reduce colic symptoms – or at least parents feel they have done something to try to help.

Bottle brush and teat brush and sterilising equipment

You should clean any bottles and teats in hot soapy water as soon as possible after using them, using clean brushes. You can then rinse this off in cold water before sterilising. You might like to use cold-water sterilising solution, a steam steriliser (such as an electric one or one you put in the microwave, or you might boil your equipment, which will wear out your teats more quickly). Whichever approach you use, follow manufacturer instructions. Remember, although a dishwasher will clean your items it will not sterilise them as it does not get hot enough.

Choosing a formula milk

There are many different formula milks at vastly different prices! Unless your baby has been diagnosed by a medical professional with an allergy or specific nutritional need, which formula milk you decide to buy is pretty much up to you – there is no one brand that is better than any other brand. Pick the one that best suits your budget and is sold locally to you.

It is important that your baby has what is known as a 'first stage' infant formula milk. These milks are designed for babies up to one year old and are the only formula milk your baby needs. Once they are 12 months old, they can move on to cows' milk as a drink (they'll need around a pint a day when they are toddlers). There is very little difference in ingredients between first stage milks. All of them have to meet certain minimum and maximum nutrient requirements by law. If any additional ingredient was shown to help babies' health or development, then by law it would need to be added to all products. So you can really buy whichever one you like. The fancy top price one is no better than a supermarket version, but will cost you *significantly* more money. If you want to learn more about this, I recommend you watch the Channel 4 *Dispatches* episode 'The Great Formula Milk Scandal' – available on demand.

You will probably notice that other milks, often known as 'second stage' or 'follow-on' milks, or milks for older children (stage three or toddler milks) are often advertised. These milks are not necessary and in fact have slightly less nutrition for your baby than first stage milks. Some have further added ingredients in them, but these have not been shown to have any benefit, and the packaging and marketing often makes very misleading claims. There is also a concern that too much added stuff actually places a strain on your baby's digestive system. First stage formula has everything your baby needs.

For more information check out the new Infant Milk Info website designed by the infant feeding charity First Steps Nutrition Trust. It includes evidence-based information on everything you need to know about formula feeding, free from industry influence **infantmilkinfo.org**.

How much will my baby need?

As a rough guide your baby needs around 150–200ml of formula per day per kilo of their body weight until they are introduced to solid foods at around six months old. This will be less during the first week of life, and it is important to build it up slowly – babies only have very small tummies. Try to split the amount of milk so that you are feeding them every 2–3 hours or so, following their cues for when they are hungry (see page 159, responsive feeding).

It's best not to get too hung up on how much your baby drinks down to the last millilitre. Babies vary in terms of size and appetite and, just like any human, vary how much they want to eat from day to day. If they are happy, healthy and hydrated and refuse to finish the bottle, don't encourage them to.

You can tell they are getting enough milk by looking at:

- The number of wet nappies – at least six a day from the end of the first week
- Regular dirty nappies – although this may not be every day in a formula-fed baby
- Their skin looks firm and hydrated and they are alert between feeds
- They are gaining weight and growing in length

Have a look back at Chapter 5 for more information on nappy contents!

Making up a formula feed correctly

It is important to follow the steps for making up a bottle of formula correctly to avoid any risk of your baby becoming ill because of dirty utensils or any bacteria or other nasty stuff being introduced. You must make sure that all bottles and utensils are properly sterilised. Unicef Baby Friendly has a great guide on their website.[1]

One of the main things to remember is that you need to make up each bottle with water that is at least 70 degrees Celsius. You should boil the water and let it cool a little before adding it to the formula powder. The reason for this is that the hot water needs to kill any potential bacteria lurking in the formula powder. Advice years ago was based around the idea that boiling the water was necessary to just kill any bacteria in the *water* but then we realized that because formula is not a sterile product – and certainly not once you have opened the packet – that there was potential for bacteria to be in the *powder*. So each bottle should be made up this way – you can then refrigerate the bottles to use later, but you must not simply boil the water and put it in the fridge to use later.

If you are away from home and unable to get boiling water, the best way to make up a bottle is to use a vacuum flask that keeps water hot for several hours. A good tip is to make sure you fill the flask full – a full flask will keep the water at above 70 degrees for around three hours, but if it isn't full it will cool much more quickly.

You can buy bottles that have a compartment in the top where you put water in the bottom and powder in the top and then click a switch and it mixes them together. However, safety concerns have been raised over these bottles. First Steps Nutrition Trust tested them and found that a 9oz portion of water only stayed at over 70 degrees for one hour, falling to 66 degrees at two hours, while a 5-oz (142 ml) portion of water stayed at over 70 degrees for 30 minutes, falling to 68 degrees at one hour and 60 degrees at two hours. Stick with a normal – and cheaper – flask.[2]

Formula preparation machines have become popular in recent years but they are not recommended. This is because it is unclear whether the way in which they add the water ensures hot enough water hits and covers the formula for long enough. There has been little independent research to establish the temperature of the water. One independent but unpublished university study found that the hot shot of water only killed 95 per cent of harmful bacteria, and that the temperature of the hot shot fell quickly. Further research is needed before anyone can really say they are safe, but it has not been forthcoming. If you do choose to use one, make sure you are scrupulous about your bottle hygiene.[2]

Don't make up feeds using bottled water – although it is okay in an emergency. This is because bottled water, or anything labelled mineral water, has a level of salt and sulphate in it that can be too high for your baby. If you do need to use bottled water for whatever reason, try and choose one in which the sodium (often written as Na) is less than 200 milligrams per litre and the sulphate (often written as SO) is 250mg or less per litre.

Feed your baby responsively – rather than to the clock

Following your baby's natural feeding cues, feeding them when they are hungry and stopping when they are full, is a really important lesson that is relevant throughout childhood and beyond. Adults who are able to stop eating when they are full are more likely to be a healthy weight and research shows that we learn a lot about how to do this – or not – during childhood.

We naturally worry about our babies and can easily get hung up on how much they have fed. But try not to worry too much. Your baby is unlikely to starve themselves and letting them follow their own internal feeding cues is really important. Don't try to get them to finish a bottle if they are full, and don't worry too much about timing of feeds – if they are hungry, let them have some milk regardless of what time it is. Research shows that when babies are bottle-fed this way it can help them stay a healthy weight.

If a baby was breastfed, they would probably naturally feed every two hours or so, taking in smaller amounts than some bottles contain. It is a good idea to try and follow a similar pattern when bottle-feeding, while looking at your baby's cues. Your baby has different stages of cues and it's easiest to feed them at the early stage before they get too unsettled.

- **Early cues:** opening their mouth, turning their head about to try to feed and licking their lips and making other sucking sounds.
- **Further cues:** putting their hands in their mouth, starting to wriggle, and getting louder.
- **Late cues:** crying, fussing and really squirming.

This might mean that you might feed them at 2pm, 4.30pm and 7.30pm, as that is when they are hungry. And the next day that might be slightly different. You will probably find your baby falls roughly into a regular routine, but remember that formula is both a food and a drink and do you eat and drink at exactly the same time and the same amount every day?

Some tips for being responsive:

- Make up smaller feeds. It can be demoralising to throw milk away, so make up smaller portions and if they want more, make them more.
- If they stop feeding don't try and encourage them to finish the bottle.
- Look at your baby for subtle signs of being full and take the bottle out. If they still want more they will tell you!
- Don't try and make your baby wait until a certain time on the clock; feed them whenever they start showing signs of hunger.

What about combining breast and formula feeding?

Of course, there aren't only two options for feeding your baby – it's not a choice between giving just breastmilk or just formula milk. Many families end up doing something in the middle, sometimes giving both breast and formula milk to their baby over the course of a day. Known as 'mixed feeding' or 'combination feeding', it is something that isn't often talked about or supported. I know from my own research that often families feel that if formula milk has been introduced, then they might as well stop breastfeeding altogether. But that isn't true. If you're able to continue breastfeeding and want to do so, then it is possible to combine both options. For example, maybe:

- You have a health issue which means you can't produce a full breastmilk supply for your baby
- You are away from your baby for work or other reasons and find it difficult to express breastmilk
- Your baby struggles to latch on or feed from the breast, perhaps for medical reasons, and you find it difficult to express enough milk for them
- You are working to build your breastmilk supply for your baby but need to give some formula at the moment
- You have health issues that mean someone else is supporting you in feeding your baby
- You've simply made the decision that you would like to combination feed for whatever reason

There are lots of reasons you might want to continue breastfeeding alongside giving formula. Breastmilk still provides your baby with immune support when you're giving formula. You may also like the closeness of breastfeeding, or the way it can be used to help support or settle your baby. You might like breastfeeding to connect at the end of a day apart. Or you might like to keep your milk supply going as part of a 'back-up plan' – breastfeeding can be very useful when your baby is sick or very clingy. Basically, there are lots of reasons personal to you and of course you don't need to justify them to anyone.

However, balancing breast and formula feeding isn't always straightfor-ward, and it's worth taking time to think carefully about how you go about combination feeding to make sure you protect your breastmilk supply as much as possible. This goes back to the simple idea of the more you feed the baby, the more milk you make (and vice versa). If you start introducing too much formula too quickly, your milk supply might drop. So, depending on your indi-vidual circumstances, it's best to take it slowly.

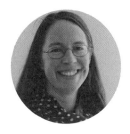

Ten top tips for combining breastfeeding and formula-feeding

Ann Bruce is an IBCLC and ABM breastfeeding counsellor. She leads South Cumbria Breastfeeding Support cumbriabreastfeeding. org.uk, which runs face-to-face groups alongside a great Facebook page www.facebook.com/pg/ cumbriabreastfeeding.

Perhaps you're thinking about combining breastfeeding and bottle-feeding, or perhaps you're already combination feeding. Perhaps this was an active choice that you made, or perhaps you've unexpectedly or unwillingly found yourself combination feeding. As an IBCLC and breastfeeding counsellor, I support many families who are combination feeding. I am constantly learning from families who find themselves combination feeding, or who deliberately choose this. I'm hugely grateful to many families in and around Cumbria, and on the National Breastfeeding Helpline, who have taught me such a lot about their experience of combination feeding. I'm still learning, and I'm glad to be able to share some of this learning with you here.

The first thing I've learned is that the phrase 'combination feeding' means different things to different people. It can mean any of these things, or more:

- actively choosing to combine breastfeeding with using some formula
- having to use formula in addition to breastmilk when you didn't plan to do that, either temporarily or permanently
- expressing/pumping your own milk and giving that milk back to baby in a bottle, or a supplementary nursing system
- completely using formula but doing that at the breast, with a supplementary nursing system
- a woman with 'insufficient glandular tissue' (IGT) or a double mastectomy who will need some extra milk for her baby in addition to whatever she can make herself

Some people combination feed through choice – it is what they wanted to do all along. However, many families find themselves combination feeding out of necessity. Sometimes this happens when there have been breastfeeding challenges in the early days, and they're not given the help that might have enabled them to continue with exclusive breastfeeding.

If you're planning to combination feed, or you're already doing so, if you've had accurate information and support, and have reached a decision that you're happy with, then I'm truly pleased for you. If you're considering combination feeding, and haven't had the chance to think about the risks and benefits with someone knowledgeable, then I hope that this section will help you to reach a decision that you feel is right for you. If you're currently combination feeding, having had breastfeeding challenges, then firstly, know that you are not alone. Also, know that it may be possible to get things back on track. It may not be too late.

Like so many breastfeeding counsellors and IBCLCs, I spend a lot of my time supporting families who are combination feeding, and answering their questions. Some questions get asked a lot. There isn't room to answer them all here, so I've picked the ones I'm most frequently asked:

1. Can I get help from a breastfeeding support group if I am combination feeding?

Emphatically YES. You are a breastfeeding parent. If you are also using formula through choice, or because you felt you had no choice, you are still a breastfeeding parent. Every breastfeeding group that I have ever had any contact with welcomes families who are combination feeding. At the groups I run, whether in person or online, many of the families are combination feeding. Some mums come to the groups for help with getting the breastfeeding back to where they wanted it to be.

2. I'm combination feeding, but I wanted to exclusively breastfeed. Is it too late?

There's rarely anything fixed or permanent about breastfeeding. Change is very often possible. If you're currently giving your baby more formula and less of your own milk than you want to, then it's very likely that change is possible. Making sure that you have access to accurate information and skilled help can make all the difference. If you feel you're not doing what you wanted or hoped for, please do reach out. There are lots of us who are ready and waiting to help you get closer to what you wanted. In the UK, a phone call to the National Breastfeeding Helpline (0300 100 0212) could be a starting point.

3. Is it normal to feel like you've failed if you end up giving your baby formula when you hadn't wanted to?

Yes. This seems to be a very common emotional experience in the UK, and probably elsewhere too. I find this very sad indeed: how awful for those mothers to feel that they have 'failed', when they wanted to exclusively breastfeed, but find themselves needing to use formula. Many mums also express feelings of guilt and shame. It's important that we acknowledge the pain, disappointment and anger that many families feel.

Let's unpack the words 'failed', 'guilt', or 'shame' here, though. I've had the privilege to support many mums who are not yet having the breastfeeding experience that they wanted to have. I can confidently say that I have never met a family that has 'failed'. For sure, something has not gone according to plan, and things have not worked out (yet) in the way the family wants, but it isn't the family who has failed. Families are failed by the system around them: by a lack of information; by 'support' that encourages them to breastfeed but which doesn't actually help them to do so; by society's expectations that babies should feed easily and then sleep for three hours. There is plenty of 'failing' going on, but it isn't within the family that is struggling with breastfeeding. For example:

- Were you told that 'the latch looks fine' when you were in pain?
- Did your baby lose too much weight or not gain weight as expected?
- Did you stop/reduce breastfeeding so you could take a medicine that you've since discovered you could have taken safely while breastfeeding?
- Were you advised to feed every three hours, and then found that baby wasn't getting enough milk?

To all of these families, I would like to say 'This was not your fault; you did not fail; you may have been let down by the system; you may have been failed.'

4. I'm pregnant with my second baby. I struggled with my first, because it was really painful. We combination fed, then I stopped breastfeeding. What can I do to get past this? I'd really like to try again with this baby.
There's every reason to think that things can be different second time round. Here are some suggestions:

- Knowledge is empowering: learn about breastfeeding from people who really understand it.
- Know how to let baby latch on deeply, so that it's comfortable for you.
- Know where to get skilled help if breastfeeding's painful, so that you can make it comfortable and enjoyable, like it's supposed to be.
- Know how to recognise when a person who is trying to help you does not have the experience or skills needed. For example, someone who says 'pain is normal' may be wonderfully supportive, but they will not be able to help you.

The chances are that by being well informed and prepared, it'll be different second time around. Just a tiny change to your breastfeeding position can help. But you need to know how, and/or know where to ask for skilled help. This is putting the ball in your court, unfortunately, but if you find that something's hurting, do ask for help until you find someone whose help makes a difference. Someone saying 'the latch looks fine' is not helping.

5. If I want to combination feed at some point in the future, can I do this? And when?
YES. It's your baby, and your body. A few things to bear in mind to help you get what you want:

- When? You might find it helpful to wait until breastfeeding, and your milk supply, is firmly established. After that, if you want to combination feed, you will have more options open to you. Combination feeding from the start is sometimes possible, and it's sometimes necessary. But it can be hard to sustain if your supply isn't securely established to start with. It's generally more straightforward to lay your foundations first, then build whatever house you want on top.
- How? There's an old saying 'Take care of the minutes and the hours will take care of themselves'. We could pinch that, and say 'Take care of the breastfeeding, and the formula will take care of itself'. For example, if your baby seems extra hungry for a few days, consider letting baby meet that need by spending more time at the breast, rather than giving more formula. Giving more formula can easily lead to a baby getting less breastmilk. If your plan is to combination feed, rather than to exclusively formula feed, then this might not be what you want.

If you're thinking about combination feeding, do think about talking it through with someone who will truly listen to you, who can give you accurate information, and who will support you to make your own informed decision. Breastmilk is very different to formula: it's a living substance, tailored to your own baby's needs. Every family deserves to have full information about the potential impact of their decisions. Some families discover, many weeks down the line, that there were actually more options available to them than anyone had told them.

People who've spent years training to support families with breastfeeding tend also to understand about safe formula feeding and about combination feeding too. But people or companies whose main experience is in formula feeding tend not to have a deep understanding of breastfeeding.

6. If I need to use a bottle, how can I do this so I can keep breastfeeding?

If you have the choice, maybe wait until you and your baby are really into the swing of things with breastfeeding. It takes a few weeks for anyone to learn how to breastfeed, and to establish a milk supply, just as it takes time to learn any new skill. Then, if you do decide to introduce a bottle, find out about paced bottle-feeding. This simple technique slows down bottle feeds, and puts baby more in control of how much milk they take. This can reduce the risk of 'overfeeding'. There are lots of great films online but, again, check the credentials of the person in the film. Who funded it...?

7. If I need to supplement, can I avoid using a bottle?

Yes, often you can. In the first few days, options can include a spoon, cup or syringe. After the first few days, when baby needs bigger volumes of milk, if they are able to latch on you could consider supplementing at the breast. Again, there's lots of information online: search for 'at-breast supplementing' or 'supplementary nursing system'. These are complicated-sounding words, but actually it's pretty straightforward. A qualified breastfeeding counsellor or IBCLC should be able to help you.

8. If I choose/need to use formula, which one's best?
Lots of families ask this question, because we all want to do the best we can for our babies, and because every formula company will tell you that their product is the 'closest to breastmilk'. It's so confusing! Well... they are basically all the same. All first stage infant formulas have to comply with the same regulations about ingredients, including supermarket 'own brand' formulas. Sometimes what's in the expensive tin is actually the very same product that's in the less expensive tin. First Steps Nutrition Trust is an organisation that can help you navigate this minefield.

9. I'm combination feeding but I want to breastfeed. Baby is three months old. Is it too late?
No, it's probably not too late. Much depends on what happened at the start: why didn't breastfeeding initially work out as you hoped? Sometimes fully breastfeeding is not possible – if mum has a diagnosis of IGT (insufficient glandular tissue), for example, it may not be possible to increase supply. But it might be. Most likely, your body is perfectly capable of making plenty of milk, and you'll be able to make changes, with the right information and, if you want it, skilled help.

10. Is it true that lots of mums can't make enough milk?
This is a biggie... so, here we go... I'm going to say it as it is: NO, IT'S NOT TRUE. This is a big old myth, misinformation, fake news, lies, bunkum, twaddle, cobblers.

But many families aren't told how to establish their supply, and there are many mums who felt, or feared, that they didn't have enough milk. Maybe something went awry with breastfeeding and no one gave them the right help. Maybe a family hadn't expected a newborn to do the things that newborns do, i.e. to feed frequently and to want to be held a lot, and this made them doubt their supply. Most mums could make plenty of milk for twins or triplets, if only they'd been told how.

Writing this, I find myself longing for a society where if a family is combination feeding they are doing it through active, happy choice, not out of necessity, and feeling that they have failed. As a breastfeeding counsellor and IBCLC I'm proud to be working to get us to that place.

Chapter eleven

Introducing solids

$\rightarrow$ Once your baby is around six months old it's time to move to the next stage – introducing solid foods. This can sometimes feel a bit complicated – but it really doesn't need to be. If you are looking for inspiration there are lots of baby cookbooks out there, but really, as long as you're eating a healthy diet yourself, there is no reason why your baby can't start to join in family mealtimes when they are ready.

However, just like feeding your newborn, you might find that suddenly everyone has an opinion about when you should start giving solids, how you give them and what foods your baby has. You'll probably hear lots about how solids will miraculously help your baby sleep, ignoring guidelines around timing, or scare stories about choking. Take them all with a pinch of salt. This stage really does not need to be overwhelming – after all, we survived for many thousands of years without weaning schedules, cookbooks or special baby foods.

So what are the main things to know when it comes to solids?

1. Wait until around six months
This is because research has shown that your baby is less likely to get a number of illnesses if you wait until this time. The main protection is against gastrointestinal infections, but there is also some evidence that they may

be better protected from other infections and it can help them stay a healthy weight. Giving your baby solid foods before they are around six months old hasn't been shown to have any benefit.

You might find that people tell you that the 'guidelines keep changing' on when to introduce solid foods, but this isn't really true. They last changed (to become six months) in 2003 (those babies are now adults, or close!) and before that they changed in 1994 (to 4-6 months). The guidelines were changed to six months in 2003 because researchers found that compared to four months, babies were more likely to have the protection against infections that we just discussed. However, research also shows that there is a bigger risk of introducing solid foods before three months. If you do decide to introduce solids early, wait until at least four months (and preferably as close to six months as possible).[1]

It is likely that people will tell you that if you give your baby solids earlier it will:

- Help fill them up
- Help them if they are a bigger baby
- Help them sleep

There is no evidence that solids will help with any of these things. If your baby is hungry and feeding lots, giving them more of their usual breast or formula milk will help more than solid foods, because milk is higher in energy than most foods. 'Big' babies also don't need many more calories than smaller babies as most of their energy goes on growing and brain development. Again a little extra milk will do more to help them.

You might find that your baby suddenly starts feeding lots, and maybe waking up more, at around four months. This is often taken as a sign that they are hungry and need solid foods, but actually it is normal and is usually because they are having a big growth. Research has shown that if you just keep on giving them milk feeds, they will settle back to fewer feeds again, but if you are concerned do check with your health professional.

Food will also not help your baby sleep. I mean, it's a nice idea, but why would it? If they were waking because they were hungry, milk would be the best solution. It's more likely that they are waking for all sorts of other reasons – they're cold, need a nappy change or just wanted a cuddle. Carrots won't fix it.[2]

You may also be told that early introduction of solid foods helps reduce the chance of your baby developing a food allergy. Although there is some interesting research happening in this area, it does have a number of limitations and the latest review of all the research into timing of solid foods, by the Scientific Advisory Committee for Nutrition in the UK, concluded that there was no rationale for suggesting early introduction of solid foods. The review found that the best protection for your baby comes from waiting until around six months.[3]

One last point: the guidance suggests at 'around six months', not bang on

180 days. Just like with any other developmental skill, some babies will be ready a little earlier than others. However, 'around' means a couple of weeks or so on either side, rather than months... which brings me to my next point.

2. Look at your baby's physical development

Your baby will give you signs that they are ready for solid foods. These do not include waking up at night or feeding lots. Nor do they include watching you eat (your baby just likes watching you) or growing teeth. Their physical development is what will give you signs that they are ready for more than milk.

Very simply, if your baby can pick up food, put it in their mouth and chew it themselves, then they are probably ready for food. For most babies this will happen at around six months old. Some might be a little sooner and some might be a little later. What I find really interesting is that research shows that these external signs of being ready for food seem to match changes in your baby's digestive system. By around 4-6 months your baby will start making different enzymes to help digest food – with most finishing this process by around six months. Some might have finished sooner, but you can't tell by looking, so waiting until six months means you can be sure. Signs your baby is ready include:

- They can sit upright for a few minutes, perhaps with some support.
- If you put food in front of your baby they can pick it up and put it to their mouth.
- They eat food they put in their mouth rather than push it back out.

Before this age, babies have something called a 'tongue thrust reflex' that pushes out things put in the baby's mouth. This is there to protect them from choking before they are ready to handle solid foods. If you see a younger baby being fed you might see them pushing puréed food back out of their mouth – this is the tongue thrust reflex and a sign that the baby isn't ready for solids (not something cute or funny, as per many YouTube videos).

3. Start small – milk should still play a major part

Your baby doesn't need ginormous amounts of food at the start. Start off with small tastes and remember that solid foods are called 'complementary foods', meaning they are there to complement the milk not replace it. Milk should still be a major part of your baby's diet until they are one and your baby's usual milk will still offer lots of nutrients and energy, including protein, fats, calcium and vitamins. Breastmilk doesn't suddenly become weaker overnight at six months (no matter what some people tell you) and still provides your baby with immune protection, so it's worth continuing for as long as you want to do so.

Guidelines suggest that babies aged 6-9 months need approximately 200 calories a day from solid foods, rising to 450 at 10-12 months. Remember that this should be a gradual increase, so you don't need to give them 200 calories on day one of weaning and keep it that way until 10 months when you suddenly up it. This is a learning and gradual process, slowly replacing milk with solid foods. These are really quite small amounts.[4]

4. Offer lots of different tastes, textures and variety

Think of introducing solid foods as a learning experience for your baby where they get to try all the different tastes and textures. Some parents prefer to offer puréed foods, and some prefer to give their baby family foods that their baby self-feeds (known as 'baby-led weaning' – more on this in a bit). Whichever you decide to do, guidelines recommend that if you give puréed foods you should also offer your baby finger foods.

Don't worry too much about what your baby actually eats, but let them play with different foods, lick and squish them. Try different coloured fruits and vegetables. If you are giving your baby purées, try making lots of different tastes for them. If you are using shop-bought jars, make sure you alternate different varieties.

Also make sure you offer some iron-rich foods. These include red meat, egg yolk, beans and lentils, fish and dark leafy green veg. You might also offer iron-enriched cereals, but the iron in these is not actually that well absorbed (despite manufacturers pushing the idea). Iron absorption is highest from fish and meat, and when you eat these foods alongside vegetables, iron absorption increases even more.

There is no need to follow a particular order to introduce solid foods. You might like to offer vegetables first rather than sweeter fruits, as there is some suggestion it might help babies get used to more bitter-tasting vegetables.

You should avoid giving honey before one year old as there is a small chance it could cause botulism. Also avoid any food that could be a choking hazard such as whole nuts (wait until they are five years old), raw jelly cubes, marshmallows and foods that might snap off in their mouth (hard carrot sticks or apple slices).

Keep an eye on the salt too. Don't add salt to baby's food (if you share food and want salt yourself, add it afterwards). Be careful with some everyday foods too. Just two slices of bread a day would take your baby over their recommended salt limit, which is easy to do if you give toast or sandwiches. Avoid things that are typically high in salt that your baby doesn't need, such as gravy.

5. Be responsive in your feeding

This means looking to your baby's cues for whether they are hungry or full rather than thinking they should eat at a set time or eat a set amount. Trust them to recognise their own internal cues of hunger and help them follow those – this is a really important skill for life! Think of it as being your role to offer them the food and your baby's role to eat as much or as little as they need.

We know from so much research with older children that being responsive is really important. Offering your child healthy options, but letting them explore and decide when they are full, leads to the best outcomes in terms of weight and how adventurous your child is with different tastes and different foods. Forcing them to eat more when they are full is a fast track to them either learning to overeat because someone else said they should, or deciding they don't like that food (or both). After all, if you were forced to eat more of even your most-loved food by a giant human, you'd probably go off it too.

Babies rarely starve themselves, so trust them to get what they need. This means not forcing that extra mouthful, letting them eat slowly and not getting too frustrated if they 'waste' food. It's not waste if they've had as much as they need. Some babies take a little time to get going with solids – maybe refusing to try much at six or even eight months. If they get to this age and are still refusing, have a chat to your health visitor, but unless they have a health or physical issue affecting their eating, sometimes babies just take a little longer to get going.

6. Try not to give too many shop-bought 'baby foods'

Manufactured baby foods all need to meet regulatory and safety standards and are safe for your baby. However, your baby is more likely to get a varied diet if you try not to rely on baby foods too often. There are a few reasons for this. Firstly, some manufacturers can be a bit misleading in what they call foods, making them out to sound more nutritious than they are. For example, they might call it a 'beef dinner', but the amount of actual beef might be very small – always check the labels!

Secondly, many shop-bought baby foods are very high in sugar, even if they don't sound sweet from the label. It is common for many to be predominantly made up of apple or pear purée with small amounts of other added ingredients – usually those that sound healthier, like spinach or mango. Although everything is okay in moderation, babies really like sweet tastes and will probably eagerly wolf down sugary purées and then start refusing more bland or bitter-tasting vegetables.

Beware of things like fruity baby biscuits – they have five times the level of sugar in breastmilk. Rusks are another problem – they have ten times as much sugar as a slice of toast and butter. Also, it's worth comparing the labels of everyday foods that have 'baby' versions. For example, baby yoghurts often have far more sugar than adult versions and are more expensive per gram.[5]

Avoid letting your baby suck directly from pouches, even though they look like they are designed for this. Food should be chewed, not simply swallowed. Okay, some foods might be swallowed without chewing, but not all the time as these pouches seem to encourage (despite warnings on the side not to do this). Sucking food means babies aren't developing their chewing skills – which are important for speech development. The sugar in the product also ends up getting sucked across their teeth. And your baby misses out on smelling the food. And they are expensive... and they end up in landfill.

7. If your baby refuses a food, try again

Although some babies seem to accept new foods with ease, others can be a bit more cautious. This is thought to be protective – after all, you wouldn't want your baby crawling off into the wild and chomping on some poisoned berries! But this means babies will sometimes refuse new foods, especially vegetables as they are more bitter tasting than breastmilk – sometimes many times.

Research shows that sometimes you need to offer your baby a new food 8–10 times before they accept it. Start with small portions so you're not worried too much about waste, then simply stop and try again another day if they refuse. Don't force them to try it or get upset with them.[6]

Don't worry too much about people telling you that there is a 'window of opportunity' for getting your baby to eat. There is no real evidence for this. One study found that if babies weren't eating lumpy foods by 10 months they were less likely to be eating family foods at 15 months. But it didn't look at *why* they weren't having lumpy foods by 10 months, at a time when most babies were having solids by four months. Similarly, a study in the 1960s reported on babies who were not eating solids by six months (guidance at the time suggested introduction at six weeks!) who then had later feeding issues. But the sample was based on babies who actually had learning or physical disabilities that would likely have affected their feeding skills.[7]

Finally, until around 1930, babies typically had solid foods at the end of the first year. If there was a window of opportunity at six months, this would mean we would have seen considerable feeding difficulties in those generations! Did we? No. Incidentally we started introducing solid foods earlier than around the first year because of the development of the baby food industry in the 1930s. Make of that what you will.[8]

8. Most of all, relax

Yes, seriously. Do not over stress. Offer your baby a range of healthy foods, incorporating different tastes, textures and nutrients. Go slowly, at their pace, gradually moving from them just having milk to having three meals a day (plus some healthy snacks if you like) by the end of the first year. Don't focus too much on the day-to-day, but rather the bigger picture over a week, a month, half a year. Follow their lead and enjoy it!

What about baby-led weaning?

Baby-led weaning, when babies self-feed family foods rather than being spoon-fed purées, has risen in popularity over the last 15 years or so. Some people say it is simply how babies were fed many years ago and certainly, before the concept of jarred baby food was invented, babies were given family foods at the end of their first year.

Whether you decide to baby-led wean or spoon-feed is a personal decision. There is no real evidence to suggest one is definitively a better option for all babies than the other, as long as you follow the steps above, waiting until around six months, following your baby's cues and letting your baby experience a variety of foods. As noted previously, the Department of Health does recommend babies have finger foods from the start of weaning, regardless of the method being followed.

Personally, I am a big fan of baby-led weaning – or rather a relaxed version where you don't worry too much about sometimes giving your baby a purée or spoon-feeding them. Maybe you are out and about and don't want to risk a mess, or prefer to spoon-feed yoghurts or give the occasional shop-bought purée because your baby likes it.

The reason I like the baby-led weaning approach is because it naturally encourages a lot of what we know is healthy for babies. It means you're more likely to wait until around six months, introduction will be more gradual as they learn to master eating, your baby can join in mealtimes more easily, they can play with and experiment with different foods and textures and they are ultimately the one in control. It also means you are less likely to rely on 'baby foods' that might be high in sugar and instead your baby gets to experience the tastes and textures of real foods rather than purées.

However, those things can very much be applied to spoon-feeding too, as well as letting your baby set the pace and not rushing to try to get them to eat too much. The important thing is that your baby gets at least some opportunity to enjoy finger foods and that mealtimes are relaxed. To be honest, one of the main reasons why I liked baby-led weaning with my own children was that it just felt so much easier – no worrying about making specific meals or feeding them separately. They could just sit at a family table and join in – which seemed to make things a lot less stressful (if you ignore the inevitable mess – it's learning, learning I tell you!).

There is some evidence emerging that babies who follow baby-led weaning are less likely to go on to be fussy eaters. This does make sense – being able to feed themselves, eating a variety of tastes and textures of foods in their whole form, and joining in family mealtimes likely promotes good eating habits. But it could also be that those babies who are adventurous eaters are more likely to follow baby-led weaning. If you were worried about your baby you might start spoon-feeding them to try to get them to eat more.[9]

The evidence on whether baby-led weaning helps your baby stay a healthy weight is mixed. Some research suggests that babies who follow baby-led weaning are less likely to be overweight. But this is based on babies whose parents decided to follow baby-led weaning, so again it might be something about who decides to follow the approach. One trial of baby-led weaning versus spoon-feeding found no difference in weight at 12 or 24 months, but not everyone who took part stuck to the group they were put in. Overall, it makes sense that baby-led weaning would encourage healthy weight gain, as babies are in charge of what they are eating and the pace of the meal is slower – which we know helps us stop when we are full. But again, you can make sure you pace a meal slowly and follow your baby's cues if they are being spoon-fed. The main thing really is being responsive.[9]

Basically, the key things to think about when introducing solid foods are:

1. Start at around six months, looking at whether your baby is physically ready.

2. Start slowly, remembering milk is still the main part of their diet.

3. Offer lots of tastes and textures, including finger foods. Remember introducing solids is as much about learning as it is about nutrition.

4. If possible, don't rely too much on commercial products.

5. Be responsive and let your baby set the pace.

All in all – remember to enjoy it!

Further reading
Some books you might like to read about the ideas behind starting solids and baby-led weaning – other recipe books are available, take your pick:

- *Why Starting Solids Matters* – Amy Brown
- *Baby-led Weaning: the essential guide* – Gill Rapley and Tracey Murkett
- *Crying Babies and Food* – Maureen Minchin

Some useful websites:

- Child Feeding Guide www.childfeedingguide.co.uk
- First Steps Nutrition Trust www.firststepsnutrition.org
- Kelly Mom kellymom.com/nutrition/starting-solids/solids-how
- Infant Feeding Matters infantfeedingmatters.com
- NHS weaning guide www.nhs.uk/conditions/pregnancy-and-baby/solid-foods-weaning

Chapter twelve

Your baby's sleep

→ Ah sleep. Remember that? On a serious note, understanding your baby's sleep and getting as much as possible for all of you is one of the major challenges of the first year. This chapter will look at realistic expectations, safe sleep, whether sleep training 'works' and how you can gently encourage your baby to sleep for longer.

How much can I expect my baby to sleep?

Babies actually sleep a lot more than it might feel like. The main problems parents face are that those hours are rarely in a long stretch without waking, and that babies prefer to sleep on you if possible. So, while they might be getting lots of sleep, you probably won't be.

As a rough guide you can expect your baby to sleep:

- Newborn: 8 hours in the day and 8-10 hours a night
- 1 month: 7 hours in the day and 8-10 hours a night
- 3 months: 4-5 hours in the day and 9-10 hours a night
- 6 months: 4 hours in the day and 10 hours a night
- 9 months: 3 hours in the day and 11 hours a night
- 1 year: 3 hours in the day and 11 hours a night

Those are estimates. Also remember that 'night' is probably not what you think of as night. They might spend most of the time between 7pm and 7am technically sleeping, but they will likely wake regularly for feeds or for other reasons throughout the first year (although this will probably reduce as they get older). It's absolutely normal for young babies to wake every 2 hours or so or even more frequently during the night for the first few months. Most babies age 6–12 months still wake once or twice a night, with many waking more often than that.

One reason for this is that until around three months babies have much shorter sleep cycles than adults and spend more time in light sleep. This means they can appear to be asleep, but stir as soon as you try and put them down. It also means that they are at risk of waking up at the end of each sleep cycle – which lasts just 45 minutes. By around three months babies start maturing towards an adult sleep cycle of around 1.5 hours, so should begin to start going longer between wake-ups.

This is obviously going to leave you exhausted. There is a daft phrase that you will hear often: 'sleep when the baby sleeps', to which I suggest you reply 'Shall I also vacuum while the baby vacuums?' but the underlying principle is sound: use any opportunity you can to look after yourself. Maybe your baby naps on you or in a sling during the day, but there is no need to frantically use that time to do loads of housework. Prioritise your own rest. Do stuff that nurtures yourself while they sleep, however mindless it might seem – it's all about self-preservation.

People might suggest you go to bed early. These people usually haven't just spent all day taking care of a baby. It is *so* common to get into a routine of staying up late when you have small children. You spend most of the day caring for someone else and their needs, and the temptation is to somehow carve out a tiny bit of time alone (but waste most of it on social media). For your own sake, try and compromise with yourself and find a balance between this and sleep. No, I don't have any tips for how you do this. Yes, I still do it even though my youngest child is now 10 years old. Yawn.

Where should my baby sleep?

Your baby is safest sleeping in the same room as you for at least the first six months of life. This is because research has shown that your baby is at a lower risk of sudden infant death syndrome (SIDS) if they are in the same room as you. SIDS is the label given to an unexpected death of an otherwise healthy baby.[1] Most cases of SIDS (almost 9 in 10) happen in the first six months of life, which is why the guidance is to room-share for six months.[2]

That statistic should be placed in context: babies do not accidentally die simply because they are in a different room. SIDS is thankfully very rare in the

UK. Around 200 babies die each year of around 700,000 babies who are born. However, given that we know that room-sharing helps reduce risk, and the consequences are so severe, this is a guideline worth following for many parents.

Why might sharing a room reduce your baby's risk of SIDS? No one is entirely sure but there are lots of ideas:

- You are aware of what is happening around them and are more likely to realise when something is wrong, such as your baby being unwell.
- You are aware of the temperature in the room. A room that is too hot – or too many layers on your baby – is a risk factor for SIDS. A baby who is too cold may wake and cry but a baby who is too hot may not.
- You being in the room, making small noises, means that your baby doesn't sleep too deeply. Research suggests that babies sleeping too deeply and for too long may be a risk factor.

You might come across some articles that suggest that having your baby sleep in a different room helps them sleep for longer. There are a few things to think about when reading the headlines compared to the research. One study, for example, was reported as showing that putting your baby in another room before six months helps them sleep longer.[3] Great headline! However, this study:

- Found no difference in sleep between babies who were placed in their own room before four months and those who room-shared for longer than this at four months old.
- Found babies appeared to sleep better at nine months old if they had slept alone from before four months old. They found a difference of 40 minutes on average. However, most babies slept well – the average sleep time of those who were placed in their own room early was 627 minutes, compared to 601 minutes for those who moved to their own room at 4–9 months and 587 minutes for those still room-sharing. That equates to almost 10 hours sleep at night even for the shortest sleep group.
- Found that by 12 months there was no difference again.

The study also relied on self-reports of infant sleep, which we know are inaccurate and can be affected by factors such as wanting to justify your decision to put your baby in another room. If your baby is in a different room to you, you will probably naturally overestimate sleep as you will become aware of their waking later than you would if they were in the same room.

Finally, although the study itself was a trial (of an educational intervention) parents were not told to put their baby in a separate room or not – it was their choice. So it could well have been that babies who slept well naturally due to some stroke of luck were more likely to be moved to another bedroom as they were no longer waking so much at night and there was less need to get up and settle them.

Another thing to think about is how you will care for your baby when they wake up if they are in a different room. How much your baby sleeps or wakes is not the only indicator of a good night's sleep. Some parents might feel happier to be woken more often by a baby in a bedside crib, who they can pick up with ease, compared to having to actually get out of bed and go to a different room to settle their baby. As the saying goes, it might be more about quality than quantity when it comes to sleep!

Sharing a room with your baby also seems to be protective of breastfeeding. If you are breastfeeding, then you are more likely to continue if you share a room with your baby. Of course, it may be that if you're breastfeeding you're likely to keep your baby close to you at night, but there are plausible reasons why room-sharing helps breastfeeding. You are more likely to spot their early feeding cues, meaning they are less likely to be frantic once you get to feed them. Given you don't need to get up to make a bottle, keeping them close is easier as you can just pick them up and feed them.[4]

How should I put my baby down to sleep?

One of the biggest simple interventions that helped decrease rates of SIDS was the discovery that putting babies to sleep on their backs starkly reduced the rate of SIDS. In fact, rates dropped from around 2,000 babies dying of SIDS per year to around 10% of that figure today. In around 1990 research in several countries showed the impact of putting babies on their back to sleep. In 1991 Anne Diamond, a British TV presenter, tragically lost her baby to SIDS after he was put to sleep on his front. She started a major campaign to get the idea of 'back to sleep' into UK policy and it has had a tremendous impact over the years, saving literally tens of thousands of babies' lives. You can read more about the research and story on the Lullaby Trust website **www.lullabytrust. org.uk/the-lullaby-trust-celebrates-25th-anniversary-of-back-to-sleep-campaign**.

No one quite knows why putting your baby on their back to sleep helps reduce SIDS – the important thing is that it does. However, research has shown that your baby is in a better physiological state when they are placed on their back. They are more easily arousable (can be woken), they are less likely to overheat, they have better blood pressure and heart-rate readings and better oxygen levels. It also means they are less likely to have their face pressed against a mattress. There is also some evidence that it helps reduce stuffy noses and ear infections, which might be protective against SIDS, and no one wants their baby to be poorly anyway.[5] So always put your baby on their back to sleep, but don't worry if your baby is older and can roll onto their tummy in their sleep. Remember the SIDS risk is biggest before six months, and most babies won't start being able to roll in their sleep until around six months old.

What should my baby sleep in?

In terms of what your baby will sleep in there are several options:

- A Moses basket in the early days – you can move this around to different rooms with you (ideally not with the baby in it) and it also makes a great by-the-bed storage unit if you end up bed-sharing.
- A small side cot with three sides that clips to your bed. Your baby is close to you without being actually in your sleeping space. However, you must be very careful to make sure the cot is level with your bed and there is no gap in between for your baby to roll into or get stuck in. If your baby sleeps alone in one, there should be an option to bring a fourth side up so your baby is safe.
- A cot – although this is more difficult to fit in a bedroom with you, you can't move it around and your baby just looks so tiny in it. If you do use a cot, never use cot bumpers as they place your baby at risk of suffocation or strangulation if the ties come loose.

With both Moses baskets and cots it is important to make sure the mattress is firm, flat and has a waterproof cover. It is advised that ideally the mattress should be new and not second-hand, as there is a very small increase in SIDS risk with second-hand mattresses. However, as long as it is clean, has no rips in it and comes from a smoke-free household the increased risk is minimal and is certainly safer than other unsuitable sleep locations such as a sofa or car seat.

- Your bed – more on this to follow, as it is vital that if you do bring your baby into bed with you that you are aware of the risk factors and ways to make it safe. If done safely, up-to-date research shows there is no increased risk from bed-sharing, especially if your baby is breastfed. However, it is vital that guidelines are followed.

Any other device – and there are many out there on the market – is best avoided. The Lullaby Trust has clear guidance warning against devices such as baby hammocks, in bed 'pods' or baby sleep nests, or anything that wedges a baby, which increase the risk of SIDS. Items such as pods, wedges or hammocks are often soft and can increase the risk of suffocation. Anything around your baby's head or too close around their body can also increase the risk of them overheating. There is no British Standard for these items, unlike cot mattresses, to help you to assess whether they are high quality and safe. The Lullaby Trust has produced a factsheet on safer sleep that I recommend you download as it gives lots of information on ensuring your baby's sleeping environment is safe. **www.lullabytrust.org. uk/wp-content/uploads/The-Lullaby-Trust-Product-Guide-Web.pdf**.

You should also avoid sleeping with your baby on your chest while you are also asleep – and no one is around to keep an eye on you both. This position is great for naps when you are awake but your baby is asleep, or if another adult is close by and can make sure you don't move and drop the baby or they slip into an unsafe position. Your baby may love it as they can hear your heart rate and feel your breathing and will feel safe and calm. However, it is not advised while you are sleeping alone because you may drop your baby or they may be pressed against your chest so they cannot breathe properly. When you hold a baby on your chest it is also likely they are on their tummy, which is not advised for long sleep periods. Again, the Lullaby Trust has a clear statement on this **www.lullabytrust.org.uk/our-response-to-the-recent-articles-advising-mums-to-sleep-newborns-on-their-chest**.

What about bed-sharing?

From a global perspective, bed-sharing, or more accurately 'sleeping surface-sharing' with your baby at night is a normal practice which is not seen as a risk.[6] There are many reasons why you might choose to share your bed with your baby. These include:

- Convenience: your baby is close by at night. If you are breastfeeding, there is little need to move to feed and settle your baby.
- Your baby is more stable lying next to you: research has shown that when babies co-sleep with their mother their breathing, temperature and heart rate are more stable.[7]
- Babies who co-sleep breastfeed for longer: this is likely to be bi-directional in that mothers who want to breastfeed are more likely to co-sleep, but co-sleeping also helps you breastfeed for longer. You are next to your baby, spot their cues earlier and when they are older they can even help themselves. Mothers report breastfeeding to be much easier when co-sleeping.[8]
- Connection: you may simply like being closer to your baby at night.

However, there has been a lot of debate over the safety of bed-sharing in a Western context. For years, it was discouraged by health professionals, who believed that if no baby bed-shared, then no baby could die in a parent's bed. However, that logic was deeply flawed, in part because it meant that parents did bed-share but without professional advice or guidance, and partly because research shows that when bed-sharing is done safely there is very little, if any, risk for your baby.

Research has now recognised the importance of talking to parents about safe bed-sharing and safe infant sleep. In 2020 the American Academy of Pediatrics updated its protocol to include this recommendation.[9]

The key words are 'done safely', and my reference to 'sleep surface-sharing' rather than 'bed-sharing' is important. This is because many sleep surfaces around the world are much safer than many Western beds. They are firm (ish) surfaces without loads of fluffy pillows and big thick duvets. They are not water beds or high beds with a drop to the floor or between the bed and a wall. So the first rule of safe bed-sharing is to make sure your bed is safe! Also:

- Put your baby to sleep on their back.
- Do not put your baby under a duvet or other cover with you. Keep pillows away from them. Many parents use a baby sleeping bag for their baby to keep them warm (but not too warm).
- You will probably find that you naturally lie on your side, facing your baby and curled in a C shape around them. This is one of the safest positions to co-sleep in.
- Make sure your bed is not overly soft or a water bed.
- Make sure you do not have any toys, extra 'stuff' or any bedclothes with cords, etc.
- Do not put your baby between you and your partner. Make sure your partner knows they are in the bed. Some couples choose to sleep alone for this reason.
- Do not have other children or pets in the bed too.
- Make sure they cannot fall down between the bed and the wall. You might like to put something soft by the bed just in case they fall out.

The second rule (or set of rules) is to make sure you do not bed-share with your infant if you:

- Are taking medications that might make you very sleepy.
- Have taken recreational drugs.
- Have drunk alcohol.
- You or your partner smoke or did during pregnancy.
- You are *very* tired.
- You have a very high BMI.

These factors increase the chances your baby will die of SIDS if you bed-share because they may affect your awareness of your baby, meaning you might be more likely to smother them or not sleep safely, or it might mean that you are breathing chemicals from smoke close to your baby's face at night. A recent review found that the risk of SIDS is:

- 1 in 3,180 for all babies
- 1 in 174 co-sleeping after a parent has consumed alcohol or drugs
- 1 in 787 co-sleeping with a regular smoker

Although most babies in those circumstances will be okay, the increase in risk is very large. Around 90% of babies who die in a bed have these risk factors or their sleeping surface was unsafe.[10]

You might also like to consider how you are feeding your baby. Research has shown that breastfeeding is one of the protective factors against SIDS. Babies who are breastfed are less likely to die of SIDS (although again the individual risk to your baby is very low). The longer babies are breastfed for, the greater the protection.[11] Guidance also states that in the absence of other risk factors and done safely, co-sleeping doesn't present a risk to breastfed babies.[8]

Why are breastfed babies at a lower risk? Well, when it comes to co-sleeping, observations of mother-baby pairs show that mothers who are breastfeeding act differently in their sleep to those who are not. They are more likely to form a protective C shape around their baby and react to their baby's movements. Whether it is lighter sleep from more feeding at night, or the role of hormones connecting mother and baby, is unclear. But what is clear is that it seems to be a very different experience for breastfeeding mothers. This is one reason why co-sleeping with your baby if you are not breastfeeding may present an increased risk – a small one, but a higher one.[12]

Never sleep with your baby on a sofa or chair

Sleeping on a sofa or chair with your baby is risky because there is a chance you will drop them, and they will fall down a gap or become pressed up against cushions and suffocate. While the risk as stated earlier of a baby dying of SIDS is 1 in 3,180, the risk when sleeping with a baby on a sofa is 1 in 174.[10]

Unfortunately, sometimes parents with the best intentions worry about co-sleeping with their baby and instead of bringing them into bed get up with them and take them downstairs to the sofa, or sit with them in a chair, to try and settle them. They then run the risk of falling asleep themselves and either suffocating the baby or dropping them. It's best to think ahead about what you will do in the night in these circumstances.

Does how I feed my baby affect their sleep?

There is a very common belief that what you feed your baby will help them sleep. People will tell you that stopping breastfeeding, introducing formula, giving your baby solids early or filling them up before bed will make them sleep. Is this true? Not really.

Some studies show that in the early days and weeks babies who are formula fed do sleep a little longer. This is because they get a little more milk and formula milk is more difficult to digest than breastmilk. However, once babies get to around 3–4 months this difference goes away. It should also be pointed out that the real difference is small. It's not as if breastfed babies are awake all night and formula-fed babies have a deep 10-hour sleep. The difference for the average baby is a matter of minutes.[13]

Other studies show no difference, especially when you use devices that measure sleep rather than rely on parental self-report. For example, in one study mothers were asked to a) report how much their baby slept and woke up and b) for them and their baby to wear an actigraph – a device that measures sleep. Measurements from the actigraph showed no difference in total sleep time or longest sleep period duration between babies who were exclusively formula fed and those who were exclusively breastfed at any time point from 4–16 weeks old. However, at 10, 12, 14 and 16 weeks postpartum, mothers who were exclusively formula feeding reported that their baby slept up to almost an hour longer per night than the exclusively breastfed mothers did.[14] They also estimated their baby's longest sleep duration was around two hours more than mothers who were exclusively breastfeeding. This was despite the actigraph showing no difference. And in fact, at 18 weeks, the actigraph showed breastfed babies actually had a significantly greater longest sleep duration – 55 minutes longer than for formula-fed infants, with an overall increased total sleep duration of 74 minutes (but this wasn't statistically significant).

Introducing solid foods doesn't help your baby sleep either. My own research has shown that in babies 6–12 months old, how much solid food you give them in the day doesn't link to sleep. Other research has shown that giving rice cereal before bed or in a bottle (which isn't recommended as babies can choke) doesn't help either. Although you can buy formula milks marketed as helping babies sleep for longer, there is no evidence that these work and they may be more difficult for your baby to digest.[15]

Some studies claim that introducing your baby to solids early will help them sleep longer. Headlines from one recent study claimed that babies slept significantly longer if you did this, but a) the data was based on self-report and b) it was only a six-minute difference on average.[16] Other research has shown babies get less sleep if they are introduced to solid foods earlier, although it could be that if parents have a baby who doesn't sleep well and they are told solids will help them sleep, they might try this, hence the association.[17]

Overall the key thing is to think about whether there would be any reason why formula milk would help babies sleep after those early weeks, or why solids would have a sedating effect. There is no logical reason. Breast and formula milk have similar calories in them and typical first foods are low in calories, meaning babies can even end up getting less overall energy as they fill up on bulky low-calorie fruits and vegetables. Meanwhile, we know that babies wake up for all sorts of reasons other than being hungry – needing a nappy change, being cold, needing a cuddle or just waking after a sleep cycle. Food won't solve that.

You could argue that although breastfed babies don't wake more, if you bottle-feed, your partner can help and you will get more sleep. I think this is a nice idea... in theory. In reality you will probably find that you wake up when your baby wakes up even if you're not feeding them. I don't know if any research has been done, but anecdotally lots of women tell me that even on their 'night off', or when their partner is sharing feeds at night, they still wake up first and can't settle back to sleep. It also relies on your partner taking responsibility for those feeds and whether you believe they will do this.

Other studies have suggested that breastfeeding mothers actually get more sleep. One study estimated around 45 minutes more of sleep for breastfeeding mothers.[18] Another study found that mothers who breastfed felt more rested than if they were bottle-feeding or mixed feeding.[19] Why? Because babies are easier to breastfeed at night (after those early weeks when you're getting the hang of it). Especially if you are co-sleeping, it's often a case of reach over, feed baby and then they fall asleep again – without having to move. If you have to get up to make a bottle it disturbs you more. One study found that breastfeeding mothers feed more at night even though their babies didn't wake more, suggesting breastfeeding can also be used as a tool to help their baby back to sleep.[15]

You might also like to take into consideration the bigger picture, and many couples find that on work nights at least they prioritise the working partner's sleep. This can change if you also return to work. In this scenario, think about how, if you are doing all the night feeds, your partner can support you in other ways. These could include getting up once your baby wakes at 5am for the day so you have some sleep then, or making sure they take the baby once they come home. Expressing some milk is another option, perhaps for them to give as a late-night feed so you can go to bed early to get a head start. Try to work together as a team supporting each other.

What about sleep-training? Does that work?

You'll find lots of books that suggest that if you follow certain instructions you will be able to get your baby into a routine for sleep and feeding that suits you and can give you some well-deserved down time. It's very, very understandable why many parents turn to these books in the hope that they can get a bit of predictability back in their lives. The question is, do they work?

The answer is probably not.

The problem with a lot of books that suggest you can get your baby to act in a particular way is that they take quite an extreme approach. There is a big difference between gently watching your baby's natural routine and signs they are sleepy or hungry and gradually encouraging those into a pattern that is easier for everyone, and suggesting you can strictly shape your baby's behaviour. The first is kinder all round on everyone and more likely to work, while the second can leave everyone feeling very frustrated.

I want to emphasise that if you do decide you want to follow any of these

books, trying to get a baby into a strict routine or sleep-training them is not a good idea with a baby under six months old, and really should not be tried until they are more like a year old. First of all, sleep-training generally uses techniques that require your baby to be in a separate room at night. As previously discussed, it's safer for your baby to share your room for the first six months.

Second, babies under 6–8 months have not developed a sense of 'object permanence'. They don't realise that when you leave the room you are just next door and will return. They think you have disappeared. Forever. They are not just demanding your attention – they're actually freaked out you've disappeared, and no one is there to protect them. Again, imagine you couldn't move or escape from discomfort (or a perceived predator): you would want to be close to someone.

Third, young babies really need to have their needs met. They can't sort them out themselves so they need you. And you responding to them is all about developing that close and loving relationship that helps you both thrive. Babies don't wake up frequently for kicks. They wake up because they have shorter sleep cycles, are programmed to not want to sleep for a long period away from everyone and because they need support to sort out the reason they woke up and get back to sleep again. Understanding why babies are like this, and that waking up through the first year and beyond is common, helps manage your expectations and frustrations. There are many gentle ways to encourage your baby to have longer periods of sleep and fall asleep more easily, and we'll look at some of them later.

You probably know someone who says they followed a book that used quite strict routines and it worked for their baby. It might be that it did. We did some research a few years ago that asked parents who tried to follow these types of book whether it worked to change their baby's behaviour.[23] Around 15–20% said that it did. Why? Well it might be that they had a baby who was more amenable to naturally following a routine. It might be that they found they could put the routines into place despite their baby's protests because they really wanted them to work.

The remainder of the parents in our study said that they found the routines didn't work.[20] Either their baby flat-out refused, or protested so much that the parents became distressed. While there are books that suggest more gentle settling behaviours, others encourage leaving your baby to cry for increasing amounts of time to 'learn' to self-settle. Some babies might reluctantly agree to do this, but others will not and will cry more and more furiously. This is understandable – babies have needs and patterns to their behaviour and a parent deciding they aren't going to respond is unlikely to make the needs go away. In fact it's more likely to make the baby even more unsettled and distressed.

Our finding that trying to get babies to follow a routine mostly didn't work reflects the wider evidence we have. The results of sleep-training research trials are mixed and those that suggest that training works often have a lot of limitations or 'buts' in their conclusions. Some might work for some babies, or work initially but not last.[21]

One of the main reasons why parents don't follow through with sleep-training is that they find listening to their baby cry too distressing.[22] We are programmed to find our babies' crying distressing – it's a protective mechanism.[23] Research has shown that if you listen to recordings of various crying babies you can a) recognise your own and b) find it far more distressing than the others.

In our research we also found that trying to get your baby into a routine and not being able to was associated with increased risk of postnatal depression and lower confidence as a parent. Although it could be that those who are already feeling low might struggle further to implement routines, we also found that parents who couldn't get their baby to follow the routines reported feeling more frustrated, anxious and even like a failure.

Crying is also not great for babies. Although no one is suggesting that your baby having an occasional cry for a few moments when they wake or settle to sleep is going to traumatise them, leaving them to cry for longer periods, or not responding to their needs, can raise their levels of stress hormones,[24] whereas responsive interactions can help decrease them.[25]

What about gentler methods?

There is a whole spectrum of different sleep-training approaches. I don't want to tell you that any one way is right or wrong for your family, but rather manage your expectations about what might work and what might not – and why. Experts are pretty much in agreement that approaches labelled as 'cry it out', where you simply put your baby to bed and ignore them if they cry (not returning because this is perceived to teach them that you will if they cry hard enough), are not helpful for either babies or their distressed parents. A variation on this is 'controlled crying', where you leave your baby to cry for a few minutes before returning and reassuring them. Again, this has very mixed results and depends on your baby and how you feel.

Another approach is a gentler version where you stay with your baby, gradually retreating a little further each night. So the first night you might be right next to them in their crib, with your hand resting on their tummy. Over the next few nights you progress to not touching them, then move further away until you're basically out the door. The idea is that your baby gets used to this gradual retreat little by little. Others suggest that you put your baby down to sleep and stay near them, but pick them up if they become distressed to calm them again. Just like with other approaches, it all depends on how your individual baby reacts. Some will be fine with this, some won't.

A note on 'put them down drowsy but awake'
At some point you'll read something that tells you to do this. The idea is that you soothe or feed your baby almost to sleep and as they are passing into sleep you put

them down, as it teaches them to do the last bit of falling asleep by themselves.

This might work.

Or, you might laugh hysterically at the idea as of course your baby protests at their soothing being removed just as they're about to drop off. In fact, it can just make them even more awake and irritable – as you would be if something disturbed you just as you were falling asleep. There is even some suggestion that the feeling of being put *down* makes babies think they are falling.

There is no research to show that putting babies down once they are properly asleep causes long-term sleep issues. Think of sleep as a developmental process, and as babies get older they learn different skills to help them get to sleep. Many an adult was put down asleep and now manages to go to sleep without someone rocking them.

Does it matter if I feed them to sleep?

No and especially not if you are breastfeeding. Breastfeeding is as much about your baby's comfort as it is nutrition and it's very normal to feed them to sleep. In fact, it might be protective against SIDS. Guidance now suggests that your baby should be settled to sleep with a dummy – so why not a breast? Yes, it comforts them and helps them sleep, but there is nothing wrong with that – it's an evolutionary mechanism designed to help babies sleep. Why fight the tools Mother Nature gave us? Babies will grow and develop and over time they simply won't need this anymore. Many, many babies are fed to sleep. You don't see many teenagers needing the same.

If your baby is a bit older and you are ready for them to stop feeding to sleep or need them to, then you can work on ways to replace it. It's all about creating different sleep associations such as a favourite cuddly toy, falling asleep to you singing a particular song or a soothing bedtime story. Elizabeth Pantley, in her book *The No-cry Sleep Solution*, recommends feeding your baby to sleep but watching them closely. As they fall asleep you gently remove your nipple by using your little finger to break the latch. You gradually remove your nipple earlier and earlier over successive nights. If your baby wakes and searches for the breast, you may gently place your hand on their chin to see if they settle. If not, and they wake further, you latch them back on again and try a few moments later.

But I'm *exhausted*

Having a baby who doesn't sleep can be absolutely soul-destroying. Sleep deprivation is a form of torture, and it can really start to mess with your mental and physical health. It can feel like you are very alone and that this is going to go on forever. So what can you do?

Maybe you decide as a family that trying controlled crying is worth a shot.

If you do this it's important to have your partner on board *and* approach it with an open mind. Whether you continue with it will depend on your baby and you. You may be one of the lucky ones who finds that your baby drops off after crying for a few minutes and not getting too distressed. Brilliant. But you may be one of the larger group of parents who finds that their baby is either going to cry for a lot longer, or flat-out refuse no matter how long you continue. This will be hugely distressing for both you and your baby. Many, many parents who try controlled crying stop on the first or second night.

So what *can* you do that will be more likely to work and won't emotionally destroy you? Try an approach that combines looking after yourself, trying some gentler tips and seeking support from professionals:

1. Talk. Talk to other parents to get a sense of how normal it is for babies to wake at night. This won't make you less exhausted, but it will help you realise how common it is. People saying on Facebook that their baby sleeps all night are likely lying, bending the truth or it was a one-off. I have a recurring Facebook memory that pops up every year declaring that my youngest, who was about eight weeks old, slept all night. I seem to remember 'all night' actually meant from about 11pm–5am, which I no longer consider to be 'all night', and he didn't do it again for several months.

2. Seek support from a professional. It could be your health visitor, or you may like to work with someone independent. You could try a postnatal doula for emotional support and someone to hold the baby while you sleep for a bit. Or you could try a gentle-sleep coach who can talk you through some ways you *can* make a difference to your baby's sleep. Have a look at the holistic sleep coaching website and register of coaches for someone who will work gently with you, rather than telling you to do things you might be uncomfortable with. www.holisticsleepcoaching.com/holistic-sleep-coaching-register

One trial that looked at encouraging sleep-training methods concluded that teaching parents about sleep-training helped improve their mental health and baby's sleep. However, if you read the study closely you find that not only were parents in one group taught about sleep-training, but they were also taught about realistic sleep for babies, encouraged to take self-care and given the opportunity to regularly talk through how they felt with a nurse. At the end of the study their mental health and perceptions of sleep problems had improved compared to the group who had no input. Was this down to the attempts at sleep-training, or their improved expectations of normal sleep and self-care? I suspect the latter, because the number one thing parents rated as important was the opportunity to have someone to talk to.[26]

3. Rest as much as you can and look after yourself. I know this will depend on your circumstances, but don't put additional pressure on yourself. If you have a non-sleeping baby and are awake frequently in the night, consider how you would treat yourself if that was a paid nightshift caring for someone. You'd try and sleep in the day, and generally not expect to be up all night and all day. What needs doing? What can wait? Is sitting staring into space with a cup of tea or watching Netflix really being lazy? No, it's self-care and much-needed down time.

4. Pull in as many favours as possible. Those people who want to help? They can hold the baby for a bit while you sleep in the day. If they're a long way away they can order you in some meals, or pay for a (well-paid) cleaner or childcare for your eldest. Make sure if you have a partner that you are balancing the load. Again this will be individual, but if, for example, you are protecting their sleep on working days, then they can help protect yours on their days off.

5. Do whatever makes you happy and calmer. And is legal, obviously. But seriously, babies pick up on emotional states. If you can stay calm, they will be calmer. So do whatever helps, whether that is going for a run, a bath in peace or indulging in a favourite snack and drink. If it makes you happy it helps them too.

6. Remember this is most likely going to pass. It feels in the moment as though things will be like this forever. But babies who wake frequently in the first year do not necessarily go on to be poor sleepers as toddlers and children. Many improve as their sleep cycles lengthen and they become more efficient at soothing themselves. It is *really* hard. But it is not necessarily a sign of something being wrong.

7. Don't let other people decide whether you have a sleep problem. It is only a problem that needs to be fixed if *you* think it needs to be fixed. It doesn't matter what your mother/friend/woman in the grocery store thinks about your baby's sleep. This works both ways: don't let them tell you there is a problem when you don't think there is, or that everything is fine when you say you need help.

Some gentle ways to encourage your baby to sleep for longer

There are some things you can do that fit within a responsive, gentle-parenting approach that meet your baby's needs while also encouraging them to sleep for longer. There will be less crying involved, which is a win-win situation all round.

- Establish a gentle routine. Bed at a similar time each day. Naps at a similar time each day. You may well need to bring bedtime earlier. Yes, *earlier*. The optimal time is 6–8pm. Later bedtimes don't seem to result in longer lie-ins, although there will be exceptions to this.

- Watch your baby. What cues do they start making when they are becoming tired? This is the time to start winding down and encouraging sleep, not when they are *overly* tired. A strange lesson you'll learn as a parent: over-tired children do not sleep well.
- Create a calming bedtime routine (that isn't overly long). Try and do the routine every night where possible, hence the not making it too long or you'll start regretting it. What you do will depend on your baby. Many like a soothing bath with some baby-skin-friendly lavender scent. Others scream the place down, which isn't conducive to the whole relaxing thing. You might try a certain song or tune, calming music, massage, gentle lighting, calming scents, a certain outfit or toy... whatever works.
- Keep your baby's room cool (16–20 degrees C) if possible. Make sure they aren't too cold - your aim is to have a cool room but a baby that is still warm enough. Cooler air helps with sleep. Use light bedding or a well-fitting baby sleeping bag at around 2–3 tog. For safe sleeping recommendations check out the Lullaby Trust website **www.lullabytrust.org.uk/safer-sleep-advice/ baby-room-temperature**.
- Try playing 'pink noise', which is a bit like white noise but more soothing.
- Try not to set a precedent of everything being too dark and quiet. If you're reading this in advance of your baby being here, it's a myth that babies need pitch black and silence to sleep. It will drive you mad trying to make sure no one makes a noise at bedtime. And they can become accustomed to it, waking at the sound of anything.
- Encourage your baby's natural circadian rhythms. Get outside during the day in the bright sunshine if possible (we can only hope, right?). As it draws closer to bedtime, dim the lights (easier said than done in summer, but even closing the blinds can help).

Read up on techniques from experts in gentle sleep. Some great recommendations include:

- *Let's Talk About Your New Family's Sleep* and *Holistic Sleep Coaching* – Lyndsey Hookway
- *The No-cry Sleep Solution* – Elizabeth Pantley
- *The Science of Mother-infant Sleep* – Kathy Kendall-Tackett and Wendy Middlemiss
- *The Gentle Sleep Book* and *Why Your Baby's Sleep Matters* – Sarah Ockwell-Smith
- *Safe Infant Sleep* – James McKenna

If you search for these authors they also have great websites and blogs full of further information. The Baby and Sleep Information Source (BASIS) at Durham University is an excellent source of reassuring and evidence-based information on normal and safe infant sleep **www.basisonline.org.uk**.

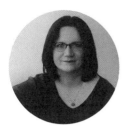

Five top tips to support your baby's sleep

Caroline Zwierzchowska-Dod is a newborn and parenting specialist and trained as a holistic sleep coach with www.holisticsleepcoaching.com. She can be found at www.doulamamababa.co.uk

'Do they sleep well?' is one of the top-two most-irritating questions a new parent can be asked (narrowly pipped to the number one slot by 'are they good?'). The truth is that most babies can fall asleep pretty easily, just not necessarily where, when or how their parents want them to! Whether it's a crib, a Moses basket or a cot, your new baby may not want to sleep in it – at least not for very long, and almost certainly not when you want them to go to sleep. Most babies will sleep very well indeed as long as they are either attached to a boob or are snuggled on your chest. The struggles can come when parents' needs and wishes don't quite align with what baby is expecting.

Tip 1: Understand baby behaviours

The first and most important thing to help you and your baby sleep is to understand why babies behave like they do. We are 'carrying mammals' and our babies are not born expecting to be put down. Sleeping on their own in a crib, cot or basket triggers their most basic response, which is to cry to tell their parent that they are alone and the sabre-tooth tigers might attack. Research shows that babies' inner ears can detect when the parent holding them sits down, and when they are put down on their backs, babies are hard-wired to wake up. Unfortunately what kept cave-babies safe doesn't fit well with modern lifestyles, where parents have to cope on their own instead of in large tribes. So remember, neither you nor the baby are broken, we just don't have the extended family or tribe of sisters, aunties and grannies to help us through the tough times.

Tip 2: Read the baby not the books

I see many parents struggling to decide which 'expert' to listen to. Should their baby wake up at 7am and sleep for 12 hours by 12 weeks? Should they co-sleep till their child starts school? And what about the celebrity influencer whose nanny swears by an eat/play/sleep routine with in-built gym and shopping breaks? No one who has ever written a book about babies – including the authors here – have ever met YOUR baby, lived in YOUR house and shared YOUR values and challenges. You are the best expert on your baby, so trusting your instincts is really important.

Tip 3: Think about naps

Getting enough sleep during the day can really help things to go smoothly at night. Getting the nap timings right is generally the first thing to tackle before thinking about how baby falls asleep, and then finally where baby naps. How many naps a day depends on the child's age, temperament and family lifestyle, so keeping a rough diary for a few days can help you to see patterns of sleepiness and wakefulness to help guide you towards a flexible daily rhythm of nap times.

Tip 4: How baby falls asleep can be key

You may want to think about the cues that help your baby to fall asleep. We all have these cues: I can fall asleep really quickly if I put on an audiobook that I know really well, and I rarely sleep well if I don't have 'my' pillow. There is absolutely nothing wrong with feeding your baby to sleep – it is usually the most reliable way to trigger sleep, especially for breastfed babies due to all of the lovely sleepy hormones in breastmilk and the soothing suckling feeling.

If you would like to support your baby to have other cues to help them to fall asleep, then you can start to layer comforts such as lullabies or soft white-pink noise, patting or stroking, or a small comfort item alongside the current comforts such as feeding. Once your baby has started to connect sleep with these new comforts, then you can gently finish feeding just before they are asleep, while continuing with their new comforts. Over time, you can finish feeding earlier in the process and continue their new comforts in their sleep space to help them fall asleep in the same place as they will be waking up. Whatever you decide to do, doing the same things in the same order in the same way can help babies of any age settle ready for sleep: consistency supports sleep.

Tip 5: Consider where baby should sleep

Many families across the world would wonder why we rush to put our babies in a cot, and then after six months into their own room. In fact, bed or room-sharing well into childhood is really common both historically and worldwide. Bed-sharing, where safer sleep guidelines can be followed, is a life-saver for many new breastfeeding mothers' sleep (**www.lullabytrust.org.uk/safer-sleep-advice/co-sleeping**) and side-car cribs which attach to the parental bed can be a good halfway house to give baby a safe sleep area but allow for comforting and contact throughout the night. Slings can help with daytime naps and having a nap in the pram on a walk gets both parent and baby out in the open air while utilising movement to get a good nap in. Floor beds can be a useful way of supporting older babies and toddlers to become familiar with sleeping in a separate room as and when you choose to make this change. With a floor bed, you can put a mattress on the floor that you and your baby share, which avoids the dreaded 'put down' when many children will awaken no matter how asleep they appeared to be before. You could use a Montessori-style floor bed until your baby is old enough for a junior bed. Alternatively, you could move from a floor bed to a cot, with the parent first napping next to the cot. With this approach you stay close to your baby for reassurance, and then gradually move further away or exit the room for longer periods of time as your child grows to feel safe and secure in their new sleep space. The key with this approach is to go at your child's pace and not to be afraid to go back to an earlier stage if this seems to be what your child needs for a while.

Just because it's normal for babies of all ages to wake through the night doesn't mean it's easy. It's okay to say that you're finding your baby's sleep tough going. Be kind to yourself! Responsive parenting takes into account both your baby's needs and your needs, so ask for help, rest when you can and remember you are doing the hardest and most important job in the world: keeping a tiny human alive!

Part three

"Let's talk about your mental health – how are you feeling?"

No really, how are you feeling?

Resist the British temptation to say *'I'm great, thank you!'* (which in reality we know can mean anything from 'everything is genuinely great' to 'my arm just fell off').

I bet you're actually feeling a whole host of emotions since becoming a new parent – good, bad and ugly. You might feel like you're on a rollercoaster, up and down and sometimes wishing you could get off. You might be thinking that you should hide how you feel and tell everyone how happy you are. I'll tell you now – all these emotions are normal and common.

But what about when these feelings are stronger or don't go away? If you're feeling this way, don't panic: there is support out there. And don't feel alone. It's estimated that around one in five new parents experience some kind of mental health issue and that is probably a huge underestimate, as many parents try to hide things out of misplaced fear that they will be judged.

Postnatal mental health is not about some black or white world where you are either 'unwell' or on top of the world. Mental health is a spectrum that we all fall somewhere along. It can change every day (or seemingly every hour). Nor does any illness have defined symptoms – you might feel just a few or a mix of different emotions. It also doesn't mean you can never be happy or experience positive emotions, just that darker emotions are often also there or just under the surface.

It's important to reflect on feelings of anxiety, depression or anger and think about whether they are simply normal reactions to stressful events. I would argue that a lot of postnatal mental health issues are. You're exhausted, perhaps worried about money, maybe physically in pain and so on – not feeling great is a normal reaction to all of that, especially if you're not getting the support you deserve. We should open up about normal 'bad' emotions that come with parenting – most of us have them, many of us hide them and lots of us worry that there is something wrong with us for feeling this way.

This is why different approaches to supporting mental health are important. Often you might just need to talk or offload to friends or a trusted individual. Sometimes a GP might recommend medication, which can help or just give you the small boost you need to try other ways to feel better. Other times it might be focusing on talking therapy, a nutritious diet and opportunity for exercise and relaxation. Obviously, those are the very things that are often missing or feel impossible when you've had a new baby. But it's why looking after and investing in yourself is so important and not being selfish.

Some important things to remember:

- Feelings like shock, anger, anxiety or wanting to run away are actually quite a common and normal part of being a new parent – it doesn't mean you don't love your baby or want to harm them.
- Experiencing mental health issues is not a weakness or something you are ultimately in control of. You are no more responsible for feelings of anxiety than you are a broken leg.
- Your mental health does not define you. You are still you, however you feel. Your illness is not you. You are a person experiencing symptoms of depression, not a 'depressed person'.
- You don't need to 'deserve' feeling unwell. Mental health is completely individual to you and your circumstances. In the 'old days' of psychology we used to measure stress and mental health triggers by set events. Things like getting divorced or being in debt were worth points on the stress scale. Now we realise that different people react differently to different circumstances (or a combination of them), so looking at how people feel is more important. You can certainly have a very privileged life and still experience mental health issues.
- Mental health is not always logical – there might not be an obvious 'reason' for feeling depressed or anxious. Your brain is just making you feel that way. What's important is not the 'why', but how we can support you to feel better.

- You can experience mental health issues and still function normally in society - at least on the surface. You can have a job, a good relationship, lots of friends and still experience anxiety or depression. People might not even ever know.
- It's not just women who experience mental health issues after birth - men do too and more are opening up about it. Postnatal anxiety, depression and anger are not just hormonal or caused by physically giving birth - they can be a reaction to your change in circumstances, increased responsibilities and worries.
- Sometimes your feelings are about what's happening now, and sometimes they are about things that happened a long time ago. Perhaps you had a difficult relationship with your own parents, a stressful childhood or a loss. Maybe those things had been buried until now. Maybe you have a way of responding to stress that is linked to those early experiences. Talking through your story can really help and many counsellors now use this as the basis for starting a conversation. Rather than asking about symptoms, they ask 'what happened to you?'
- Apart from the most extreme circumstances, there is no link between how you feel and how you care for your baby. You are still a great parent if you have mental health issues. In fact, the worries and anxieties of many parents with mental health issues mean that they interact with their babies more responsively and often. Your baby will be fine - this is about getting you well.
- Finally, there is support out there. Don't be afraid to open up and ask for help.

Chapter thirteen

Normal emotions on becoming a parent

→ How are you feeling? I mean really, how *are* you? Has anyone asked you lately? Of course, the first rule of parenting club is that there are no rules about how you should feel. I mean, if you believe what books and films tell us, we should feel nothing apart from overwhelming love, gratitude and excitement. Never again will we have a negative emotion, and we must show this to the world by spending our days posting on social media about how #SoBlessed we are and how we just can't believe our luck.

But what's actually normal at this time? What are people really feeling?

Anything! Pretty much anything. And sometimes all at the same time. First up we have the emotions that we spend a lot of time talking about – happiness, love, gratitude and so on. All the great stuff (although if you talk openly to people, you discover that many find these emotions actually take a while to arrive). But there is also a whole range of emotions that you might not have been expecting, which are not entirely positive and might not feel acceptable. You might feel overwhelmed. You might feel regret. You might be a ball of anxiety and rage. You might be missing your old life. You might wonder if you've made a big mistake. And then you feel guilty on top of it all.

I'll let you into a well-kept secret - these emotions are absolutely normal and nothing to worry about unless they last for a very long time and/or are having a negative impact on your mental health or how you feel you care for your baby. Feel like you want to get up and run away and leave your baby sometimes? Fine. Normal. Nothing to worry about. Actually getting up, running away and leaving your baby is more problematic (but also, don't panic, there is support out there!).

So why don't we talk about the not-so-good stuff if it's so common?[1] I think we're stuck in a cycle where people think everyone else feels really happy and that we therefore shouldn't say anything. In our darker times we might worry that these feelings are wrong and someone will take our baby away. We might think everyone will judge us if we say something negative. Or that they will think that we don't love our babies or aren't grateful that they are here. Research has shown that women in particular are often sold the idea that new motherhood should be an entirely positive experience and feel ashamed or hesitant about openly challenging this status quo.[2]

But it's important to remember three main things here:

1. Negative and mixed emotions are a very normal part of life.
2. Having negative emotions about people and things we love is also normal. Who can genuinely say they've never thought a bad thought about a partner, family member or friend... that they actually do love very, very much?
3. People lie on social media – that's just generally a good life lesson.

Stop and imagine for a moment that this baby was your job. A job that never ends, from which there is never a holiday and you don't get paid. And your co-worker keeps crying, refusing to be put down and is frequently sick down your arm. You'd complain, right? Or at least want a pay rise and extended holidays rather than the 24/7 shift you seem to have signed up to. And I bet when you did get a moment to complain, you'd vent away even if you did go back the next day. And the next.

In short, having negative emotions and complaining does not mean you don't love your baby or actually want them to go away forever. Emotions aren't an either/or thing... you can experience multiple emotions at once. They can also be passing, while things like love are much deeper.

Isn't becoming a parent meant to make you happier?
Advertising certainly tells us that it does! It claims having a baby makes you perpetually happy, happier than before and certainly happier than people without children. But what does the data – people's real-life experiences – actually have to say? Turns out it says... possibly... maybe... eventually.

Possibly?! Maybe?! This may be a shock. But looking at the bigger picture of happiness and babies the story isn't straightforward. On the one hand, becoming a parent in itself, on average, makes you happier. You love your baby very much and wouldn't actually want to give them away.

But unfortunately, life isn't simple. For every action there is a reaction, and what many parents find is that while they love their baby, all the stuff that goes along with them can be very stressful indeed. Having a baby makes work, money and relationships suddenly more complicated. And when you look at this bigger picture, happiness doesn't increase. In fact, things get a bit worse in the early years, before equalling out again and possibly rising as children become more independent (well, until they become teenagers – but let's not talk about that here).[3]

Of course, if you're in a secure position, with fewer money, work or relationship troubles, you're probably going to be happier than you would be if you did have these issues. Your circumstances when you have your first baby can also have an effect – it can feel particularly frustrating if you're older, used to a high-powered job, and you have had a considerable drop in income.[4]

Happiness is also gendered. Overall, women are less satisfied with their life with a baby than their life before than men are. The reasons are pretty obvious: more women bear more of the brunt of growing the baby, giving birth to it, feeding it and caring for it. A common pattern is for women's satisfaction with life to rise during pregnancy, peak in the days after birth and then slowly fall to lower than it was before she got pregnant as reality (exhaustion!) kicks in. Again, this isn't to be confused with not loving your baby or wanting them to go away, but is more about wanting the other stuff to get easier (or in other words to have a good night's sleep and some peace and quiet on your own). As the author Adrienne Rich said back in the 1970s: *My children cause me the most exquisite suffering of which I have any experience. It is the suffering of ambivalence: the murderous alternation between bitter resentment and raw-edged nerves, and blissful gratification and tenderness.*[5]

Women are also fed a whole load of nonsense from the media telling them what a good mother is – supposedly someone who sacrifices her whole life to motherhood and is grateful for the opportunity to do so. Men can feel pressure to work more, but their day-to-day life often doesn't change so completely. This tension between loving your baby but also missing your life is a common feeling and one that leaves some women worrying that they're not a good mother for feeling that way. Again – you're allowed to both love your baby and miss your former life![6]

This difference in experiences (typically) between men and women makes small things feel so much more important for whoever is at home with the baby all the time. A key sticking point for women is how much they feel having a baby has impacted on their ability to have quality time with their partner, whereas men don't seem to be as affected by this. If we look at the common pattern of a woman staying at home, at least for maternity leave, and a man carrying on working, the social contact the parent at work typically gets acts as a buffer. Their whole day isn't about the baby with no other adult contact.

This can make a huge difference – especially if the conversation they have is nothing to do with babies.[7]

So although you love your baby and having them makes you feel happy, this isn't a magic bullet that makes the whole of your life happier. And that's okay. Don't beat yourself up because you are not skipping through fields, overjoyed by life. You're exhausted and have more responsibilities. Happiness in life is not synonymous with love for your baby.

But aren't I meant to love my baby immediately?

Nope. Not necessarily. A range of emotions are reasonable. You may fall instantly in love with your baby and feel like they've always been here. But it's also entirely normal to look at them and think 'Argh, what have I done?' Or in my own case 'Where did that come from? I knew I was pregnant, but no one told me I would have a baby!' Bonding can take time, and if it doesn't happen in the early days and weeks, that doesn't mean it never will. I've always thought that just after birth is a pretty odd time to bond with anyone. You've just created a human and everything that entails, are sleep deprived and keep having to care for someone's demanding needs. And you're meant to fall instantly in love with them?!

Bonding – or more a lack of it – is one of the first big emotional elephants in the room when it comes to 'feelings about parenting we don't talk about'. I bet if you asked around, lots of people would tell you that they took a while to bond with their baby. In case you don't feel comfortable doing that, I did it for you, and not only did many of my friends say 'Oh yes, actually now you mention it, I did feel that way', but many also said 'I thought it was just me and was too embarrassed to say'. As one friend said:

It's hard to put it into words but I was surprised to feel somewhat discon-nected. I didn't have that movie-style rush of love and it was like meeting a stranger. One I was so glad to meet and desperate to get to know, but still, I didn't feel instantly like I knew her and I was jealous of everyone cooing over her because I felt like they seemed to be bonding with her more than I was.
Hannah

Perhaps instead of instantaneous love you feel that you are on auto-pilot or going through the motions, knowing what you have to do to care for your baby and maybe even acting like you think you should – smiling and telling everyone how lucky you are.

With my first I didn't feel that overwhelming rush when she was born that
you're 'supposed' to feel. Every day I was just going through the motions of

taking care of her but it just took me a really long time to fall for her. <u>Rosie</u>

This might be exacerbated if you had ideas about what your baby might look like or be like, which turn out to be different – it can be a shock when there is a disconnect between expectations and reality. Again, this is *so* normal:

I remember feeling shocked, and actually slightly horrified when I first saw my newborn because she didn't look how I imagined my baby looking. For some reason, in my head I thought I was going to have a blonde boy. We ended up having a 10lb, 7oz black-haired girl, who was very red and very angry! <u>Alice</u>

The type of birth you had can have an effect. If it was long, painful or complicated then of course it is normal not to feel love and devotion immediately. Imagine coming round from any other operation or procedure and being handed a baby you hadn't met before to take care of!

I thought the pain of labour would stop, and I would immediately be filled with love. I thought I'd want to hold him. In reality, I was in so much pain and so traumatised from labour, I couldn't hold him. It took a while to process the birth, and eventually feel that rush of love. <u>May</u>

You might find that this is exacerbated if you have experienced a previous loss or you had complications that made you worried about your baby. It is likely that this is protective - your body's way of protecting you in case something terrible happened.

After losing two babies prematurely, when my third was also premature, I found myself very unattached in the early days visiting in NICU, just going through the motions almost like playing a role in a play. To the point that when she was allowed home I wasn't sure I wanted to take her home. This sounds terrible now! I almost couldn't bond with her because I felt I shouldn't just in case something went 'wrong'. After a rocky start we have a lovely relationship now. Not really aired these thoughts before (she's 30 now!), so thank you. <u>Liz</u>

Sometimes, events around the birth and in the early days can play a part. Having a baby who needs to be taken away after birth, is in NICU or has a lot of medical intervention can mean that you feel disconnected and that they are not quite yours (see Chapter 6):

When my son was born he did not cry loudly but just made soft baby noises. It was a lovely birth but he had a slight fever and my water had broken right around 24 hours before so he went to the NICU. I remember thinking when going in to nurse him that I had no idea which baby was mine because I'd never even heard him cry! I think I was a little in shock from managing the separation (I got discharged but he stayed in the NICU for a week). The whole thing felt more like 'he was the baby assigned to me' to care for and I was just mechanically following instructions. It was all very business-like with the pumping at home and going back and forth to the hospital. Things got better when he came home and we were able to relax. <u>Maureen</u>

Remember, as with anything to do with having a new baby, things change. How you feel today is unlikely to be how you feel forever. It might take days, weeks, months or even longer, but as you spend more time with your baby that bond and connection will grow (if it doesn't, and you are still struggling see Chapter 20 for more support). Give it time.

Eleanor's story

My first baby was what everyone around me said was 'a good baby', as he slept well and breastfed really well. I had heaps of milk and he was happy to cluster-feed from 6–10pm then pass out for 7–8 hrs from day 11.

That first night when he slept through I couldn't go to him to see if he was okay, I thought he had died in his sleep. My husband went to him while I lay in bed feeling quite calm and disassociated. Baby was okay and I just 'plugged him in' at the breast to feed. I was pleased he wasn't dead as that would have been dreadful, but not overjoyed that he was fine.

I thought I was a good mother: I fed on demand, lots of cuddles, sang to him heaps, but he sort of didn't quite feel as though he was mine as he was never really awake – he literally just fed and slept. Friends and family visited, I went out and about, but felt I was a 'false mother' as I didn't feel overwhelming love for my baby.

Then at five and a half weeks my exclusively breastfed baby became sick. To this day, I cannot explain how he got Campylobacter. His belly was so distended, he had frothy, foul green poo and was a poor little miserable baby. As a nurse and midwife I knew he needed hospitalisation and investigation as his bowel sounded like a drum.

I felt totally disassociated from him still. He was now a patient who needed rehydration and decompression of his bowel to prevent NEC. He was on the breast and utterly miserable. He was admitted with me and the poor little thing was so dehydrated they found it really hard to get a capillary for his IVI – he ended up with one in his scalp and one in his foot, really awkward for feeding. One of the paediatricians, who I knew as they were the team I worked with as a midwife, told me he would have died if I hadn't been breastfeeding him. I felt efficient and pleased I had recognised he was really sick. It had been a battle via my GP to get to see a paediatrician urgently. But I still didn't feel that bond.

Then out of the blue, five days later we were home and he looked up at me from the breast and he smiled. Really smiled. That lovely 'I'm enjoying this feed and don't want to let go of the breast, but as I'm stabilising it with two hands and she's never whipped it away before, I'll let her know I love being here and I'm safe and happy'... and I just totally fell in love with my son at that moment. He became my reason for existence almost! He was the sweetest baby and I just adored him totally.

He is 33 now and I have two grandchildren from him. We all live together in a huge house as they couldn't afford to buy yet. I have a daughter too, who I fell in love with immediately - home birth. I love them both so much. But if it is possible to say the happiest thing that I've ever experienced, it wouldn't be my wedding or my births. It would be Jonathan's smile and my stomach turning over with this huge surge of love for him and life becoming normal for me. I became a mother at that point and all the strange feelings went away.

I've never told anyone this before. I don't think I was postnatally depressed as I was pleased with my baby, my husband was supportive, everything was fine - apart from the Campylobacter - but I felt almost as though he wasn't mine and I was acting the mother role.

What else is normal?

Alongside the shock and feeling like things aren't quite real, there are a whole host of other emotions you might be feeling that no one really warns you about. These might be unexpected, feel awkward or you might worry that you're alone in feeling them. I asked parents on social media about their most unexpected emotions or ones they felt they should keep quiet. The list was longer than I expected and goes to show just how varied things can be and how there is no one right way for everyone. Here are 10 really common but not often discussed emotions:

1. Stunned that this baby is yours - and they're going to trust you to take care of it

I just couldn't believe that the hospital were expecting me to take the baby home and look after her all by myself. I remember feeling the most incompetent and incapable that I have ever felt in my life. Jackie

We spend a lot of pregnancy thinking about our baby growing, the birth and a

205

vague future. But a really common experience when actually handed your baby is to feel shock: they are your responsibility, with very little 'training', and it turns out 'they' are just going to let you get on with things. Have they not seen what you do to houseplants?!

2. Overwhelmed by responsibility
It was like I grew up within minutes. There was the old me and then sudden-ly a baby and then the new me. It hit me like a truck. It wasn't just me now.
Craig

The responsibility can feel overwhelming when you suddenly realise that this very small person is your responsibility and they are relying on you to meet all their needs. Gulp.

3. Horror at what you've done to your life
The first night home when she wouldn't settle, and we were both exhausted. We sat and talked about what the hell had we done to our lives!! Heidi

At some point either during pregnancy or after your baby is here you will most likely have *the moment...* when you suddenly realise the finality of all of this. You have made a baby and now you need to look after it. For at least 18 years or so. Eeek. This emotion is totally normal, and you will get used to your new life, I promise. But it really helps to hear that other people feel this way too, as it's not exactly a Hallmark slogan, is it?

4. Grieving for your old life
I think I spent some time mourning what had been to be honest. I didn't discuss it as who says that out loud? But I missed the things I used to be able to do with ease like heading off on a long bike ride all day Sunday. I wasn't going to be that idiot who left my partner to it but it felt like I had lost some-thing. Oliver

Closely related to the previous point, it's actually completely normal to grieve your 'former' life while still being happy you are in your current situation. Things have changed and will be changed for a very long time. Recognising that even though you have different positives in your life now, that you have had to leave behind some things you love is healthy and normal. It's okay to grieve.

5. Shock at how much there is to learn
I can remember feeling shock. As a midwife, I naively thought that I would find caring for a newborn easy and I should know what I was doing, but I really didn't! Yes I knew the basics, but it suddenly dawned on me that I had to learn to get to know my baby, learn how to breastfeed, how to be a mother! Lilly

During pregnancy all the focus can be on that and the birth, with little thought about the practicalities of actually keeping someone alive and healthy. Then they're here and suddenly you realise just how much you don't know. Don't panic. Feed them, change their nappy regularly, cuddle them and keep them vaguely clean and you're doing fine!

6. Feeling trapped but also not wanting to be separated

I felt trapped and confused – desperately wanting to get away from my baby and not have to hold him or feed him again, but being paralysed with fear if I left him with his dad for 10 minutes. <u>Charlotte</u>

Ah, this gem! Just. Ten. Minutes. PLEASE. Yup… while you're with them you are desperate to get away, feeling trapped and like you're never going to get a break. And then someone offers to take them for a walk or suggests you pop out to the shop alone and suddenly panic arrives on horseback, and you're physically terrified about being apart. You might also be furious about how much freedom your partner has to just get up and leave the baby and go to work… yet not actually want to leave the baby yourself.

7. Feeling like you have lost your own identity

I felt like I had lost myself, I wasn't me anymore and it took me a while to accept who the new me was. Everybody knows life will be different, but nobody tells you how much you will change and how quickly too! <u>Amy</u>

This is another really common feeling. Who are you now? How has life changed? Will you ever be the same? Just breathe… you will feel like you again, albeit perhaps a different version. You're just growing, changing, metamorphosing.

8. Outrage at the inconvenience

I felt completely outraged when she wouldn't go to sleep at 'bedtime'. The first night I got back from the hospital we settled down with a meal and a video and put her in her cot, but of course we ended up having to press pause and go through to settle her and then bring her through to be with us. I knew she didn't know night from day but my level of resentment was huge and unexpected. Didn't she know how tired we were? How we deserved some adult time alone? It was the first wake up call to 'life will never be the same again' and for a few hours when I was stuck in some kind of ego battle, I really fought it. Then I remembered how small she was, gave in and prioritised doing what worked, and what she seemed to need over what I thought she should do. <u>Alice</u>

Let's face it, babies can be awkward little things. Content to sleep when you've nothing else to do, but the minute you want to do something for yourself, they immediately want attention. It is inconvenient. It's a good job they're cute.

9. Feeling incompetent

I remember looking out of my living room window a few days after having my first and seeing people just going about their day and all I could think was how is life still just going on? I saw a woman walk past pushing a pram and thought I'd never be like her, I'd never be able to leave the house and push my baby in his pram! Obviously these feelings didn't last long but they did last longer than I thought. I think we had all settled into life a little bit by eight weeks. Michelle

Especially when you look at other people going about doing their thing. Just like that. In public and everything. When you can't think past leaving the house.

10. Sometimes you forget that you've even had a baby or what they look like...

I also had several minutes each day where I'd completely forget I had a baby at all! Once I was driving and completely freaked out when I glanced in the rear view mirror and saw a baby safely strapped into the back seat. There were several times where he'd be asleep in his Moses basket and he'd stir and I'd get a fright because I'd forgotten he was there at all. Melissa

This one is surprisingly common. Yes, it is possible to feel overwhelmed, like you're never going to get a break and shocked at what has happened to your life... and then simultaneously have moments when you somehow forget your baby exists.

Remember, life is a rollercoaster

I gave birth to my first baby five weeks ago. The first few weeks we had a few nights where she didn't sleep at all and so the next day, overtired and over-emotional, I couldn't stop crying and just wanted to run away and let someone else be the mum. I felt so guilty for feeling like this. Luckily she slept well that night, and the next day I felt much better. I think all new mums have their 'good' days and 'bad' days. Caitlin

Remember it's perfectly normal for your emotions to change from day to day and even hour to hour. There will be good days when you feel on top of the world and bad days when you're wondering what you have done. These emotions aren't necessarily due to anything particular happening either. You could have an easy day and still feel terrible, or a day when everything seems to go wrong but all you feel is happiness and love.

In the early days and weeks your feelings will be hugely affected by hormones if you are the parent who has given birth. Straight after birth your levels of oestrogen and progesterone will drop dramatically, most likely leaving you feeling tearful and anxious at around day three or so. This usually goes away, but if it doesn't and you find yourself feeling low, anxious or on edge most of the time, do speak to your health professional (and see part 3). It can take 2–3 months for these hormones to get back to pre-pregnancy levels if you're not breastfeeding.

If you have any underlying issues related to your blood sugar or thyroid hormones, or have become deficient in some vitamins during pregnancy, you might also be feeling low, anxious and fuzzy-headed. If you are worried about this, speak to your health professional and see Chapter 24 for more info.

You'll also have other hormones sloshing around. Oxytocin from all the cuddles with your baby, which can make you feel calm and loved-up. And if you're breastfeeding more oxytocin again, alongside prolactin, which can also make you feel calmer and help you sleep.

There is some evidence that men experience hormone changes too – notably a small drop in testosterone levels and an increase in oxytocin as long as they are spending time cuddling their baby. Although the research has only been done in rats, male rats have an increase in the hormone vasopressin while their partner is pregnant and after birth. This hormone is associated with an increase in protective behaviour and being aggressive towards any threats. It's thought that this is designed to help bond fathers to their family and to take a more nurturing role that isn't focused just on sexual attraction.

It's also possible to feel everything and anything at once and not know what to do with yourself. It can feel frustrating, but be reassured that there is no need to worry about this – it's so normal.

A word on IVF guilt

I used to feel really guilty and angry at myself because I felt like I put so much effort into having her and I felt so lucky that it actually worked and I had the privilege of affording it that I felt I should never feel anything negative about being a mother. Joanne

Feelings about being a mother when you have had IVF, struggled to conceive or perhaps your baby was born very sick or premature are not often talked about. A lot of parents feel like they should be grateful for every moment because it so nearly didn't happen for them. Again, cut yourself some slack. Of course you can complain about the difficult parts! Just because it took you a while to get here doesn't make the experience any easier. Maybe you do feel more gratitude than if it had been easier, but remember, you can have more than one emotion at the same time. It's fine.

Research shows that most parents feel a mixed bag of emotions and find settling into parenting a challenge, and there is no difference in that whether you have IVF or fall pregnant in two seconds flat.[8] Remember that IVF is stressful – you're allowed to feel shell-shocked by the whole experience.

> Motherhood is a bittersweet rollercoaster of these opposite emotions – so lonely at times while never alone. Desperately needing a hug while being so touched out. Needing a break but not wanting to be apart. It's so overwhelming. I'm on week five of my third child and bloody hell it's a journey.
>
> Sarra

What about when it's your second (or more) baby?

There are so many potential emotions to be had in this scenario, and often not what you would expect. All the things above apply a second (or more) time around, but there are also some very common additional things you might feel:

- More confident because you've done this before.
- Less confident because things are different.
- Caught off guard by a more difficult experience.
- Realising how difficult things were last time by a better experience this time.
- Feeling irritated by or resentful of your older child.
- Feeling angry that the younger child has turned up.
- Feeling it's not as special as last time and feeling guilty about that.
- Feeling split in two.
- Regretting adding another child.

It's also common not to know which child to feel most protective about. Some parents find that they feel more protective towards their tiny baby, while others feel almost resentful of them and as though they are missing out on being with their older child. Relax. Both are normal (and again can change from day to day). Everything is new and unusual right now and just because you've done it once before doesn't mean you are expected to know what to do this time round – it's a brand-new situation for you!

I missed my son so much when my daughter was born and felt like I was getting a raw deal having to look after her (random baby who I didn't know, cried all the time and caused me pain) while my mum or husband spent more time with him (wonderful child who loved me totally and had spent nearly every day of his life with me for two years). Also the total sensory overload of having a baby crying in your face for three months and inability to deal with anything the poor older child asked for or did wrong because it was just one more thing in my ears. <u>Ilana</u>

It's also perfectly okay to feel disappointed with the experience the second time around, because it's not as new and exciting as the first time. Yes, you have a brand new baby, but look at parenthood as the bigger picture. It's not just the baby, it's what changes in your life. And other things haven't changed. It's not new. Some stuff is just carrying on as before.

I also think there's a lot to be said about becoming a mother for the first time and that 'rush of love' not just being about the baby but being about falling in love with being a mummy and then being able to call partner daddy and parents granny and grampy and all the pride and fun which is involved in that and going to baby groups etc. Subsequent babies are no less magical but you don't get the same changes and all of that seemed somewhat old hat so for me the rush of feelings wasn't as uplifting and energising and exciting and cloud 9 didn't last so long, but I think cloud 9 for baby #1 is made up of more than just love for your baby. <u>Marianne</u>

Emma's story

I think a big thing that I wish was talked more openly about is the change in your relationship with your other kids when you have a new baby. I spent years thinking there was something wrong with me after my second child was born. Before she was born I had this unshakable bond with my first. There seemed to be no limit to my patience with him. If you could see a physical connection between us you would have seen it stretch and thin towards the end of pregnancy but it was still firmly intact.

The moment my second child was born it was as if that bond, that connection was abruptly cut and I didn't have that unconditional patience and empathy that had always been there for my first child. My attention has switched to the needs of my second. I spent years worrying that I had broken that bond, that I didn't love him as much as his sister, that I was a 'bad mum' because of how my feelings towards him had changed so abruptly. I had to work harder and dig deeper to find the same level of patience for him. I had to make a point of remembering to give him physical affection, some days needing to even set an alarm as an external reminder.

When I had my third baby the exact same thing happened to that unshakable bond I had with my second child and I realised how normal it was. All that had happened was that my attention had shifted to the new baby who needed more of me because of how vulnerable they were in comparison. I now think it's a biologically normal rewiring that happens to ensure the survival of the baby, who really does need more of us. There are other examples of this such as how our body prioritises making milk appropriate for the younger child when you become pregnant or are tandem feeding.

I wish I had been able to hear others' stories of how their relationship with their older child changed when they had a new baby and that it was normal to have less patience and empathy for them despite still loving them unconditionally. That both things can occur simultaneously. I think it would have been a lot less confusing to hear that it was normal and okay. That then opens up space to find solutions that help you continue being the parent you want to be for your kids rather than being hindered by shame.

If you need some further reassurance, I can recommend:

- Following Kristina Kuzmic on Facebook www.facebook.com/KristinaKuzmic
- *The Mask of Motherhood* – Susan Maushart
- Following the poet Hollie McNish on her website and social media. Her book *Nobody Told Me* is a brilliantly raw and funny series of poems about motherhood holliepoetry.com
- Buzzfeed is amazing for honest parenting moments www.buzzfeed.com/asiawmclain/100-hilarious-parenting-tweets

To sum up, what you are feeling is perfectly normal and okay. It's a time of huge change and transition and reality is often very unlike our expectations. It's okay to be exhausted and desperate for a break. It's okay to have those moments of panic and wanting to run away. None of it means you don't love your baby.

Chapter fourteen

Am I a good enough parent?

→ If you're even thinking about this question, then yes, of course you are... despite what the small voice in your brain tries to torment you with late at night. You are doing enough and absolutely are enough for your baby. And no matter how serene and calm and together other parents around you might look, they're thinking about this too. And if you're still doubting it, remember hamsters often eat their babies if they're feeling a bit stressed. You're definitely doing better than that.

I'll let you into another well-kept secret – it's actually okay to just be an 'okay' parent. You don't have to be perfect. You don't have to be calm and engaged and loving all the time. You don't have to feel exhilarated and exude love and energy all day long. It's okay to be watching the clock until bedtime. While there are certainly parents out there that are not good parents, they are those who abuse and neglect their children – and by neglect I mean leaving them to forage food out of the bin, not just trying to get ten more minutes' sleep in the morning.

The idea of being 'good enough' is actually supported by science. There's a whole body of research that has looked into what babies and children need, based around the idea not of perfect parenting, but parenting that was 'good enough'. This phrase was coined by Donald Winnicott, a paediatrician and psychoanalyst, back in 1953. He spent many years watching mothers and babies and concluded that sometimes not being able to meet your baby's needs immediately and perfectly might actually be a *good* thing.[1]

Bear with me for a moment here, as that sounds a bit crazy at first. But by 'not responding to your baby's needs' he didn't mean things like beating them, leaving them alone in the house while you go out partying or slipping gin in their bottle. He meant things like not always knowing why your baby is crying, or not being able to respond immediately, actually being an excellent example to your baby.

By responding to your baby's needs your baby learns that someone loves them, cares for them and helps them (see Chapter 5). All good things. But Winnicott believed that if you were 'too perfect' it could backfire. When your baby has small 'disappointments', such as you not quite knowing why they are crying, or indeed leaving them to cry for a few minutes as you're just trying to finish something else, they learn that although they are very much loved the vast majority of the time, the world is not in fact a perfect place.

These experiences help them learn in very soft ways that the world doesn't actually revolve around them and sometimes they might need to wait a little. It is their very first lesson in resilience. It is important to add that Winnicott stressed that for very young babies these 'disappointments' should be very minor – i.e. occasionally having to cry for a few minutes will do no harm, but much longer periods could have a negative impact. As babies get older, they will be able to understand more and wait longer (at least in theory), but young babies have little sense of time. He also stressed it was very much about the overall pattern – not being able to respond immediately sometimes is fine, but it might become an issue if you *never* responded quickly.

This doesn't mean that your baby's early years are not important, or that any investment in them in terms of time and love is pointless, but is more a reminder to look at the bigger overall picture and what you are doing rather than what you aren't. We know that responding lovingly to your baby, talking to them and making sure their physical needs are met sets the scene for their later years and development. Helping babies learn they are secure and safe and loved is the foundation for an older child, teen and adult who continues to feel secure and confident.

But no one says you have to be Mary Poppins every second of the day (and night) to make that happen. Do you expect perfection in everyone else? Do you expect perfection from your children? If your partner leaves the dishes in the sink one night, do you pack your bags and leave even though they usually clean up after everyone? Do you bin years of friendship after one trivial argument? I mean... is perfection actually possible in anyone? (Spoiler – no).

Learning about this balance is good for children. I really like the opening line of this article entitled 'The Good Enough Parent' in *Psychology Today*, which you might like to look up: *If we define parenting as caregiving to one's child, then the best parent is not the one who parents most, and certainly not the one who parents least, but the one who parents just the right amount. That's the parent Goldilocks would pick, if she had tried out three different parents along with the three different bowls of porridge, chairs, and beds. It's the one most children would pick if they had the power to choose.*[2]

I still don't feel like I'm good enough

I hear you. And this is such a common emotion to feel. But it can help to step back and think objectively about what your baby needs and what you are actually giving them. It can also help to reverse things and look at yourself as you would a friend – do you think they're doing well? I'm sure you're much kinder to them than you are to yourself.

So what do babies actually need (and what do the media and those selling stuff try to tell us that they need)? They need food, they need hugs, they need to be kept clean (ish), and they need to feel loved. Giving your baby these things most of the time makes you a good parent. Other stuff is not essential, so you're not a bad parent if you...

- Look forward to their nap
- Take them on a really long walk just because they sleep
- Entertain them by a screen sometimes
- Some days spend all day in the house seemingly doing nothing but feeding and holding them
- Haven't bought them the latest overpriced supposedly educational toy
- Haven't read any of the 'my baby day-by-day' books you were given that told you how to apparently support their development
- Pass them over to someone so you can sleep/have a bath/whatever
- Want to reclaim some of your old life and go for a date night or out with friends (as long as someone is looking after them!)
- Have to go out to work to pay the bills, keep sane or just because it's important to you

And you are certainly not a bad parent based on how you choose to feed them – those decisions are complex and personal and you're doing your best.

We all think and feel these things some days. We just might not say them out loud or post about them on social media. In fact we're all so worried about what everyone else thinks and posts on social media, we post made-up stuff on there instead, about how we've had a blissful afternoon and are so happy. When actually we've been hiding in the bathroom, eating chocolate spread out the jar, and crying for half of it. It's not real and if you ask close friends they will tell you stories of all the supposedly 'bad' things they have thought.

I've had some really off days lately...

As Winnicott said, it's all about the bigger picture and how you usually respond. Don't believe me? Well luckily there has actually been research conducted on just how often you need to get it right for your baby to be okay. How often do you think that is? 99% of the time? 90%? 80%? No! Drum roll...

It's just 50%.

Yes. 50%. Get it right at least half the time and your baby will most likely be fine. But let's be sensible: if you let them smoke and drink and play with knives 50% of the time, you run the risk of things not quite turning out okay, even if you meet their every need the rest of the time.

That 50% figure comes from a study conducted with low-income mothers in Washington during their baby's first year. Researchers examined mothers' reactions to their baby's crying and not crying, i.e. whether they could understand what the baby needed, responded calmly and appropriately (i.e. not overly roughly) and were able to soothe their baby if they were crying. They then measured whether their baby displayed positive attachment behaviours. They found that as long as 50% or more of the mothers' reactions were supporting her baby's needs, then her baby was more likely to show a secure attachment to her – something which we know helps children feel more confident in later life. The researchers concluded that responsive reactions help a baby learn that their needs will be met and they can trust you... but that doesn't need to happen every single time. You get to have bad days, or days when everyone is pulling you in different directions, or days when you just don't know what's wrong, and that's okay.[3]

It's also worth pointing out just how much has changed over the last few decades in terms of how engaged we are with our babies and children. We've never been more engaged... or worried about how engaged we are. A survey in the *Economist* found that across 10 countries, we all spend far more time interacting with our children now compared to 1965 (apart from France). The UK showed one of the steepest rises, alongside Italy and Denmark, with mothers now spending around 155 minutes per day with their children compared to just 35 minutes in 1965. For fathers this has risen from barely anything in 1965 to around 110 minutes per day.[4]

We have also become far more risk averse – things that would have been acceptable in the 1960s, 1970s, and 1980s are now viewed with horror. Some are welcome changes – seatbelts for example – but we also feel a lot more anxiety that we must be watching and engaging with our children every moment of the day. We worry far more than previous generations that we have to stimulate and educate even very young babies and that we are wholly responsible for their development and wellbeing.[5]

The sociologist Sharon Hays wrote about this back in the 1990s, particularly about the pressures on women to *'expend a tremendous amount of time, energy and money in raising their children'*, in a way that simply isn't expected of men. Although it is very much recognised that engagement and care during the early years play an important role in helping children develop the confidence and security that will serve them well in adult life, there is increasing pressure to ensure that this engagement is perfect all the time - as if stimulating activities and never letting them cry will guarantee that your baby will be successful and happy throughout life (or doomed if you don't do it). And that's just not true.[6]

" We've never been more engaged... or worried about how engaged we are. "

I still feel really guilty and ashamed that I'm not good enough

Despite all of this, you may still have niggling doubts. First, be reassured by how common this is. But if you are really struggling it is worth seeking support - perhaps from good friends who'll no doubt tell you they also feel that way. I've never come across a single parent who says they always feel like a good parent. In fact, some of the best parents I know, in terms of how they respond to their babies, are those most likely to say they are plagued by these thoughts. You are enough. In fact, I'd say that if you are worried about being a good parent, then that pretty much makes you a good parent.

You might also like to talk to your health visitor, or even, if this is really taking a toll on you, seek some counselling support. This is absolutely a topic you can take to a counsellor or psychologist. Look for one who specialises in supporting new parents through the transition to parenthood.

It's not so much guilt... I just feel pressure to be *perfect* all the time

Maybe you don't feel guilty or ashamed that you're not doing well enough, because you always try to make sure you do things perfectly. Perfectionism - the tendency to hold yourself or others to impossibly high standards - is common, and especially so when it comes to parenting as you have a constant barrage of voices in the media, maybe from your own family and your own internal voice telling you that *you need to do better*.

As you probably know, trying to live up to your own high standards (or those you perceive others have of you) is not the route to a calm existence... instead it's

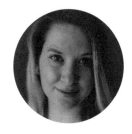

An interview with Dr Marianne Trent

Marianne is a clinical psychologist with Good Thinking Psychological Services and also the creator of the 'Our Tricky Brain' kit. She has experience of working with many families during the perinatal period and finds feelings of guilt and shame around parenting are surprisingly common. You can find her at www.GoodThinkingPsychology.co.uk.

How common are feelings of guilt and shame in the new parents you work with?

In my role as a clinical psychologist it's a rare day when I'm working with parents and guilt and shame aren't mentioned, even if that's not the reason they have come to see me. In my work now I only tend to see parents when things get to clinically significant levels of concern, but it would certainly be great to get the word out there that guilt and shame are completely normal human reactions and that they are not going to suddenly stop showing up just because we become parents.

What are some of the most common things they feel guilt or shame about?

Honestly and unfortunately, it may be easier to compile a list of things parents don't feel guilt or shame about! Finding labour/birth problematic, not finding labour/birth problematic compared to others, gender disappointment, bonding not being as hoped for, wanting a sibling, not wanting siblings, wanting to breastfeed, not wanting to breastfeed, being able to breastfeed, not being able to breastfeed, being able to have your own children, not being able to have genetically related children, wanting to see extended family, not wanting to see extended family, feeding taking too long, feeding not taking long enough, baby sleeping too long, baby not sleeping long enough, finding their baby boring compared to an older child, finding their baby boring compared to their old life, wondering whether they are cut out to be parents or even should have had a child at all – the list goes on! When I tend to see families in clinic it can be about people taking and inferring meaning from intrusive thoughts such as dropping or harming their baby and/or not feeling a rush of connection for their baby or babies.

Where do these feelings often come from?

The short answer is that they come from our incredibly complex, but normal, tricky human brains! Here's the long answer to explain the short one though. Our brains have gone through changes to make us top of the food chain; first our brains were reptilian, then mammalian and then human. It means we have a whole host of uniquely human states, traits and thoughts, but these brilliant brains of ours are not all sunshine and roses.Let me explain. Imagine a group of zebras. Suddenly a lion appears and the zebras scatter. The slowest zebra somehow manages to get away and is not harmed. Following the escape, and once it has caught its breath, that zebra goes back to doing whatever it was doing before it laid eyes on the lion. That might be feeding its baby or grazing or having a drink... normal zebra things. It wouldn't think about lions again until it next encountered one.

However, when humans encounter danger and risk our brains operate in an entirely different way. The initial fight or flight bit is the same, but everything which comes after is different. We'd be retelling tales of the lion and likely crying and shaking and off our food for quite some time. Sleep might well be problematic and our intrusive thoughts of lions and our hypervigilance for growling sounds or footsteps and lion smells would be off the scale. Hours, days, and likely weeks and years later we would likely be recalling snippets of our close shave with the lion.

Danger is everywhere for a human with such fantastic brain capacity. We have the ability to activate our threat systems by just thinking about or watching scary stuff, and our bodies respond accordingly by increasing our heart rate and getting us ready to react to save our skins. The old, reptilian parts of our brain which control our fight and flight responses don't get the memo that there is no active threat and we are just triggering ourselves with memories, ideas or intrusive thoughts.

A biggie for parents is that we overemphasise the importance of the completely normal intrusive thoughts we have, like throwing our baby out of the window. As humans we have hundreds of non-intended intrusive thoughts per day. We are natural scientists and our brains have the ability to wonder and imagine what might happen in a host of scenarios. It's part of being human and we must try not to judge ourselves for it. Our brains are naturally going to offer intrusive thoughts to us along the line of dropping or throwing our baby down the stairs, crashing the car with them in it, finding them unresponsive in their cot... the possibilities are limitless and often grisly.

They are grisly thoughts because as humans we have the power to imagine awful things. We need to remember that this is the way our brains have wired us up to be; zebras do not have this capacity. It does not mean that we have plans to do the things we have imagined, nor that we want to do them. Things become more problematic for us as humans when we begin to believe that because our brains have conjured up these macabre ideas we must want to follow them through. In the vast majority of cases that's just not true: there is most certainly a difference between thinking about something out of the blue and actually doing it.

Another part of being human is the power of social threat. We can get ourselves in quite a state wondering what others would say or think about us. A zebra with its purely mammalian brain doesn't care that its baby has been eating the same type of grass for days or done a runny poo or that it's wearing the same outfit as all the other babies.

Our wonderful human brains also have the ability to read, plan and hope. Therefore, we can come to this parenting game with ideas about being a gold medallist at x, y, z, and yet that's not the same expectation we would place upon ourselves on day 1 in a pole vault class. However, there's less social threat involved in pole vaulting, we probably don't know many pole vaulters and people don't talk much about it or post pictures on their social media of them nailing pole vaulting! If we met a friend, family member or stranger and told them we had just had our first pole vault class they would likely listen in rapture and just be keen to soak up our experience. However, if we meet that same person in the street and tell them we have just become a parent then it's far more likely that advice and comment will start to be offered and our human brains, especially in their sleep-deprived state, can interpret this as criticism or a suggestion that we are not doing it right. Even if we don't at the time it might come back to us later in the form of intrusive thoughts and memories. Honestly, it's a minefield. Pole vaulting or grazing sound appealing in comparison.

How do you support parents to work through these emotions?

I would do exactly as we have described above and normalise the experience and explain the way that our human brains work and why. In no other relationship in our lives do we place as much pressure upon ourselves as we do with our newborns. Once parents start talking and being honest about their thoughts and feelings and feel validated and heard it can be like a pressure valve has been released. The early days and weeks of parenting can leave a couple wondering what on earth has happened to their previously very satisfying relationship and often to worry that this is their life now for the next 18–25 years! The process of bringing a baby into a relationship was described very well by an actor in the 2020 BBC programme, *Taboo*: '*Think of it as like adding a baby to a marriage. All was ordered and now there is this thing that demands attention, stops you sleeping, belches, farts, screams...*

and she's going to make this whole process louder and wilder, more insane, more impractical!'

This chap was actually describing making gunpowder, but I think anyone who has scraped baby poo off shoulder blades would surely agree a baby is no less explosive. When parents are feeling stuck or being dragged back to previous times it can be a sign that there is some trauma in need of processing. Once we have processed those traumas with the appropriate talking therapy we will hopefully have freed parents up to live in the moment, they then have flexibility and an ability to breathe and focus on the here and now without judgement or excessive self-criticism.

Sometimes processing traumas can be as simple as discussing what their hopes, dreams and fears would have been, and helping them compare and contrast to what they actually got. It's important to de-shame and de-guilt and that's why the explanation of human brains can be so powerful. We are only experiencing this variety of complex feelings and events because we are human, and being human is most definitely not our fault. It can be incredibly beneficial for parents to know that health professionals are hard to shock and just want to help support you to optimally parent your children, however that looks for you and your family.

What would you say to any parent feeling guilty that they're not a good enough parent, or shouldn't have certain thoughts?
I would say that they need to be more compassionate to themselves. Parenting is a never-ending job which we can enter into without so much as a job interview or reference check. Expecting ourselves to willingly and enthusiastically parent for the rest of our lives is unrealistic. A lot of the time, especially in the early days, parenting can feel like a pretty ungratifying job. It's normal and understandable to find it tough and want some peace and quiet and time for yourself. Expecting every moment of parenting to feel like a blessing for which we ought to be grateful is like publicly declaring that from now until the end of time we are going to make all meals from scratch, using the finest, freshest most nutritious ingredients and taking the utmost care. We all know that sooner or later, despite our best intentions, we are going to be out of time, patience or ingredients and just fancy chicken Super Noodles!

I've now made you imagine Super Noodles. It doesn't really matter whether or not you like Super Noodles, but now you are thinking about them all the same. Maybe you can even imagine what they smell like and would feel like in your mouth? Intrusive thoughts are just the same as this. Suddenly you have these thoughts in your mind and can even imagine yourself doing these things you didn't invite into your head, but it doesn't mean you actually want to do them. You are a human and as such you are in no way any more responsible for your intrusive thoughts than you are for your very recent exposure to the words 'chicken, 'super' and 'noodles'.

Parenting is the toughest job any of us will ever do and we need to allow ourselves to grow into it, to get to know our little person and get to know ourselves as parents too. Think of your very best friend or the person, other than your child, that you most like to spend time with. Imagine how they make you feel and how nice and fun it is to spend time with them and what adventures you've had together. Yet sometimes you have a desire to sit in silence and be by yourself and do your own thing without this perfect person. To want and need to do this is entirely normal and entirely human. This urge to be you, with your entirely normal selection of urges, impulses and desires won't suddenly stop showing up just because you've become a parent.

Be kind to yourself, be careful who you take advice from and be careful who you take criticism from too. 'Don't accept criticism from someone you wouldn't ask for advice' can be a useful mantra to adopt.

pretty damn exhausting. But when it comes to parenting, the need to be perfect is yet another emotion you can just chuck in the bin right now.

Great, I hear you say. But how? And indeed, the special trick of perfectionism is to give you the fear that everything will go wrong and everyone will hate you and you're a total failure if you don't perpetually overachieve. The twist is that as a perfectionist you will never achieve enough to feel like you have achieved, because as soon as you do achieve something amazing, you spend approximately three seconds feeling pleased with yourself before setting yourself the next goal to strive towards... and the next... and the next. You will never get to a place where you are happy enough. Sorry, do you feel personally attacked right now?

Seriously, this is why many people high in perfectionist traits are also prone to score highly on tests of anxiety, depression and low self-esteem, with a favourite pastime of dwelling on their perceived failures. So the only way out of perfectionism is to try and break up with it. More on this in a bit, but I'll just repeat again – you do not need to be perfect to be a good parent.[7]

Am I a perfectionist?

If you're reading this rather than skipping forward you've probably already got an inkling that you might have some perfectionist traits that niggle away in your mind. Broadly speaking, there are three types of perfectionism:

When you hold *yourself* to perfectionist standards, including things like:
- Feeling upset when criticised
- Obsessing about small details
- Feeling you can't meet others' expectations
- Finding it difficult to make decisions
- Feeling devastated when you have made a mistake
- Worrying about stuff a lot
- Avoiding trying things you might not be good at
- Feeling awful if you miss a deadline or let people down

When you hold *others* to perfectionist standards
- Being critical of others
- Being accused of being controlling
- Being told you are judgemental
- Getting irritated when others don't do things right
- Finding it difficult to trust people or delegate tasks
- Getting upset when other people don't meet your standards
- Hating being interrupted

When you feel pressure to conform to society's standards
- Worrying what others think of you
- Finding it difficult to say no
- Feeling guilty if you take time for yourself
- Not complaining about things out of fear
- Feeling anxious if other people feel badly about you
- Nervousness when meeting new people
- Thinking people will look down on you if you're not perfect

Recognise yourself?

One problem with perfectionist thinking is you might find yourself being an 'all or nothing thinker'. Either you succeed or you fail – to you there are no shades of grey when it comes to success. Obviously, this doesn't work particularly well with caring for a baby – no one gets it spot on all of the time – and it also doesn't fit well with the good enough parenting idea of cutting yourself some slack occasionally. And it can be particularly tricky because how on earth do you measure whether you have been successful or not when it comes to your baby? Speed of nappy changes? Number of naps? Angle of first smile? There is a potentially endless list of things you could choose to measure success... or use to condemn yourself as a failure.

Perfectionism in relation to parenting has been measured in the handy Multi-dimensional Parenting Perfection Questionnaire (which you can find online at **www.ravansanji.ir/?9305230852**). It covers things like:

- Needing to parent perfectly to feel like a good enough parent
- Setting yourself overly high standards
- Feeling like you must always be 'successful' as a parent
- Feeling pressure from your partner to be a perfect parent
- Feeling that you need to be a perfect parent to be seen as a decent human
- Pressurising yourself to be as perfect as possible
- Judging your partner by how perfect a parent you deem them to be
- Placing a lot of value on being a very organised parent
- Feeling like a failure for a tiny parenting slip-up

Parenting perfectionism is split into the same types as mentioned previously, i.e. holding yourself to account, thinking society is holding you to account, or holding others to account. Research has shown that the type where you worry about doing everything perfectly because society will judge you as a parent and a person is particularly associated with feeling like a failure and not a good enough parent and having high anxiety levels.[8] Most of the research in this area has been done with women and new mothers, but it would equally apply to any men feeling this way.

The issue is that no parent is perfect, yet the media devote vast amounts of column inches to suggesting that this is possible. Social media is particularly bad for this, with posts that encourage the belief in perfect parenting – mothering in particular. We all know how many followers the *'perfect'* mummy bloggers have on Instagram with their *'perfect'* figures, *'perfect'* life and *'perfect'* babies. And research has shown that the more time we spend looking at these women, the more we feel under pressure to have that ourselves (even if we know it's all set up for the camera) and end up feeling like failures.[9]

Research has shown that the more time new mothers spend looking at idealised images of motherhood on Facebook, the more they post idealised images themselves in order to try and get confirmation from others that they are a perfect parent. You know the type of post... photo of baby engaged in artwork or something followed by numerous *'you're such a good mum, hun'* comments. When in fact the artwork session most likely ended in tears and the house covered in glitter.[10]

We all go along with this, creating a false impression of motherhood on social media by either just posting the best bits or even just making stuff up. But it seems that even when we know we are posting lies, or at least glossed-over versions of the truth, we still get validation from people's reactions.[11] We know social media is terrible for making us compare ourselves to others and ending up feeling awful and lacking because of it.

Research has also shown that this relationship is increased among mothers with higher levels of society-focused perfectionism. The more mothers worried about how society judged them, the more their use of Facebook increased their symptoms of anxiety and depression. The researchers traced this back to being down to increased comparison of the mothers to others they saw on Facebook.[12]

Tackling perfectionism as a parent

There are a number of ways you can try and help yourself heal from perfectionism. I won't lie, it can be tough and if you are struggling it might be an idea to explore these issues with a counsellor. But here are some quick ideas for how you could work towards reducing the pressure you put on yourself.

- Try an experiment of not being totally perfect and look at your baby at the end of the day. Are they still okay? Still happy? Of course they are.
- Try saying no to new added pressures, or stop doing some of the time-consuming things. Make a list of how much time you spent on these things. Was it worth it? Or do you prefer the break?
- Try and think about why you feel this way. Who told you that you weren't good enough? Who are you trying to prove things to? Or who told you that you were only good enough if you were overachieving? Understanding why

we are this way helps us stop and think.

- Cut yourself some slack. Think about this from your baby's perspective. What do they really value? Cuddles? Warmth? Love? Make those your sense of achievement. If they're covered, then you're doing a great job.
- Pretend you are your friend. Do you judge them as not good enough? Or think of a parent you admire - are they really running themselves ragged each day?
- Some psychologists suggest personifying your perfectionism. Make it a funny or pitiful character. Now when you find yourself thinking perfectionist thoughts, imagine it in a squeaky or daft voice. Surely you can't take orders from that?
- Take very small steps to change - try being 'good enough' a little bit at a time.
- Try activities that help you relax. Research has shown that things like meditation and yoga can actually lead to drops in perfectionist thoughts. This is a good trick if you are feeling overwhelmed by such thoughts.[13]
- *The Good Mother Myth* edited by Avital Norman Nathman is a reassuring read.

Chapter fifteen

Spotting the signs of postnatal depression

→ The previous chapters have covered difficult emotions that many parents have. But what about when things become more serious and have more of an impact on your life? How do you spot those signs and how do you get help?

One of the most common mental health challenges new parents face is the experience of postnatal depression. Feeling depressed in the year after having a baby is more common that you might think. Estimates are that 15-20 per cent of women and men have symptoms of depression in the months after birth.[1] However, research has shown that lots of people hide their symptoms of depression. They worry they will be judged as a bad parent or have their baby taken away. Some will worry they don't 'deserve' to feel depressed or feel they shouldn't admit to it as the other parent has it worse. This really isn't true - as discussed earlier, how you feel is how you feel and you deserve support for that. Please open up and tell someone that you trust and take it from there. Whether that's a health visitor or GP, a confidential listening service such as the Samaritans or Mind, or a friend or colleague, just take that first step and talk.

When we think about depression, we might think about the stereotype of someone being very miserable or morose. Depression is not just about feeling 'sad'. If you are feeling depressed you may be low and tearful, but depression can also show itself in signs of anxiety, sleeping and eating too much or too little, or feeling completely overwhelmed. If you're feeling depressed, you'll probably experience these symptoms most days and for at least a couple of weeks or so. They might be better in the day and worse at night (or vice versa). Some days you might feel better than others. It's about looking at the bigger pattern.

A common tool for exploring feelings of postnatal depression is a questionnaire known as the Edinburgh Postnatal Depression scale. This explores how often you are experiencing a number of different thoughts and feelings and adds this up to give an indication of whether you might need more support. It is not considered to be 'diagnostic' in that it doesn't tell you whether you have depression or not, just that you might be experiencing feelings that resemble depression. Although there is a cut-off score that suggests depression, many practitioners dislike that idea as it suggests that just one more frequent occurrence of one feeling could determine whether someone was depressed or not.

You can have a look at the scale online and use it to start a conversation with your health professional **www.fresno.ucsf.edu/pediatrics/downloads/ edinburghscale.pdf**. It explores things such as how often you have felt low or tearful, your sleep and eating, feelings of anxiety and overwhelm and whether you have ever considered harming yourself. However, if you are experiencing any worries at all about your mental health you don't need a scale to validate that for you – don't be afraid to reach out to your health visitor or GP. Note that this scale can be used by women or men – it's relevant to all parents.[2]

It's normal to sometimes feel some of the symptoms of depression. When a health professional uses the questions, they ask how frequently you have been feeling them. There are different response options for each question, but they basically go from 'never' to 'all the time'. For example, feeling sad or miserable is a very normal emotion to feel some of the time or in relation to specific events. But if you're feeling it all the time, particularly if nothing major has happened in your life that sadness would be a normal reaction to, then it can be a sign that there is a problem.

Sometimes professionals will use other scales. I really like what is known as the Whooley questions. These are two simple questions which have been shown to be a good predictor of depression:

- During the past month, have you often been bothered by feeling down, depressed or hopeless?
- During the past month, have you often been bothered by having little interest or pleasure in doing things?

Again, it's about how you feel more generally. There is no cut-off that says you have to experience something every hour to be depressed and need support.

Occasionally women can experience a more intense mental health issue know as puerperal psychosis. It is rare but serious. If you are aware of yourself, your partner or any new parent experiencing symptoms such as hallucinations, delusions, extreme mood swings, losing all inhibitions or behaving in a way that is very confused or out of character, get medical support immediately. This may include an emergency GP appointment or ringing 111 for further advice.

I love my baby, so why am I feeling depressed?

There is a stereotype that suggests that if you're feeling down and miserable after birth you must regret having your baby. This is absolute nonsense and fortunately an idea that few people would now hold. It is, however, something that many new parents beat themselves up over, thinking they must be ungrateful, or something is wrong with them. With kindness, never ever think that. Depression is not something you 'choose' to have happen to you. It can strike out of the blue, or be related to stuff going on in your life that is in no way linked to your feelings for your baby.

So why does depression happen to so many new parents? It's usually a combination of things. Physical exhaustion and depletion after a long pregnancy, birth and sleepless nights. The relentlessness of caring for a small baby and not being able to care for yourself. If you are having any difficulties in your home, work or social life these can be exacerbated by the stress of caring for a small person. Relationship difficulties can flare, money worries appear for the first time or become more of an issue or you may feel more uncomfortable living in not such a nice area now you have a baby to care for. You may feel vulnerable in your job or miss the connection you had with colleagues and your role every day. Is it any wonder you feel depressed and overwhelmed?

Depression is also much more common if you are lacking a good support circle around you. Going back to the idea that many new parents feel isolated and alone, it's not surprising that we have much higher rates of depression than countries where new parents are cared for and supported to rest and recuperate. Personally, I think many cases of postnatal depression are simply a reaction to how we expect many new parents to live.[3]

The experience of becoming a new parent can also throw up all sorts of emotions from your past. Having a baby and becoming a parent may make you reflect on your own childhood or relationship with your parents. For some people this might be a positive thing. You might have really great memories and see how much your parents did for you in a new light. Or it might be the opposite and bring back difficult memories, or you might question why your parents treated you in a certain way. If you've lost a parent, especially recently, this might bring up a whole load of memories and emotions around your relationship and them no longer being here.

There is increasing research into the impact of difficult or traumatic experiences during childhood and the impact that these can have upon our physical and mental health in later years.[4] Known as 'Adverse Childhood Experiences' (ACEs), research has shown that if you experience more than a few significant predictors of trauma during your childhood you are much more likely to experience mental health difficulties and chronic illnesses in adulthood. These experiences include:

- Experiencing emotional abuse such as being sworn at, insulted or humiliated regularly by an adult in your household.
- Experiencing physical violence from an adult in your household.
- Being sexually abused.
- Feeling that no one in your family loved or cared for you.
- Not having clean clothes, enough to eat or feeling your parents couldn't care for you.
- Divorce or separation.
- Domestic violence occurring in your home.
- Having a parent who was an alcoholic.
- Having a parent who was depressed.
- Having a parent who went to prison.

Having one of those experiences is not uncommon; only around a third of people experience none. Around 26% of people experience one, 16% two, 10% three and 13% four or more. But the more you experience, the greater your likelihood of experiencing mental health difficulties, physical illnesses such as heart disease or adopting addictive behaviours as an adult. Among women, around 17% of those with no ACEs will go on to develop depression at some point in their life – a level much lower than the population average. But among those with more the rates get much higher: 22% for one ACE, 33% for two ACEs, 41% for three ACEs and 59% for four ACEs or more. Levels are a little lower in men but still follow the same pattern.[5]

Why? Researchers think that it is because the stress of experiencing these events in childhood, which is often long term or continual with bursts of intense stress, actually changes the way the brain develops, making you more prone to depression. Also, if you spend a lot of your childhood scared or worried about things this can affect how you behave. You might find it difficult to trust or make friends, you may find your confidence takes a knock, or you spend a lot of time feeling ashamed. This can impact upon your education and how your life turns out.

Adverse early experiences and stress can also explain a lot of addictive behaviours. Addiction is often about using substances to ease pain, distract you or comfort you. Obvious options are alcohol, smoking or drug use, but people can also use food and overeating as an emotional crutch. Others might

> **"For many women, their first or strongest experience of depression comes after having a baby."**

use very restrictive diets as a way of trying to regain control. It might seem counterintuitive at first, but overworking and overachievement is also often a sign of childhood trauma – work serves as a distraction or an attempt to feel accomplished and confident (it rarely works).

Newer research into the causes of depression also suggests that it is a stress-related inflammatory disease. Stress, whether that is physical or emotional, increases inflammation in the body. When you are stressed your immune system starts working overtime. A side effect of this is inflammation. This is why when you experience a lot of stress you may also have aching muscles, joint pain, or headaches. The risk of developing autoimmune disease is also linked to chronic stress and inflammation. Our bodies were never meant to deal with stress long term. Our stress response is all about flooding the body with a response to deal with a short-term stressor such as an animal attacking us, so any adverse effects of that stress response were worth it because they weren't long-lasting and were much better than being eaten. Now our stress is more chronic and long term and our bodies suffer from it.[6]

If you had a stressful childhood, you may carry stress in your body. You may always have felt on edge at home, and over time your body adapted, thinking that you always needed to be stressed just in case. As an adult you might find yourself feeling very tense, maybe startling or jumping easily if you hear a loud noise, or feeling very stressed by shouting or tension. But this stress also appears to increase your risk of depression, through the increased levels of inflammation that go alongside chronic stress. Research is showing just how intertwined these reactions are: antidepressants not only reduce the experience of depression, but can also reduce chronic pain and even the risk of someone developing an autoimmune disorder. Therefore seeing depression as a stress-related disorder and treating the stress rather than thinking it is depression can have really good results.

For many women, their first or strongest experience of depression comes after having a baby. ACEs predict an increased risk of depression during pregnancy and after birth. If you think about the relationship between ACEs and health described above, you can see why. Inflammation often increases after birth because you are likely to be sleep-deprived, may be in some pain and feeling stressed or overwhelmed. On top of existing tension and stress, this can push you over the edge, increasing the inflammation in your body to levels that lead to depressive symptoms.[7]

You can read more about the research into ACEs, calculate your own ACE score and learn about how you can develop resilience against these previous experiences here: **www.acestoohigh.com**.

Getting help

The first step is to speak to someone and start a conversation. Ideally, speak to your health visitor or GP who can explore your feelings more deeply and decide with you what the next steps could be. These might include:

1. Medication

You might be prescribed antidepressants. Whether you are or not depends on how you are feeling, whether your GP thinks they will benefit you, and whether you want to take them. The evidence about whether antidepressants work to improve depressive symptoms is mixed. This is because they affect people in different ways. Sometimes just doing something and taking them might help you feel a little better, which helps you take other steps to feel even better. Most people who take them say they are not immediate happy pills, but give them a small boost that enables them to do other stuff to improve things. Some people might experience a more significant boost.

Antidepressants will take a little while to work because they don't just give you more 'happy hormones', but work on the receptors in your brain to keep better levels circulating. Some people feel much better on them, but unfortunately others do not. Some people have side effects which make them feel that it's not worth it, like weight gain, not being able to sleep or sometimes erectile dysfunction in men – but many people are fine or feel these side effects are better than the depression. Some people don't like how they make them feel, reporting that although they no longer feel sad, they don't really feel anything.[8]

You might decide that you will try antidepressants and see what happens. It's not a case of having to take them forever if you try them – you're allowed to stop if you don't like the side effects or don't feel they are working (although do talk to your GP and cut down gradually). You might also be able to try a different type that might suit you better. Don't worry that you'll be stuck taking them forever. They are not addictive and most people can wean themselves gently off once feeling better.

There are antidepressants that are safe for breastfeeding. There is no need to stop breastfeeding to take them. A lot of research now shows that being able to continue breastfeeding if you want to do so can be really helpful for your mental health. Alongside the psychological benefits of being able to continue doing something that is important to you, breastfeeding can also help protect you physically. Women who breastfeed have lower levels of inflammation; the hormones of breastfeeding appear to dampen down your immune response to stress, decreasing the risk of depression.[9] The Breastfeeding Network has a factsheet about research into the safety of antidepressants here: **www. breastfeedingnetwork.org.uk/antidepressants**.

2. Talking therapy and counselling

There are a number of different options for supporting you to talk more about how you are feeling. Different therapies work in different ways. Some may explore with you why you are feeling how you feel – is there something in your current set-up or past that might be making you feel low now? Some might focus on your relationships with others and how that might be affecting how you think. Others might focus on ways to change your thought processes, such as trying to stop negative thoughts and replace them with more positive ones. Sometimes just listening can be enough. Different people are comfortable with different approaches, and different therapeutic approaches lend themselves better to different experiences. A good counsellor will work through this with you and work out what approach might be right for you.

You can ask your GP to refer you for counselling. There is often a long waiting list but it's worth getting yourself on it. They may be able to refer you to group counselling or support in the meantime. You don't have to take this offer up – some people might really benefit from such a group, while others would feel worse. It really is up to you. Research is also showing promising results from interventions that you work on yourself at home through the internet.[10]

You might also like to pay someone privately. This can be an expensive option but one that has very positive results. Make sure you check their qualifications before agreeing to any payment. A good counsellor will also let you have a first session before booking any more to make sure you are a good fit. Different people will take different approaches and it's important to find one you feel comfortable with. The British Association for Counselling and Psychotherapy has a search tool where you can find local counsellors in your area. They check qualifications and hold counsellors to high professional standards so you have peace of mind **www.bacp.co.uk/search/Therapists**.

If your feelings are in relation to being a new parent, it's a good idea to search for a practitioner who specialises in mental health during pregnancy, birth and the postnatal period. This will ensure that your practitioner specifically understands the challenges of being a new parent, what can trigger difficulties and how to best support you.

Another option is to work with a doula. Some postnatal doulas might have qualifications in counselling or particular skills, but all will be trained in postnatal support and talking openly about experiences. You might work with one to talk through how you feel and think about the next steps. Again check out Doula UK **doula.org.uk** or Abuela Doulas **abueladoulas.co.uk** to find one close to you.

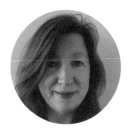

The Parenthood in Mind practice

Julianne Boutaleb is a consultant perinatal psychologist who has worked for over 18 years in the NHS and private practice. She set up the Parenthood In Mind practice in January 2018.

We are a team of 16 practitioners, all of whom are specialised in working therapeutically with parents and parents-to-be and their bumps and babies up to one year post-birth. We offer a range of therapeutic approaches to individuals, couples and families across London, and are all accredited psychologists and psychotherapists.

The journey to becoming parents is not always easy, and some individuals and couples may face unforeseen challenges. For example, while the announcement of a pregnancy or birth may be a joyous event, it also involves huge shifts in identity in the parent-to-be and in the couple relationship. Then once your baby arrives, you may find yourself struggling with the exhausting reality of sleepless nights, the demands of breastfeeding, and getting to know your baby. Lots of parents find that talking through these normal emotions, or more challenging experiences, with a specialist can be really helpful.

Based on this we offer therapeutic support to individuals, couples and parents and infants presenting with a range of issues including: perinatal depression and anxiety, birth trauma and tokophobia, fertility issues, OCD and PTSD, pregnancy loss and miscarriage and other psychological issues as they arise in the perinatal period. We also offer specialist consultation, supervision and training on perinatal mental health issues to individuals, teams and organisations.

Please see the Parenthood in Mind website for more information **www.parenthoodinmind.co.uk** or for more information contact Julianne on **jboutaleb@ parenthoodinmind.co.uk**.

There are also a number of charities that offer support and information. These include:

- Association for Postnatal Illness (APNI) helpline on 020 7386 0868 (10am to 2pm, Monday to Friday) or email info@apni.org or look on apni.org.
- Pre and Postnatal Depression Advice and Support (PANDAS) helpline on 0843 28 98 401 (9am to 8pm, Monday to Sunday) or look on www.pandasfoundation.org.uk.
- Mind the mental health charity – infoline on 0300 123 3393 (9am to 6pm, Monday to Friday) or email info@mind.org.uk or look on www.mind.org.uk.

Some people might find it difficult to start a conversation about mental health with friends, medical professionals or supporters. You aren't alone and ironically your depression can make this harder. Knowing this, Mind have launched a campaign called 'Find the Words' to help people through this. More info here on opening up: www.mind.org.uk/information-support/guides-to-support-and-services/seeking-help-for-a-mental-health-problem/talking-to-your-gp.

Finally, it can help to read about others' experiences of postnatal depression (or depression in general) and how they recovered, or books that help you think and work through your feelings. Some really good ones include:

- *Down Came the Rain* – Brooke Shields
- *Reasons to Stay Alive* – Matt Haig
- *Jog On: How Running Saved My Life* – Bella Mackie
- *Eyes Without Sparkle* – Elaine Hanzak
- *This Isn't What I Expected* – Karen Kleiman
- *Surviving Postnatal Depression* – Cara Aiken

Reading more widely about postnatal depression itself can also help you understand how you are feeling and why. Some good recommendations here are:

- *Why Postnatal Depression Matters* – Mia Scotland
- *Daddy Blues* – Mark Williams

3. Take the time to put yourself first

Research consistently shows that things that make you feel better do indeed make you feel better! Have a look back at Chapter 3 on self-care and putting yourself first. But here are some evidence-based things that can help reduce symptoms of postnatal depression. Not all of them worked for every participant in the research and not everything will work for you, but they are worth a try:

- **Exercise** – the impact of endorphins, strengthening your body and time to focus on you.[11]
- **Yoga** – the calm, the focus on the power of your body, the time to yourself all help relax and heal the body. Yoga can also reduce the impact of stored tension in your body, whether that is recent or carried from previous experiences.[12]
- **A balanced, nutritious diet** – there is some evidence that nutrient deficiencies can exacerbate depressive symptoms. These include zinc, magnesium, calcium, folate and riboflavin. These can all be boosted through a balanced diet or a high-quality multivitamin.[13]
- **Fish oils** (*possibly*) – the evidence for these is mixed but some studies suggest they can help improve depressive symptoms. Given fish oils can generally help with other things such as inflammation and are inexpensive, they might be worth a shot. Look for ones with EPA and DHA.[14]
- **Music or art therapy** – again, simply time to spend doing what you like, focusing on working through your emotions.[15]
- **Meditation** – calm and the chance to focus on yourself.[16]
- **Baby massage classes** – the connection with your baby, calmness of the classes, time out and meeting other new parents. It also increases oxytocin (the feel-good calming hormone) in you both and can help relax your baby, so a win-win all round.[17]

Those are the healthy and evidence-based options. I couldn't find anything on the benefits of being brought a decent gin and tonic in a sunny garden at 6pm each evening while you have an hour's peace and quiet to yourself, but I suspect if I could get funding for that trial it would work. It's about doing something you enjoy, that is calm and restoring and gives you some time to just be you without being talked to or touched.

In summary, feelings of depression are common, not your fault, and not indicative of how much you love and care for your baby. Open up, talk to someone and get the support you need. It will pass and you will feel better. You're not alone in this.

Chapter sixteen

Coping with anxiety and intrusive thoughts

When we think about postnatal mental health, we often immediately think of a depressed woman who is low and miserable. But as we have seen, not only is anxiety often a core feature of postnatal depression, but it is also a common diagnosis on its own among new parents. Being worried or anxious about your baby and being a new mother is normal. It's when these symptoms start to become more problematic that they need to be addressed. Maybe they affect your sleep or they don't go away if you sit and chat your worries through with someone. Maybe you have specific recurring or intrusive anxious thoughts that you don't want. Or maybe you might feel agitated, wired and on edge all the time without really having any specific thoughts. Be reassured you are not alone.

Some signs of postnatal anxiety include:

- Not being able to sleep at night, even though you are absolutely exhausted. Maybe you can't fall asleep or maybe you wake up at 2am panicking about things happening. Maybe you wake for the day at 4am.

- Worrying a lot about things happening to your baby. Every new mother worries about their baby, but if you are worrying about things that are unlikely to happen or have no indication of happening then you might have anxiety.
- Needing a lot of reassurance that you haven't done anything wrong and everything is okay. This works briefly, then the feelings of anxiety return.
- Feeling overwhelmed when you leave the house, particularly in crowded places such as shops or a café. Equally you might feel overwhelmed by being left alone.
- Feeling restless, perhaps pacing around and feeling that you can't settle – again, despite being absolutely exhausted.
- Having 'whirring' thoughts in your mind – the sort where you feel you can't stop thinking, or having multiple thoughts. Maybe your thoughts feel particularly noisy or relentless. One woman described it to me as a 'tape stuck on fast forward' (remember tapes?!).
- Feeling physical symptoms of anxiety such as trembling, a racing heart or sick to your stomach, but being unable to work out why you feel that way.
- Panicking about the future or having catastrophic thoughts such as feeling genuinely scared if your partner is 10 minutes late home (they must have been in an accident/left me for someone else/are being held hostage/have lost their job and are too scared to come home).
- Reacting very strongly to small things. I do not want to use the words 'over-react' because to someone with anxiety they are not an overreaction.

Getting support

Support for postnatal anxiety is similar to that described in the previous chapter on depression, so have a skim over that too. You might also find the books listed helpful, as there is such an overlap between experiences of depression and anxiety.

1. Medication

You and your GP might decide that anxiety medication might help you. There are a number of options including those you take regularly and those you can take in response to a panic attack. Some medications labelled as antidepressants can help reduce anxiety too. Some of these medications reduce the physical signs of anxiety but might not necessarily fix any thoughts. Talk to your GP about how you feel and what might work best. A number of treatments are listed on the NHS website **www.nhs.uk/conditions/generalised-anxiety-disorder/treatment**.

2. Talking therapy

Again, therapy can be great for feelings of anxiety, helping you work through what might be causing them, understanding why you might react like that and helping you develop different cognitive strategies for changing your thought patterns. Remember to seek out a qualified counsellor – the BACP website has a list www.bacp.co.uk. There are also some great resources online for helping you work through your anxiety. Anxiety UK has a number of resources, including some free to download, on its website www.anxietyuk.org.uk/product-category/free-resources. Very Well Mind also has a list of supportive online groups for people experiencing anxiety www.verywellmind.com/best-online-anxiety-support-groups-4692353.

3. Trying to calm your thoughts and physical symptoms

There are a number of techniques that can help you deal with symptoms of anxiety in the short term.

These include:

- Grounding. When you feel symptoms of anxiety look for things in the environment around you. Try and find five things that are blue. Or five things that are soft. Count them and say them out loud.
- Breathing exercises. Anything that stops you and focuses your breathing, making you breathe more deeply and evenly. There are lots of apps for this online.
- Telling yourself you are okay and safe. Sometimes we feel symptoms of anxiety and desperately try to label them. A common pattern is to feel the physical symptoms and for your brain to immediately start scrolling back through your day wondering what on earth you are anxious about. It digs and digs and digs until it finds something to blame, when actually they weren't connected at all. Your brain just wanted to think your anxiety was logical... but oh look, now you're worrying about something you weren't actually worried about. Sound familiar? One way of reducing this is reassuring yourself that everything is okay. It's just physical symptoms. Nothing is wrong.
- Deliberately do something to change your thoughts. This might include focusing on something physical such as colouring or a jigsaw or building something. It might be going for a walk to change the scenery.
- Try a meditation or mindfulness app. These apps help you pause, relax and reduce anxiety. Some of the best include Headspace, Calm and Breethe. Many are free so experiment with what works for you. You might find some relaxing sounds, colours or phrasing more useful than others.
- Exercise can be brilliant, especially forms that either calm you, such as yoga, or really help burn off excess energy and raise endorphins. It can feel

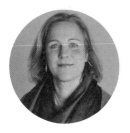

How mindfulness can help calm anxious thoughts

Sophie Fletcher is a perinatal hypnotherapist with over 15 years' experience of teaching and training people all over the word in hypnosis and mindfulness tools for birth and beyond. She is founder of Mindful Mamma, author of *Mindful Hypnobirthing* and *Mindful Mamma* www.mindfulmamma.co.uk for coping as a new parent.

Mindfulness is something that can really help you, as a new parent, to navigate day-to-day life while at the same time supporting your emotional and mental wellbeing. It's all about staying in the moment, accepting what is in the here and now. It can be tricky to do this when you are a new parent, there is so much to do! But this is exactly why it's so important. Mindfulness allows your mind to rest even in the moments when you are not resting. You can choose to be mindful in your day-to-day life – noticing small moments that may otherwise be missed or dismissed in the everyday chaos of parenting. Mindfulness is a kindness to yourself and your family, it reduces stress, and can switch on your soothing system – this will help you feel calmer and less anxious. It's really important that new parents learn that by taking this approach it is possible to support changes that are happening in body and mind at a hugely transitional time.

Little preparation is given to emotional wellbeing in the first days, weeks and months of parenting. It can feel far from relaxing if you haven't prepared and even if you have prepared! Yet we know from research that when you are more relaxed it can make feeding easier, and when you are calmer you are able to pick up on small unconscious cues from your baby, for example when they need sleep or when you are feeding them.

Importantly mindfulness allows you to rest your mind. You are essentially learning a new job – your brain is processing all these new skills, and you are learning and juggling a lot of information. This, coupled with baby's sleep patterns, will mean that you can feel exhausted. In my book *Mindful Mamma*, I talk about the difference between sleep and rest. While you may not be getting much sleep, you can learn how to create moments of rest so your mind isn't juggling so much. Small pauses, mindful moments, can give your mind an opportunity to let go and breathe. This can be simple things like a mindful walk with your baby or paying attention when you are feeding your baby. Some audio tracks can help you to feel rested in a short amount of time; there is evidence to show that we can sleep dynamically when listening to some types of relaxation tracks, getting the equivalent of three hours' rest in just 30 minutes.

Remember that mindfulness is also about your baby and can have an immensely powerful impact on how they respond to the world within them, and around them. When you learn ways to regulate your emotions and are able to adapt and respond to the emotional demands of parenting in a gentle way, your baby learns to mirror you. Being aware of your own emotions and feelings and being able to respond to them kindly will teach your baby to regulate their own emotions. That may take a few years, so be patient, but every single time you choose to breathe, meet your own difficult feelings and respond to them with loving kindness you are teaching your baby to do the same. This is a very powerful gift you can give your child.

If you are feeling frazzled and the opposite of calm, how do you get there quickly? I'll use crying as an example of when you can connect with your own feelings, so you can help soothe your baby.

First of all, if your instincts tell you that something isn't right or you are unsure, trust your instinct and ask for help. Your baby isn't crying because they don't love you or are rejecting you. Surely you have had moments in your life when you have felt the need to sob into a friend's arms: you may not have stopped sobbing, but you would have felt loved and supported by the friend hugging you. When your baby is crying and you are able to be calm, it will be helping them even if you think it's not making a difference.

I invite you to try this exercise:

The CALMER way is a simple process that helps you to respond to your baby's feelings and crying in a gentle loving way. Remember that they are learning how to be human; they are learning how to respond to the experiences they are having. When you respond in a calm way, you are showing them how they can learn to soothe themselves.

Check in with your feelings
Accept and name them
Let them be
Mindful deep breath in
Exhale
Relax

You can continue to breathe deeply: you may notice your shoulders, arms and body soften. Your thoughts may run off – 'Why won't they stop crying?' 'What do I need to do differently?' 'Am I getting it wrong?' If you feel your mind wander like this, name the feeling that sits beneath that thought; it may be fear or anger, then come back to your breath with the words, breathing in 'I relax', breathing out 'I let go'. Your baby will sense you are calm, that your body has softened, and this in itself is incredibly soothing.

This is just one example of many exercises in my book that are purposely designed for different situations you might experience as a new parent in the first year of your baby's life. It's a complete toolkit of practical techniques for the first year. My focus is on you, the parent, and my aim is to help guide you compassionately. You are so important; your needs are important. This isn't just self-care, it's an approach that nurtures and supports your incredible brain and your body as you transition into parenthood.

Mindfulness has been amazing for me as a parent and these words just scratch the surface of how it can be used in daily life to help find calm amid the chaos. You can find more tips, tools and support on Instagram **@sophief-letcher_author** or on my website **mindfulmamma.co.uk**. You can download the MP3s that accompany *Mindful Mamma* for free at **penguin.co.uk/mind-fulmamma**. I have also recorded a contribution on mindful parenting for the audiobook *The Here and Now, an anthology on mindfulness for life*.

like the last thing you want to do but try it – research shows that about 30 minutes of medium-intensity exercise will give you a boost in endorphins that will make you feel calmer, more energised and happier. www.wellandgood.com/endorphins-and-exercise

- As in the previous section on depression, take time to do stuff that helps you feel good and calms you down. Anything that lets you focus, feel happier, calmer or distracted from thoughts helps. Massages or reflexology or any therapy that focuses on you are an excellent idea (if you enjoy them).
- Focusing on self-care can help – more sleep, better food and chance to relax where possible. Although it won't work for everyone there is some evidence that increasing your levels of vitamin D, selenium and potassium might help. Any food that reduces inflammation is also beneficial, such as turmeric and fish oils.[1] Foods high in tryptophans can also calm your mood and boost your sleep, such as turkey, milk, cheese, eggs, fish, pumpkin seeds and chicken – which are all just basically healthy foods in moderation anyway.[2] Research has also shown that eating dark chocolate might help – surely worth a shot whatever the outcome?[3]
- Finally, two really good books to read include Sophie Fletcher's *Mindful Mamma* – perfect for anyone needing to slow down and relax their thoughts – and *Mind over Mother* by psychotherapist Anna Mathur.

A note on intrusive thoughts

Have you ever had a thought that seems to just pop into your mind that you can't control? One where your baby, you or someone you love is harmed or in great danger? Maybe the thought is about you harming your baby?

The good news is that these thoughts can be completely normal and that many mothers have them – it's just not the sort of thing you post on social media or bring up with your new baby group mums over that first coffee.

Intrusive thoughts can include things like

- Your baby being hurt in an accident by someone or something else.
- You accidentally hurting your baby.
- You deliberately hurting your baby.
- Something happening to you and you not being able to save your baby.
- Something happening to your partner or other loved one.

Just so you know that you are not alone, some of the most common images include imagining yourself shaking your baby, hitting your baby too hard during winding, throwing them on the ground or against the wall, puncturing the soft spot on their head, drowning them in the bath, smothering them or letting go of the pram at the top of a hill or into traffic.[4]

And they really are very common – a quick post on my own social media page brought lots of stories from women talking about how they had these kind of thoughts. Here are some examples – sound familiar?

The most unexpected thing for me was the feeling of the 'what ifs' and the anxiety. Sometimes I would have a 'What if I crashed the car?', 'What if I dropped the baby from the first floor window?', 'What if I have a brain injury and forget who my baby is?'. All these weird and quite scary thoughts that had about a 0.003846483% chance of actually happening. Jessie

On a practical note after having my baby I could never leave her out of my sight. I checked where the emergency exits were in every new place and I would not go into a lift (unless she was with me) in case I got trapped and couldn't get back to her. Deirdre

I had a food processor in the kitchen, when I was sitting breastfeeding I would get really vivid day dreams about my babies (twins) being all chopped up in there. It was like a recurring nightmare but otherwise I was totally fine, no depression/anxiety. Maybe due to sleep deprivation. (Looking back, why didn't I move the damn thing into a cupboard?) Jayne

I kept imagining driving the car into the ditch as well. I only learnt a long time later that it's completely normal, and possibly your way of dealing with the immense responsibility. Megan

I remember a friend saying 'I read this book that said to put baby in the cot if you feel like hurting them, but what sort of parent might hurt their baby?!' And I was nodding along thinking 'I must never tell her I contemplated dropping mine out a first-floor window last night...' Lucy

I used to get an overwhelming sense that I might throw him out of the window by mistake. I didn't want to (bloody hell, I really didn't want to), I wasn't depressed or especially anxious. I think it was because he was so tiny, weirdly. At no point did I ever come even close to actually doing it (god, the horror!), but I just had this overwhelming sense that I might do it by accident/mistake. It haunted my dreams when he was first home and eased as he got bigger. Jane

It's likely that these intrusive thoughts are a strange product of our brain trying to make sure we are vigilant and take care of our babies. We are programmed to be aware of dangers that are around us. This is good. But sometimes this system seems to go a bit wrong - probably not helped by our perpetual exhaustion. Your brain starts looking at things that are unlikely to harm you or happen and makes you think about them just in case. This is obviously distressing, but they are *just thoughts*. They are not a sign or premonition that you are about to throw your baby down the stairs or whatever your brain is choosing to depict today.[5]

In the vast majority of cases, parents who have these thoughts are highly unlikely to ever come close to actually acting them out. They are *not* a sign of being a 'bad parent': in fact it seems that some of the most engaged and caring parents are more likely to have these thoughts. The potential harm is to your mental health – women who have these thoughts often feel intensely guilty and anxious about them, worrying that it means that they are indeed a 'bad mother'.

The thoughts can be extremely scary – what if I actually do these things? In reality the fact that you are worried about the thoughts means that the risk of you ever carrying them out is very low. In the rare cases something does happen, research has shown that it's those with extreme mental health difficulties, who feel completely unaffected or even enjoy such thoughts, that are more likely to do something dangerous.

These thoughts can be really persistent. Sometimes they might be a one-off, but some women find they are plagued by them at regular periods during the day, or perhaps wake at 3am unable to stop thinking about them. It's not as simple as telling yourself that they're not true, or as some people's unhelpful advice suggests, just not thinking them. These types of thoughts generally feel out of your control.

It's also common to feel guilty about your intrusive thoughts, as if somehow you are responsible for them. You're not. It's your brain doing weird stuff from a mixed-up evolutionary perspective or because you're exhausted. Thoughts are just thoughts. They are not actions. Your baby will never know.

In terms of managing your thoughts, or more likely trying not to react if your brain pushes them into your mind, there are a number of things that might help you:

- Recognise that these thoughts are more common than you think. You're not alone, weird or unusual. Ask a friend – I bet they have them too.
- Keep reminding yourself that there is no link between the thoughts and carrying out the behaviour.
- Tell yourself it isn't you controlling the thoughts – it is your anxiety.
- Imagine someone else is telling you the thought – would it be scary or would you say 'that's crazy', reassure them and maybe see the funny side in some cases?
- Distract yourself. Use some of the anxiety techniques listed above to make yourself think about something different.

As always, if you find these thoughts are particularly strong, common or cause you a lot of distress rather than being momentarily problematic, do seek support from your GP or a counsellor. If you are having lots of them and they are frightening you, they can be a sign that you are struggling and may need greater support.

Further reading:
Because intrusive thoughts are common, there are some great resources written by others who have experienced them.

- 'Intrusive Thoughts: My Journey With Postpartum Depression' www.huffpost.com/entry/intrusive-thoughts-my-journey-with-postpartum-depression_b_58b86a04e4b0a8ded67b507b
- Check out the Postpartum Stress Center website – a brilliant resource for all sorts of emotions, particularly intrusive thoughts postpartumstress.com.
- Karen Kleiman has written two excellent books on the subject – *Good Moms Have Scary Thoughts* and *Dropping the Baby and Other Scary Thoughts*.

You are not alone with anxiety or intrusive thoughts. You are not a bad parent. Do seek support – there are people out there who can help.

Chapter seventeen

Postnatal anger and rage

→ Postnatal rage is the less-talked-about sibling of postnatal depression and anxiety, but once you start scratching the surface, it turns out it's a really common experience. If you're experiencing postnatal anger or rage you might spend a lot of your time on edge or irritable, or attacks of rage may feel like they come out of nowhere. Yes, the anger might be simmering away under the surface, but often it comes out over the smallest thing. Your partner saying they're exhausted. Shoes left in the middle of the hallway. A throw-away comment from your mother. RAGE.

Postnatal rage isn't very well understood. It's thought that the hormonal fluctuations women experience may trigger it and of course sleep deprivation can put us on edge. Really though, if you think about how isolated and overburdened a lot of new parents are, is it any wonder that this sometimes simmers over? You're not sleeping, shattered and suddenly your whole world revolves around this tiny creature who in between episodes of looking cute, screams at you and repays you with dirty nappies.

Postnatal anger is a weird one, because as with much of motherhood, some people will dismiss it, suggesting you have everything you wanted and should be happy 100% of the time. But the purpose of emotions is to signal to others

> **"The purpose of emotions is to signal to others how we are feeling and what we need."**

how we are feeling and what we need. Ever since humans have existed, our emotional reactions have been part of a communication system that helped us and others. We could express fear that would help warn others, or joy that would encourage others closer and to bond. Anger was a sign something was wrong and needed fixing – a hope that others will see this and help us fix it. But instead, we sometimes get told that we should be happy instead.

Sara's story

My second baby was born by emergency caesarean section at the end of a difficult pregnancy. Nothing had gone to plan this time even though last time things had been so straightforward. First, we thought we were going to lose him. Then I developed SPD and could barely walk and then gestational diabetes. Pregnancy was not enjoyable and I guess it was then I started to feel really angry at things. I had loved my first pregnancy but the second felt more like a psychological and physical endurance exercise. I was induced at the end because they said he would be too big and after several failed attempts and him going into distress I had to have a section with a load of people in the room panicking. Compare that to the lovely home birth I had last time and you can see how this didn't get off to the best start.

Once we were home I hoped everything would get better. I had spent a lot of time crying in hospital but figured it was the birth and being trapped on the postnatal ward for so long. I craved my bed and to see my daughter who had completely freaked out at me being away for so long. But it didn't get better, in fact it seemed to get worse. Despite me being so much more incapacitated this time (a section after having SPD is not fun) it was like everyone around me just thought I could get on with things. I'd done it all before after all.

It was the little things that got to me. I had stopped crying so much it seemed but instead was angry. Angry at my daughter for not listening. And angry at Gary my husband for not helping. And angry at my mother who had decided now was the time to go away with a friend. And angry at the never-ending stream of other visitors who just wanted to see the baby and didn't seem to care or think I was anything to do with him.

The angrier I got, the more people got irritated with me. Gary and I started bickering. And my daughter got more and more difficult in her behaviour, which of course was a completely normal reaction to her life being turned upside down and her usual attachment-parenting calm mother suddenly snapping and rolling her eyes at all times. But everything got to me. Every little thing like the way Gary breathed or loaded the dishwasher or drank his coffee. And I had ridiculous expectations about how much a three-year-old should keep things tidy or be careful. I was just so angry. All of the time.

It took me screaming at my daughter one day over a dropped glass of milk to change things. Gary had spent weeks getting annoyed at my anger and even leaving the house at my snappiness but I yelled so loud and threw the spoon I had been trying to cook with at the wall and he was stunned into silence. He realised something was wrong and long story short we actually talked. If this was a rom-com film, we would have stayed up all night chatting and that would have been solved, but back in reality the next step was to talk to my health visitor who sent me to the GP. A combination of antidepressants and some time with a counsellor (who I had to pay for privately to see at any speed, which enraged me at the time but I was so lucky to be able to afford) saw me gradually get better over time.

Looking back now I can see everything that left me feeling that way. I was feeling incapacitated by the birth (and grieving the birth I so desperately wanted). No one was helping me as I'd been the full on, competent first-time mum before who in reality was probably a bit too controlling. Everyone thought I had it sorted without ever stopping to think how difficult the pregnancy and birth was for me. I also felt trapped by having two children. Most of my friends had stuck to one at that point and seemed to be getting their freedom back while I was going backwards.

I was worried about how we would afford for me to go back to work with two children now and also didn't want to admit just how much my job meant to me as for some reason I felt I shouldn't care about that now I had two children. Gary's job wasn't the most secure and again, once we talked, I realised that it wasn't that he was abandoning me, but more that he had been stressing about his job as he was so worried about our money too.

I was really embarrassed at the time about how I felt and tried to keep it secret. I remember telling friends that everything was great and posting lots of photos on social media saying how lucky I felt. In reality I had spent the day simmering with rage or crying in frustration, but the happy photos told of a life I wished I had. I was ashamed, but now I'm out of it I can see it was just a consequence of how stressful things were. I would say to any mother feeling this way, open up, talk to people about how you feel. Ask for help and ask how they are feeling too. None of this is easy, but if people know how you feel and what they can do, it can certainly be easier.

We don't talk about it much, but anger is in fact a feature in many theories of depression. When we imagine someone feeling depressed, we imagine them being sad and maybe tired or not wanting to participate in something. But if you look back in psychology, all the way to Freud, anger is a key part of depression. Freud spoke about a lot of weird stuff, but his theory on depression and anger kind of makes sense. He saw anger as a reaction to loss. And postnatally you can feel like you have lost something – your old way of being, your old sense of self, your old day-to-day life. This doesn't mean you desperately want to go back in time and this all hadn't happened, but it's okay to grieve.

You might be worried that the anger you are feeling 'isn't like you'. Research shows that for lots of women who experience postnatal anger, these feelings come out of the blue. Many women didn't think of themselves as prone to anger before they had their baby and found that others around them ended up feeling shocked that they were acting that way. You can then end up in a vicious circle. Women face social pressure not to express their anger, especially not in relation to motherhood. So you feel angry and then end up feeling guilty about feeling angry.

At present, anger seems to be largely missing from tools used to diagnose mental health difficulties, including in the postnatal period. If you look back at the questions in the postnatal depression assessment, there's nothing about anger. However, when researchers in Canada started collating evidence about how women felt during pregnancy and the months after their baby was born, anger was a common theme and was closely linked to other symptoms of depression.[1]

A common finding was that anger was closely related to feeling powerless. Hands up who doesn't feel powerless to some extent after having a baby? We all feel powerless at some point. There's no escape from caring for your baby for the next 18 years or so, worrying about being financially dependent to some extent on someone else (or worrying about needing to get back to work), and feeling trapped with your partner forever (even if you do really quite like them) – these are all very common feelings that don't mean anything is wrong.

When feelings of powerlessness get strong or last for longer, they can be expressed as rage. There are certain life circumstances that can increase this, such as worries about money, having health issues or having relationship problems with your partner. These are all more common if you are a younger mother.

Another key point was that anger often arose when there was a mismatch between perceptions and the reality of motherhood. This again is such a common feeling. How many of us were ever truly prepared for having a baby? Even if we had lots of family experience or worked closely with babies before we had our own, that feeling of never being able to clock off or hand the baby back can be overwhelming. No one ever tells you about the little things like how much stuff you need to take with you when you leave the house or how often they will wake up.

This feeling can be especially strong if your baby was a much longed for birth. Yes of course, many women would describe their baby this way, but if you tried for a long time for your baby or perhaps had fertility treatment, sometimes the mismatch between perception and reality can feel even stronger, in part because

you might not feel like you can 'complain' about any of this. After all, you really tried for this - you must have desperately wanted it, right? Of course, but that doesn't mean you aren't allowed to have simultaneous emotions. You are allowed to be very grateful for your baby and angry at the reality.

Stress was another factor, particularly unexpected stress. Women who have had unexpected stressful events happen such as marital breakdown, job loss, illness, death, financial difficulties and so on are more prone to feelings of anger. And rightly so! Of course you would feel angry.

Anger was more common if women had a partner or family who were unsupportive, particularly if they had high hopes that they would be supportive. Broken promises, absence and generally being let down can all lead to anger. Why wouldn't they? Why are we surprised that someone who has been let down is reacting angrily? Why do we assume that motherhood is a serene, Madonna (not that one - the one with the child)-like state? Some common scenarios that are (rightfully) linked to anger include:

- Partners who don't do their fair share (especially those who get a full night's sleep)
- Sudden changes in household chores (you being automatically responsible for them all)
- Partners or family who criticise the way you care for your baby
- A partner who doesn't stick up for you when their family criticises you
- When your partner's life doesn't seem to be affected but yours has changed massively
- When everyone pays attention to the baby and ignores you (including turning up and expecting you to make them a cup of tea while they hold the baby)
- When health professionals don't spot issues or offer useful help
- Money issues

Another core trigger for anger is feeling like you've lost your old self and will never get it back. This could be in relation to all sorts of things but some common ones might be:

- Simple freedom to do what you wanted when you wanted
- Financial independence
- Relationship independence (knowing you could just leave if you wanted)

- Feeling stuck in terms of housing or location
- Job worries or wondering how you will return
- Missing your day-to-day professional self
- Your body
- Your sexual identity (especially if everything hurts)
- Your perception of yourself as a person (you're a mother now)
- Personal space, to be alone and have room to think

Supporting anger

We need to be more comfortable with the idea of anger. Everything I've described here is familiar to many women, along a sliding scale of feeling a bit angry every now and then to feeling full of rage every day. A lot of it comes down to our perceptions and ideas around motherhood. Writing this section has given *me* the rage because all these things would rightly be considered rage-inducing in any other context.

But female anger is not in line with society's view of the ideal mother being calm and loving and nurturing. Men are allowed to be angry about all sorts of things. To be completely stereotypical for a moment, think about how much anger and emotion we see on a Saturday when a football team loses. That's like a national acceptance of anger. Yet women have their lives turned upside down and we wonder why they are angry? I wonder if the reason we have so much more written about postnatal depression is because we are more comfortable at the idea of a woman being depressed. A woman crying? We can cope with that. But a woman angry? Steady now!

This of course is a simplification (and I know plenty of women can get angry when their football team loses), but this issue is continuing to harm women. In the little research that there is looking at women's postnatal anger, much of it talks about how women try and hide their rage or try to turn it into something more 'acceptable' such as saying they feel guilty or sad. Some do this out of a perceived need not to risk their relationship or even protect themselves from violence.

It is so important that we start talking about this. There is even some idea that the reason anger and depression might go hand in hand is that the act of trying to suppress anger actually leads to depression. Looking around the world, in Korea there is a type of depression known as 'Hwa-Byung' which translates as 'illness of fire'. This depression is specifically believed to be a consequence of trying to suppress anger, especially when that anger comes from inequality, feelings of powerlessness or control. It is particularly prevalent among middle-aged women – perhaps a sign that they have put up with patriarchal crap for far too long.[2]

What can you do?

- Know this is a common feeling. You are not alone. You are not weird. There is nothing wrong with you.
- Remember this is a completely normal reaction. We wouldn't be questioning this if caring for your baby was a new job you'd applied for.
- Recognise that this is most likely your circumstances and not you. Having a baby is stressful. Anger is a normal reaction to stress.
- If possible, talk to your partner. It's likely they just don't understand everything that is going on for you.
- Is there anything that can practically be taken off your plate? Childcare for older children? Someone to come and clean? Make a list of what would help and don't be afraid to ask for help. Remember, we were not meant to do this alone.
- Don't be afraid to speak up to other new mothers. The more openly we talk about this, the more it becomes accepted. But more importantly, the more you talk about it, the more you realise you're not alone. If you don't feel that you can talk to any of your friends, think about talking to someone professionally.
- Try and recognise your own trigger points. Is it specific fears? A particular lack of sleep? When your partner does something specific?

Read more

- 'Postpartum rage is real. One mum and psychologist shares her story' www.abc.net.au/news/2019-09-28/postnatal-rage-parenting-motherhood-depression-motherhood/11537916
- '"I was a charging, brutal, half-animal": The ugly truth about postnatal rage' www.irishtimes.com/life-and-style/health-family/i-was-a-charging-brutal-half-animal-the-ugly-truth-about-postnatal-rage-1.2950662
- 'Postpartum Rage Is Real, And We Need To Start Talking About It' www.scarymommy.com/why-isnt-anyone-talking-about-postpartum-rage

Chapter eighteen

Birth trauma

Birth has the power to change lives. It very literally does, bringing you your new baby, but the memories of the experience can leave you feeling empowered or they can leave you feeling floored. While many of us might look back on our births and remember feeling overwhelmed or frightened at some point, others are left with long-standing feelings of trauma characterised by flashbacks or lost memories, or intense feelings of fear coupled with physical symptoms or guilt at what happened. These feelings may constantly play at a low level in the background, or might rear their heads when anything reminds of us our experience.

Many women carry very strong emotions and memories after their birth, with around 4% having such strong reactions that they can be considered clinically traumatised, although this rises to five times as many among those who have had complicated pregnancies and births.[1] Women remember their births for a very long time. Doula and childbirth educator Penny Simkin found in research back in the 1980s that women had clear memories of their births for at least twenty years.[2] Many of us will know someone far older than that who still has strong emotions connected to birth.

It's absolutely normal to feel distressed if you had a difficult birth. Just because women give birth every day all over the world doesn't diminish your individual experience. Even after a good birth (that went how you hoped and was relatively complication free) it's still normal to feel a bit overwhelmed by it all. If you experienced that level of pain and exhaustion after any other event people would be quick to listen to how difficult you found it – think about people who run marathons or climb mountains!

Many people spend a bit of time somewhere in between awe and horror thinking back. They might talk about it to friends or family or strangers on the internet. And over time the feeling fades. Sometimes though, particularly if a birth has been very challenging, these feelings might not go away and it might be more serious.

What are the symptoms of birth trauma?

Clinical trauma is increasingly recognised by health professionals and psychologists as being something women can experience after a difficult birth. The concept of trauma historically came from symptoms that some soldiers returning from war were experiencing. They had flashbacks, nightmares and all sorts of physical symptoms, long after physical injuries had healed. To cut a long research history very short, psychologists soon realised that this was a reaction to awful events and that memories of their experience, not just physical injuries, could lead to ongoing symptoms. The idea of psychological trauma was born and expanded to other difficult events such as natural disasters, car crashes and other accidents.

To be diagnosed as traumatised, certain criteria were used. The first was that you were very scared for your own life or that of someone close to you, you witnessed someone else die or you or someone else were badly injured. Symptoms then included having flashbacks, negative thoughts, difficult memories (or memory loss), physical symptoms and emotional reactions such as anger, guilt or blame.[3]

The concept of clinical trauma in relation to birth experience first started being written about around 20–25 years ago. If you search for research on the topic, before this time birth trauma typically related to physical injury, not how a woman felt. Slowly it was recognised that women could be left with lasting emotions after birth that mirrored those of others who had experienced trauma.[4] Since then more and more research has been done and it is now recognised that women can be left with clinical symptoms of trauma after birth, especially if they were worried for their own life or that of their baby, had a lot of difficult interventions, or psychologically felt very out of control or were mistreated.

There are four key symptoms when it comes to thinking about whether someone is experiencing birth trauma:

1. **Re-experiencing the event over and over through intrusive thoughts** (thoughts you don't want to have, flashbacks and nightmares). These are

typically difficult to block out, and leave you feeling panicky and very distressed. It might take you some time to recover. Sometimes these come almost out of thin air and sometimes they might be a direct response to someone asking you about the birth. Other times small things might remind you of it like finding something from your birth bag, seeing your hospital on the news or hearing that someone else is pregnant.

2. **Wanting to block out all memories of the birth.** This can be closely linked to the first symptom. You might not want to read anything about birth or speak to friends who are pregnant. You might need to avoid the hospital or midwives that remind you of birth (or indeed any hospital or midwives). This can obviously be very tricky if you are of an age when everyone seems to be having babies or you live near the hospital.

3. **Having negative thoughts.** These can be linked to the birth or more general. You might think about your birth and become angry or sad. You might blame yourself (unnecessarily) for how things went or be really angry at the health professionals involved in your care (rightly or wrongly). Guilt is a really common feeling. Sometimes though, you have continual feelings like this... but have no idea why. It is linked to the birth but you haven't made the connection so it feels even more unsettling as you can't explain it.

4. **Having physical symptoms including being very on edge.** You might struggle to sleep (or sleep too much). You might sleep all day long then not be able to sleep once you get into bed. You might be eating all the time or hardly eating at all. You might feel exhausted or wired (or both at the same time). Many women feel very jumpy, like something is wrong. This is because their body, after going through a traumatic experience, is ready and waiting for it to happen again – it is in 'fight or flight' and adrenaline is flowing ready to either fight a stressor or run away. This is exhausting, hence the other symptoms.

If you are feeling negative about your birth and are worried about some of the symptoms you might be experiencing, you might like to have a look at one of the scales that examines different symptoms of birth trauma. One of the most recent and useful scales is known as the City University London Birth Trauma Scale.[5]
It looks at different aspects such as:

- Whether you were worried during the birth that you or your baby would be seriously injured or would die.
- Thoughts and emotions you've been having recently such as recurrent unwanted memories of birth, nightmares or flashbacks to the birth, feeling

tense, anxious or upset if you are reminded of it, trying to avoid talking about your birth (or finding you've forgotten details) or feeling anger, shame or guilt over it.

- Recent feelings such as irritability, feeling detached, losing interest in things you usually enjoy, problems concentrating and feeling on edge.

The tool is not meant to be 'diagnostic' – you do not have birth trauma if you hit a certain score, or not have it because your score is one point lower. Rather, the more symptoms you have, the more likely it is that you have birth trauma and the more important it is that you speak to someone.

What experiences can lead to birth trauma?

Research has shown that how you feel about your birth isn't necessarily directly related to what happened. Two individuals can have a very similar experience, at least on paper, yet feel very differently about it in the short and long term. There are lots of things that might have happened during your birth that you might be struggling with and can cause your body to react with trauma symptoms. These include the typical things we might focus on when thinking of a difficult birth such as:

- 'Difficulties' during the birth such as a very long labour
- Interventions or complications that happened
- Having a lot of pain

However, what research shows is that it's not just whether you can tick off the 'big things', but more about how you felt during birth.[6] This can include things like:

- Feeling worried about yourself or your baby
- Feeling overwhelmed
- Feeling poorly treated
- Being ignored or belittled
- Not getting the support or medication you asked for
- Your pain or concerns being played down

None of these experiences ranks any higher than the others. Please never feel that you have to experience certain things during your birth to be 'worthy' of a label of trauma. Often we simply can't predict who will be left traumatised and who won't. One woman could have a birth full of interventions and pain yet not have any lasting issues, while another might have a straightforward birth but something leaves her with a trauma reaction. Sometimes it can be the smallest thing. Research consistently shows that the most important thing is whether you felt communicated with and safe rather than what actually happened.[7]

Can partners experience birth trauma too?

Yes. A partner can very much be affected by birth, sometimes even more than the woman actually giving birth. It is well recognised that you can develop symptoms of PTSD if you watch something traumatic happen to someone you care for (or even a stranger) and the same goes for birth. There is limited research in this area, and what has been done has been conducted with male birth partners. It is, however, very likely that the same experiences can also affect female birth partners, so I will use the word partner here.

One of the most common reasons why partners experience birth trauma is intense fear for either their partner or child. Many then feel that they can't open up because it didn't physically happen to them and they feel unjustified or wrong in taking the attention away from the mother. Any partner experiencing feelings of trauma definitely deserves support – trying to ignore or dismiss your own feelings makes everything worse.

In two studies that used interviews with men who experienced birth trauma, a number of factors were found to have increased their feelings.[8,9] These included:

- Feeling unprepared for what birth would be like
- Feeling that they weren't involved in the process
- A lack of control over what was happening
- Being sent out of the room
- Distress at seeing their partner in pain
- Fear of their partner dying and having to look after the baby
- Not being able to look after their partner and others playing that role instead
- Feeling that they couldn't share how they felt
- Have to physically look after partner/take time off from work
- Grieving the loss of positive first moments as a family
- Expectations of birth and fatherhood not matching up to expectations

Men in both studies described how this left them with lots of different emotions. Some had a lot of anger and rage. Others felt very disconnected. Many pushed themselves back into work because they could control that. Others struggled to concentrate at work or were very preoccupied. There was an almost universal feeling of wanting to speak out and get support, but feeling like they didn't deserve it as nothing physical had happened to them.

For more information on fathers'/partners' mental health, how it can affect behaviour and where to get support, see the next chapter.

" One of the worst things we can say to women is that 'all that matters is a healthy baby'. "

Getting support

If you have any negative feelings when thinking about your birth, it's important to reach out to someone and talk to them. It might be that you simply need to talk about your experiences with friends, family or your partner. Research shows that sometimes just telling your story, letting the emotions out and have someone listen to you and take you seriously is all that you need.[10] One option if you feel unable to open up to anyone close to you is to talk your feelings through with a doula. You might do this in the weeks and months after birth, or many years later. Some women might work with a doula before becoming pregnant with another baby.

However, if you are experiencing deeper symptoms of trauma and are particularly stressed about your birth, you might find you need more help than talking can offer. In fact, if you are experiencing more complicated emotions and trauma, just talking about it rather than seeking professional support to use established therapeutic techniques to work through your experiences and reactions could actually make things worse – retraumatising you as such. If you're unsure what support you need, a first step could be to talk to your health visitor or GP or indeed seek out a doula or counsellor who may have more specific experience on this topic. They may be able to support you in working through your birth experience yourself, or help you access further support such as counselling or therapy approaches that use techniques such as EMDR or Rewind (more details coming up). For further information on counselling and support see the interview with clinical psychologist Dr Emma Svanberg below.

The most important thing though is to make sure you do talk to someone about how you feel. You might tell yourself that with just a bit of time, memories will fade and disappear. They might. But for many women, especially those with more serious trauma, this is unlikely to happen and may become worse in future as things like potentially becoming a grandmother remind you of your own trauma.

It's also really common to worry that your symptoms aren't serious enough or to think that just because you didn't have X,Y,Z happen in your birth then you don't 'deserve' to feel traumatised. This is in no way true. One of the worst things we can say to women is that 'all that matters is a healthy baby'. You immediately feel dismissed and as if no one is listening, or that you don't deserve to feel this way if your baby is healthy. Nonsense. You can feel terrible about your birth and very grateful your baby is healthy – they are not mutually exclusive!

It is especially important that you reach out and talk to someone if you don't have anyone around you that you trust to talk to, or they are trying to tell you that your experiences don't matter. One of the big things that makes trauma worse is someone trying to downplay things or tell you that you're being silly. You are not.

Further sources of support include:

- The Birth Trauma Association web page is a wealth of information, including specific links for partners who are supporting someone with birth trauma, or who are themselves experiencing symptoms www. birthtraumaassociation.org.uk/. They also have a social media group www. facebook.com/groups/TheBTA/.
- The Fathers Network also offers support to men following birth trauma www.fathersnetwork.org.uk/birth_trauma_and_timetotalk
- Mind offers support for individuals experiencing a range of mental health challenges including PTSD and birth trauma www.mind.org. uk/information-support/types-of-mental-health-problems/postnatal-depression-and-perinatal-mental-health/ptsd-and-birth-trauma/.
- Again, to find a registered counsellor, the British Association for Counselling and Psychotherapy has a list of practitioners on their website. You can filter for location and speciality www.bacp.co.uk.

If you would like to read more about birth trauma I recommend:

- *Why Birth Trauma Matters* – Emma Svanberg
- *Birth Shock* – Mia Scotland

Giving support

If you are a partner trying to support someone with birth trauma, know that you do not have to be a complete expert to help them. Just listening and encouraging them to open up and seek support is a really important first step. Some other key ways in which you can offer support are listed below:

- Don't dismiss their experiences. Listen to what they are telling you. It matters to them and you are not the one to judge whether it deserves to be considered traumatic or not. Many may already be struggling to open up or worrying they don't deserve to feel this way. You might think you are helping by suggesting it was all okay, but this can have a negative effect. Imagine being in any other traumatic situation and being told it didn't matter.
- Reassure, repeatedly. They may be experiencing physical symptoms of fear. Anxiety can lead to needing frequent reassurance. You are not repeating yourself, you are helping. Remind them that they are safe now.
- Be an advocate – go with them to appointments if that will help. Speak up and don't let people dismiss them. Find information out for them about where they can get support.

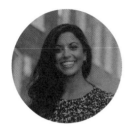

Supporting birth trauma

Dr Emma Svanberg is a chartered clinical psychologist specialising in the perinatal period, and author of *Why Birth Trauma Matters*. You can find Emma at www.mumologist.com

You're a clinical psychologist who specialises in pregnancy, birth and the postnatal period. What sorts of things do parents contact you about? Does someone need to have a clinical diagnosis of a mental health difficulty to see a psychologist?

This is a more complicated question than it seems! When I first started working in the perinatal field I was in a primary care setting (in GP surgeries and Sure Start centres). People were often referred to us with anxiety around birth, postnatal anxiety or depression, but often were referred to discuss broader issues such as navigating the transition to becoming a parent, relationship stresses and managing two children. Services have changed a lot in recent years and, while funding has gone into improving secondary care perinatal mental health services and Mother and Baby units, there is much less on offer at a primary care level. This means that, yes, usually you need a moderate-severe clinical diagnosis of a mental health difficulty and I've spoken to many people who feel that they cannot get support unless their mental health deteriorates. Perinatal mental health is also very complicated, so people are often misdiagnosed with postnatal depression when in fact they are experiencing symptoms of trauma, for example.

I now work independently and see people for basically any difficulty they may be experiencing from first-time pregnancy all the way through to having young children. My focus is on the parent rather than the child, so my experience is in adult psychology, although of course I also have experience with children and families which I draw from in my work. People might see me because they are anxious about their pregnancy, worried about becoming a parent, having relationship problems, scared of giving birth, to discuss a previous difficult birth, because they are feeling more sad, angry or anxious than they would like, or just because they would like a space to discuss what it means to them to be a parent.

You are particularly well known for your work on birth trauma and the book you have written on that subject *Why Birth Trauma Matters*. How did you become interested in that?

We never learned about birth in any of my psychology training. I don't remember it being mentioned once, except in a child assessment in case there had been any physical injury. That's not surprising considering how new birth trauma research is, comparatively, but it really is indicative of how much psychology focusing on families has downplayed the experience of mothers (there is a long history of 'mother-blaming' in some fields of psychology). It was through working with women that I started to realise one of the common experiences among them was a difficult birth experience, and in particular often this was down to anxiety and feeling unsupported around the birth. This was back in 2009, and there were very few pieces of research available at that time, but I did find the Birth Trauma Association which introduced me to the concept of birth trauma.

I trained as a hypnobirthing teacher as a way to learn some new skills to prevent anxiety during pregnancy and birth – there is a lot of overlap between anxiety management skills and hypnobirthing, although I became conscious of the 'gold standard' birth that some schools can inadvertently encourage.

My interest moved away from the purely clinical in 2018 when I set up Make Birth Better with perinatal psychiatrist Dr Rebecca Moore. I think we were both frustrated by how things seemed to be getting worse instead of better, and how often women and birthing people come out of their birth experience feeling they have failed in some way rather than that they have been failed.

How can a psychologist help people who are experiencing birth trauma? What sort of support or treatment might be available?

There is a range of different methods. The two evidence-based treatments of choice for birth trauma are Trauma Focused CBT, and Eye Movement Desensitisation and Reprocessing (EMDR). Within the NHS you should be able to access these treatments, but you may need a diagnosis of PTSD. The majority of people with birth trauma are impacted by their experience but may not meet the full PTSD criteria, so at Make Birth Better we often hear stories from people who couldn't access help. We released a report on this recently that found that only 25% of women felt they received the support they needed after experiencing a traumatic birth. It also revealed how inadequate the help on offer can be – only 13% of women who had received psychological help felt it had resolved their birth trauma.

There are new NHS England guidelines coming out this year which aim to fill those gaps, but the longer I work with trauma the more I feel that women and their partners need a lot longer to process what has happened to them than is given, especially when they have experienced trauma in their past too. There may also be some focus on repairing a relationship with a child which has been affected because of the traumatic start to their life, and work with a partner who might be vicariously traumatised. I worry that the short-term sessions which are often offered may leave some women continuing to feel unsafe. This is, of course, not everywhere and I have heard many stories of people whose lives have been transformed by the therapeutic interventions they were offered.

When we think about birth trauma we might automatically think of it applying to those who have given birth. Do you also support birth partners if they are struggling?
Yes absolutely, and at Make Birth Better we emphasise the need for support for staff too.

How do you help new parents?
I draw from a range of different psychological models and theories to meet new parents wherever they are, psychologically speaking. So often what is at the core of people's difficulties is identifying then letting go of some of the messages they were brought up with – about themselves, about what to expect from relationships and about what 'good enough' parenting looks like. I do this by using a brief psychodynamic model called Dynamic Interpersonal Therapy, but also draw from other models such as Cognitive Behavioural Therapy (CBT), particularly third-wave approaches like mindfulness and compassion, and Systemic Therapy. The latter is particularly important to me as we don't exist in a vacuum, and many of the difficulties faced by new parents are exacerbated by the lack of support parents, and particularly mothers, are given.

Do you only see people face-to-face or are there different ways people might access support? Could they be anonymous if they wanted?
Clinically, I see people face-to-face or over online platforms. I've never had a request from someone to stay anonymous: therapy does involve a certain amount of exposure and that is sometimes the hardest step. It's important that I create conditions where people feel safe to be open and honest, so knowing who they are is essential! Plus psychologists always have safety at the back of their minds; there are situations where we might feel really worried for someone and knowing who and where they are is very important to make sure we can help to keep them safe if need be.

I do a lot of work on social media, awareness raising and what would probably be classed as self-help. So much of my work with new parents is about normalising what they are experiencing, and online social communities are a fantastic way of supporting new and expectant parents. I often get contacted with questions via social media. It can be really hard to navigate services, which can be really off-putting, so I'm always happy to offer brief advice and signposting over email.

Finally, what would you say to anyone who has concerns related to pregnancy, birth or caring for a baby, but is worried about getting in contact with a psychologist or thinks that their feelings aren't 'serious enough' to take up your time?
The two things I think I hear the most are either that people worry their feelings aren't serious enough or that they will tell me the most horrifying story I've ever heard and I'll think they are very damaged. Parents also, understandably, worry about telling me how they feel about their children in case I think they are not fit to parent. Sometimes people feel all three of those things at the same time.

What I would say is that what I'm interested in as a therapist is how these feelings are affecting you. There is no value placed on the depth of your feelings or the situations you have been in. Instead, my role is helping you think about how these things have affected you and are still affecting you and how you might be able to move forward.

Chapter nineteen

Partners' mental health

→ This chapter explores the mental health of the partner who did not give birth. As we've seen, all the research that I know of has been conducted with fathers. That itself is a very new field, which has been boosted by the amazing work of Mark Williams, founder of Fathers Reaching Out. It is likely that some of the research and findings will be relevant to same-sex partners, due to shared experiences of being the parent who didn't give birth. But there are obviously a lot of differences too, from different hormone patterns, to different societal expectations and pressures and different relationship patterns (research shows that same-sex partners tend to have more balanced sharing of chores and childcare). Therefore, sometimes I refer to partner and sometimes father – based on the underpinning research. I apologise for any confusion or lack of inclusivity, and call for more research on same-sex partners' mental health.

Being the partner who didn't give birth is not always the rosy, easy experience the media often imply it to be. Statistically you are more likely to be the one returning to work in just a few weeks, with a whole new tiny person in your life and wanting to care for your partner too. It's really normal to feel pushed out or like a spare part and even to feel jealous of the bond between

> **"If you are a partner reading this, please never ever feel that your wellbeing doesn't matter at this time."**

your partner and the new baby. You've probably got less free time, less time one-to-one with your partner and you are exhausted on top of that.

For far too long, the mental health of partners was ignored. A lot of ideas around postnatal depression focused on the role of birth, physical recovery and being at home, either on maternity leave or indefinitely. Fathers or partners? Well they just hung around for the birth, popped down the pub and went back to work without a care in the world, didn't they?

Thankfully things have changed massively. I remember teaching a session nearly 20 years ago about the idea of fathers having postnatal depression after the birth and the general feeling was disbelief that it could be possible. Now, I teach a similar session and everyone takes it absolutely seriously, just as they should.

If you are a partner reading this, or perhaps a mother wanting to support her partner, please never ever feel that your wellbeing doesn't matter at this time. Okay, so you haven't given birth, but as important as giving birth is, it's not the only thing that affects your mental health after a baby is born. In fact, there's very little evidence at all that things like hormones are related to postnatal depression in mothers. Most of the focus and support has turned to realising that in fact massive life changes affect mental health, and that happens just as much for partners, albeit often in a different way.

What might mental health difficulties in partners look like?

You're probably very aware of the 'typical' image of someone who is depressed. You might think about them not getting out of bed, being very miserable and very tired. But mental health issues don't always look like this. Anxiety, for example, is a really common part of depression – yes, it is possible to feel both exhausted and wired at the same time. If you're a partner reading this have a look back through the chapters on depression, anxiety, postnatal anger and birth trauma – you may recognise some of the signs in yourself.

Research with fathers who experience mental health difficulties after they've had a baby shows that often their emotions lean more towards irritability and anger than depression or anxiety. Men are more likely to experience emotions such as:

- Irritability
- Anger
- Exhaustion

- Poor concentration
- Sleeplessness
- Recklessness
- Risk-taking
- Eating too much or too little
- Feeling overwhelmed by responsibility
- Guilt
- Physical symptoms such as headaches
- Feeling mentally drained
- Withdrawing from others
- Finding it difficult to make decisions
- Feeling alienated from your partner and/or baby
- Throwing yourself into work/hobbies, being too busy

Men are also less likely to be able to recognise they are experiencing a mental health issue.

Interestingly, research has shown that when men have a partner experiencing postnatal depression they can identify and label the symptoms. However, when they experience exactly the same symptoms themselves, they find it really difficult to label them. If you're reading this you might be thinking that 'she has it worse' so I need to 'just get on with it'. Sometimes you might think you should call it stress or exhaustion rather than thinking it is something more. Or it might come through as feeling overly worried about your partner and how she is. Maybe you don't want to tell anyone because you think you're taking time away from her? Or that men's health doesn't count?[1]

How many partners experience mental health difficulties?

How common is it to experience mental health difficulties as a new partner? Well that depends where you look for your data. Common sense suggests that it is very common indeed. After all, we know that estimates for mothers experiencing mental health challenges after birth show it is really widespread, if not always well documented. Research in this area isn't copious, but it suggests that around 10% of new fathers experience depression or anxiety in the months after birth.[2]

However, we know from research with new mums that many don't want to admit how they are feeling. Many hide it from health professionals or researchers (or indeed are feeling so awful they wouldn't take part in research at all). And we know that in general, men are far less likely to report depression or anxiety than women.[3] This means that any estimate we have is probably really low. In fact in one study of families who were in challenging situations

"It's really common for men in particular to ignore their own mental health after having a baby."

and at risk of mental health difficulties, less than 4% of fathers reported seeking help for any anxiety or depression they were experiencing, which is in line with figures for how many men are diagnosed with depression or anxiety each year.[4]

It's really common for men in particular to ignore their own mental health after having a baby. One really interesting study has a lot of quotes many fathers will identify with. Men talked about feeling that they needed to be the one to hold it all together for their partner, and being 'a rock' was very closely tied up in their image of themselves and their role as they saw it. They worried about letting people down, seeing themselves as the provider of support, not the one who was meant to receive it. Lots of men in particular say they struggle with feeling like they have to 'do it all' – keep doing a good job at work, be hands on with their baby, and support their partner, without having a support system themselves. In one study men described it as being both a 'provider and a protector'.

Another common feeling is that everyone is pulling you in every direction. You really want to be a good partner. A good parent. And a good employee. But every time you put more effort in one direction, it feels like you're letting the others down.

Others had not even considered that them having mental health difficulties could be a 'thing'. They assumed it just happened to women and that they were feeling a bit grumpy or worried compared to normal. Because of this they worried that they couldn't talk to people about how they felt, worrying that they would be dismissed as being ridiculous or criticised for making a fuss when their partner was seen as coping with so much more.[5]

What might increase the chance of partner mental health difficulties?

There are lots of different reasons why partners might experience mental health difficulties. These might include things that tend to affect both partners, such as exhaustion, a baby who cries a lot and a lack of time to yourself.[6] But other risk factors include:[7,8]

- Worrying about your job security or performance
- Working in a low-paid, unskilled job
- Having relationship problems or feeling like you have lost 'closeness'
- If your partner is having mental health difficulties – research suggests that if your partner has diagnosed postnatal depression, somewhere between a quarter to half of partners will

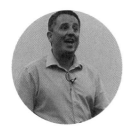

Supporting fathers' mental health

Mark Williams is founder of Fathers Reaching Out and author of *Daddy Blues* published by Trigger Press. Mark suffered from undiagnosed depression after his wife's traumatic birth which has led to him campaigning for better support for fathers after birth.

Tell us about your story

I suffered my first ever panic attack at 30 years of age and I didn't have a clue what was happening to me. It was the day my son was born. My wife Michelle was taken to theatre for an emergency c-section and I honestly thought she was going to die. I was terrified. Thankfully, both Michelle and my son survived, but Michelle was left suffering from anxiety and depression. Shortly after that we realised Michelle had actually developed severe postnatal depression. My world changed forever. Within weeks of Michelle's diagnosis, I had to give up my job as a sales rep and coach to care for Michelle and Ethan.

How did you feel?

I was busy caring for my wife and son and didn't realise at first the impact everything had had upon me. I had never really known anyone before who had depression. I was so uneducated about mental health I used to wonder: 'How can people be depressed?' But little did I know that I was actually experiencing it myself.

Looking back, it was not surprising at all. I had loved the social side of my job but now I was totally isolated. Sometimes I wouldn't get out the front door for days. I was isolating myself from people. I felt totally alone. Within months, my personality changed, and I was drinking in an attempt to cope when my family helped out. I was also experiencing awful nightmares about Michelle and Ethan dying in theatre. I would wake up in a panic thinking it was real.

I used to think people who had depression just got sad. But I also became angry. It got to the point where, if I did manage to get out with friends, I wanted to fight the doorman. I had this strange need to get hurt to try and stop what I was feeling and the thoughts that were going through my head. I didn't have the overwhelming feeling of love I was told by society I would have, and I felt I wasn't going to be good enough as fatherhood totally changed me. I began to have uncontrollable suicidal thoughts, but never acted on them. I just worried that Social Services would take my son off us, as Michelle was unwell and now I was feeling the way I felt.

As time went on my dark thoughts and nightmares just got worse and worse. It was difficult not knowing how long my wife would be unwell for. In the end, it took around 18 months before she started to feel better, but while she was getting better, I wasn't.

Did you feel you could talk to anyone about how you felt?

At the time, I felt like I couldn't talk to anyone. I was raised in a working-class community and my father and grandfather were coal miners. Growing up we looked up to 'hard men' who didn't show their emotions and now I was feeling emotional – and I was feeling weak. I kept telling myself I just had to 'man up' and everything would be okay.

I also felt that I couldn't tell my wife how I was feeling as I didn't want to risk impacting her mental health. I felt I was meant to be strong and the one looking after her and that it was women who got depressed after the birth not men. Of course, this all affected our relationship. It so often causes the breakdown of families when there's no early intervention. Michelle was back then and still is an incredible mother, but that first year was the loneliest in my life.

I had also gone back to work, this time working in mental health services as a support worker on a secure forensic ward. I didn't want depression on my medical records as I loved working and providing for my family and was worried that it might risk my job.

What changed?

I suffered in silence for around five years. And then my mother, who I loved so much, was diagnosed with cancer. Within weeks of this, my grandfather, who I cared for with my family and loved so much, was diagnosed with dementia and sadly died. The impact of this on top of not dealing with my postnatal trauma broke me. One day, while sitting in my car before walking into work, I had a complete breakdown. I just literally couldn't get out of the car. I was shaking, crying and suicidal thoughts were racing through my mind. While in the car, I phoned an organisation called Mental Health Matters Wales and was told to seek help. I was ready to embrace everything as I didn't want my son to be fatherless. He may have saved my life. As we know in the UK, the biggest killer in men under 50 now is suicide.

Eventually, I was put on medication and took a course of cognitive behavioural therapy (CBT) and mindfulness. While under the support of the community mental health team, I was also diagnosed with ADHD, which I realised I had been dealing with all my life.

During my treatment, professionals suggested that if I had been screened after my son was born I would likely have been diagnosed with PTSD or postnatal depression. I think now, looking back, if I had been screened early enough, I think I would have managed it so much better. I felt completely unprepared for the birth and I was totally unaware that fathers could even develop postnatal depression.

I also think about how it affected my relationship with Ethan. I didn't bond with Ethan during his first weeks. I didn't have the overwhelming feeling of love that I thought I would have. I felt an overwhelming need to protect him, but also felt distant, which I now know is a sign of trauma. Thankfully that all changed and our bond grew and grew. I think that actually being home with my son, being able to do things like skin-to-skin and play a big role in his care, particularly at night, really helped our bond grow.

What would you say to new dads who might be feeling this way?
You are not alone. It's not just mums who can feel anxious or depressed after giving birth, but often how dads feel isn't talked about. It's normal to find transitioning to being a dad difficult – especially if you have a lot of unresolved trauma in your history. Sleep deprivation and changes to your social life are tough. You might not know how to support your partner if she is struggling with things like breastfeeding. Lots of men also worry about their job and making enough money to support their partner. Or you might be traumatised by big events such as your partner having a difficult birth, miscarriage or your baby being born with a disability. You might feel anxious, depressed or angry like I did.

It's really important to know that lots of other men feel this way, even though many hide it due to worries about stigma. Suicide is now the biggest killer of men aged under 50, with fathers twice as likely to have depression than non-fathers of the same age, and new reports show that actually four in ten fathers say they needed more support for their mental health in the first year of fatherhood.

What is important is that you speak to someone. You're not being stupid or less of a man and it's really important you get support not just for you but for your family too. They love and need you. That's why I published *Daddy Blues*, as I want as many men as possible to know it's not just them going through this. Society might be telling us it's the happiest time of our lives, and for many it is, but for others it can be the most difficult time.

Tell us about what you're doing to get more support for dads
My story does have a happy ending. I am so thankful to say that both Michelle and I are doing well these days and have a great bond with our son. My mother also recovered and is still cancer-free today. Thankfully, once my mental health was under control, I was lucky to be able to put my energies

into making a difference for the next generation of fathers. It was clear to me that this was needed for dads, but also the whole family. If a dad is suffering, mum and baby will suffer too.

After speaking to a new father in the gym in 2011, who told me a very similar story to my own, I decided we needed something that would support new fathers who were experiencing depression and trauma so I set up Fathers Reaching Out. I started to talk to other fathers and researchers about the importance of dads' mental health, and then moved on to lobbying government to make changes. I deliver talks to health professionals, students and policymakers about how dads can better be supported. In 2012 I was also lucky enough to meet Dr Jane Hanley, an expert in perinatal mental health, who started mentoring me and trained me to deliver perinatal mental health support in 2014.

Setting up Fathers Reaching Out really gave me a purpose, another reason to stay well and a hope that I could change things for the future. I've now spent nearly 10 years campaigning to try and make governments realise how important dads' mental health is too. And we've done it – fathers' mental health is now being mentioned in policy and we now have International Fathers' Mental Health Day, which I founded.

I also started the #HowAreYouDad campaign to make sure that we have more conversations with all dads about their mental health. I want to make sure they are screened for mental health difficulties like mums, and that there are lots of resources available for them too. One of the things I am doing with the campaign is collecting together different resources to help parents at this time.

Overall, I want people – and particularly fathers – to know that there is help out there. Don't suffer in silence like I did. Ask for help, and the earlier the better. Different people might need help in different ways and that might include talking therapies or medication. Most of all, tell someone how you are feeling. Talk to other parents and your health professional. Don't suppress your feelings like many men do – they can unfortunately come out as anger.

You can do this. Don't suffer in silence. There is light at the end of the tunnel and it will make you stronger once you recover.

Find out more

You can read more about Mark's story, work and campaigning, including how to invite Mark to give a talk or workshop at **www.reachingoutpmh.co.uk**. You can find his book *Daddy Blues* at **www.triggerpublishing.com/product/daddy-blues**.

- If your partner has a better paid or more prestigious job
- If you are both working and your baby is very young
- Not feeling confident as a parent
- A difficult pregnancy or traumatic birth
- A lack of social support
- Being a younger first-time father
- Feeling really unprepared – research has shown that when dads are offered education antenatally, they are less likely to experience anxiety once their baby is here
- Having existing mental health difficulties

A lot of these risk factors are based around feelings of worry and feeling out of control. You may have become more traditional in your relationship and are now responsible for going back to work and being the main wage-earner, at least for a while. Others are linked to there often not being much support for partners so you don't have anyone to turn to or offload to.

A lack of focus on partners in antenatal education can also exacerbate feelings of being unprepared or insecurity. Unfortunately there is a really mixed bag of support out there for men in particular. Sometimes it's missing altogether and at other times it takes the jokey, inept father route, which for some could be amusing but for others might make them feel rejected and not important. Research suggests that many men want the skills to be able to support their partner and care for their baby, but find these often aren't targeted at them.[9]

Getting support

If you feel you can't seek help, or that you don't deserve to take up the time of others, firstly realise that you are just as valuable as your partner. If you really feel you don't deserve it, seek support for the sake of your partner and baby. Getting yourself better is a way of caring for your baby.

- Remember you can talk to your GP or indeed your health visitor – they're not just for mothers. Likewise you can talk to a doula too.
- Check out the sources of support in the previous chapters with regard to counselling and finding different sources of support. The British Association for Counselling and Psychotherapy has a list of counsellors – you can filter by region and speciality. www.bacp.co.uk
- The Fathers Reaching Out website has a lot of support for fathers experiencing mental health difficulties www.reachingoutpmh.co.uk.
- Dr Andy Mayers has a great resource for fathers' mental health including lots of articles you might find reassuring www.andrewmayers.info/fathers-

mental-health.html.

- You might also like to look at the Men's Sheds project – a series of get-togethers for men across the country, bringing them together to socialise and talk, usually based around an activity. The scheme has had a really good impact on mental health and wellbeing. menssheds.org.uk

Chapter twenty

I wish I'd never had a baby

→ Having moments when you wish you'd never had your baby and feeling like it has all been a huge mistake is an extremely common, yet little talked about emotion. It is particularly common in the early days and weeks as you are adjusting to life (have a look back at Chapter 13 for some very honest responses to becoming a new parent). Often these go away again, particularly after a good night's sleep or a break or a good, honest chat to someone about how you feel. But for some parents they don't go away. And then what do you do?

The first step is to think about whether your mental health might be causing you to have these thoughts. If you are in the midst of postnatal depression or birth trauma, then these thoughts can arise as a reaction to how you are feeling and what you have experienced rather than your relationship with your baby. With the right treatment and time it is possible they will pass and many women reflecting on that time talk about how when the fog of anger and depression lifted, they fell very much in love with their baby.

But for some the feelings either don't go away as they start to feel better, or they are rational thoughts that occur when your mental health is generally good. So then what?

It's important to think about the wider context here. You are not alone. A recent survey in the US found that at least 7% of adults said that if they had their time again they wouldn't have children.[1] It makes sense that some people might find the whole experience of parenting very challenging. Your life has changed, you are getting little sleep and your freedom has diminished as your responsibility has increased. You may feel that you simply don't love your child – or you may feel that you love your child but really hate everything about parenting.

Despite fewer young women actually planning on becoming mothers these days, many societies view the experience of having a baby and caring for them as the pinnacle of human fulfilment. We glamourise it by glossing over the awful bits and perpetuating pressure to conform to say you love your kids more than anything else. We present it as if it's the key to understanding life, criticising senior political figures who don't have children as if that's something they should be ashamed of, and they can't possibly understand life because of it. It is the natural order – fall in love, get married, have a baby – a timeline that is majorly pressurised in certain areas and families.[2] If anyone dares express their regret, they are held up as a terrible human being or are met with disbelief. There is vastly more societal pressure on women to feel this way – and regrets have to be hidden behind jokes about being frazzled and needing wine.[3]

Regretting the impact on your life

Some parents, when they say they regret having children, don't mean that they wish their child wasn't here, but that they wish that life was different. They feel like running away from their lives, because they are fed up of the stress and pressure, but express love for their children. This then gets mixed up with feelings of guilt and shame for feeling that way, which makes things even worse.

Strangely, the more stressful you find parenting, the more likely you are to sometimes regret your choices – who'd have thought! Women who are doing it all on their own, exhausted, juggling work and who have no time to themselves are more likely to regret the impact of having children on their lives.[4]

One really interesting study explored why parents regretted the impact of children upon their lives. They used a discussion thread on Reddit on the subject, which of course meant participants were anonymous and more likely to be honest.[5]

The first group of parents identified in the research were those who stated that although they loved their children, they did not love what parenting had done to their lives. They didn't necessarily regret having their children as such, but regretted things like:

The timing

Parents regretted when they had their child or the space in between children.

Some regretted having them too young and felt like they missed out on opportunities, while others regretted having them later, feeling that they were too old and tired to be an active parent. Some felt the timing stopped their career ever getting off to a good start, and others felt they had to step away from work just at a point where they had success or responsibility. Money played a role too – some felt they had children too young or before they had a good salary, meaning it was difficult to afford things. Others were used to a high salary and level of expectation, which was then majorly cut if they dropped their hours.

How many children they had

Again, this worked both ways. Some regretted not having another baby. Others regretted having more children, feeling it damaged the relationship with their oldest child or placed extra stress on the family in terms of practical and financial issues. This went away sometimes when their children were adults and no longer a financial or space issue.

The sacrifices they had to make to have them

Parents yearned for the things they could no longer do, or do so easily: long lie-ins, doing things on a whim, using money selfishly, moving to a new house, lazy hangovers, taking educational opportunities, travel and so on. Women often felt this more starkly than men.

A major feeling experienced by a lot of parents was that they desperately wanted their lives back and wished for sleep or travel or just time to think. Yet when they then thought of not having their child, or something happening to them, they also felt loss. Parents felt like they were stuck in some kind of no man's land where they could never really feel happy. They either felt exhausted and stuck, or horrified at the idea of being without their children.

The partner they had them with

A common emotion among parents who had split up or are simply not getting on was 'I wish my child had a different mother/father'. This differed according to situation. Some saw traits in their child that they disliked in their partner, or felt they had to stay with a partner for the sake of their child. For others their child's other parent was just completely missing from their life, or caused chaos or harm. This is closely tied to the idea of knowing that your former partner will always be part of your life, at least in some way, and the awful feeling of knowing your child feels positively about them despite the circumstances – which is only made worse by the opposite option of your child hating their parent or being let down by them. It's a no-win situation.

Regret at bringing a baby into this world

Some parents regretted the idea that they had been, in their eyes, selfish in

> **“ Children do not see the world in the same way adults do – what you may have remembered as peaceful likely brought many challenges for your parents. ”**

bringing a child into what they saw to be an awful world. Commonly they believed that their childhood had been safe and pleasant, and today's world was cruel and unrelenting. Given we have never had a time in our world when things have been peaceful and perfect, this is in part whimsical thinking or just simply different memories of events. Children do not see the world in the same way adults do – what you may have remembered as peaceful likely brought many challenges for your parents. In the 1980s, for example, we had Black Monday and the stock market crash, the 'mad cow disease' outbreak, the Aids epidemic and Pat Sharp's mullet.[6]

This feeling was particularly stark for parents of colour who were worried about having brought their child into a racist society. Particularly when their child looked like them, mothers feared they would have the same experiences.

What if you really regret ever having children?

The examples above mainly involve not necessarily regretting having your child, but more regretting the impact having them had on your life. But what if you just genuinely feel you wish you had never had a child – even if somehow the rest of it could go away?

Again this is not as rare as social media might make you think. Some parents in this category wished they could get in a time machine and 'go back'. They did not like the reality of parenting and felt that wouldn't change even if their partner was different or they had all the money in the world. They did not want the responsibility and feelings that remained outside the day-to-day drag of caring for a child.

Others admitted they did not like their children. Some disliked traits in their children or how they behaved despite every effort. Some found it difficult to cope with physical disabilities or emotional issues such as depression, openly stating that they couldn't wait for their children to be old enough to move out.

Some felt that they regretted becoming their child's parent because they did not believe themselves to be a good enough parent. This was rarely along the lines of what we all sometimes feel – that we don't say the right things or put the time in. It was more about major things such as being in prison, gambling away family money or being an alcoholic. Mental health issues in parents often featured strongly in this category. Some felt that due to their own upbringing they had no understanding or role model of how to parent, meaning life was chaotic with Social Services or others involved.

Many parents who feel this way state that they feel they have to publicly add on the tagline *'but I love him and wouldn't want things to change'*... when in fact they don't love their child and really would like things to change.

Most research in this area focuses on mothers, but the research that does open this up to both parents finds that mothers and fathers can both experience these feelings of regret. Women often find it more difficult, however. In part this is due to societal attitudes that do not censure a father who simply walks away compared to a mother.

It also stems from the fact that traditional pressures from society shape most families. Mothers feel pressure to be around and care for their baby intensively when they are born, while fathers feel pressure to work harder and earn more money. This gives fathers an 'outlet' – a reason to be away from their baby. It can be badged as providing for the family rather than having to admit that you'd really rather not be parenting.[7]

What do you do?

Know that you are not alone for a start – there are more and more articles about parents openly admitting how they feel. Take this article in the *Guardian* newspaper for example: www.theguardian.com/lifeandstyle/2017/feb/11/ breaking-taboo-parents-who-regret-having-children. There is also a Facebook page that doesn't seem active but has lots of useful posts www.facebook.com/ IRegretHavingChildren. And a Quora thread on what it's like to regret having children www.quora.com/What-is-it-like-to-regret-having-children.

Another common tactic appears to be 'fake it until you make it'... hoping that perhaps one day that if you just try hard enough and smile and engage enough that love will follow. This has mixed results but gives hope. Although if you are struggling with the demands of parenting rather than not wanting to be a parent, know that things will change and develop. They won't be this way forever.

You can also explore whether, if it is circumstance, anything can change. Are any small changes feasible that would carve out time for you or some additional distance? If you can afford it, childcare will not harm them and will give you much-needed space.

It could also help to step back and recognise that society places pressures on women in particular to feel a certain way. Feminists have long highlighted how guilt is used to shape women's behaviour, particularly as mothers, pressurising and encouraging women to think of guilt and motherhood as going hand in hand. Women are praised – subtly and otherwise – for admitting their guilt at not being 'good enough' mothers. Love for your children, alongside willingness to sacrifice everything, is seen as synonymous with femininity.[8]

Part four

"Let's talk about your postnatal body"

Pregnancy, birth and the postnatal period are not only some of the most demanding experiences for your mental health, but also for your physical wellbeing.

Frazzled by the new experience and exhausted by a lack of sleep, it's really easy to slip into a pattern where you're not able to take care of yourself. And this can have a knock-on impact on your energy, physical wellbeing and mental health.

There are many small changes you can make to help yourself regain strength, energy and thrive after you've had a baby. The emphasis is on 'small'. This isn't the time for weird crash diets and starting endurance running (unless you happened to be an endurance runner before pregnancy). It's about looking after yourself and nourishing your body with the right foods, exercise and rest (where possible). It's about being aware of symptoms that suggest something may not be quite right and finding the support you need to fix that.

Never feel guilty about taking the time and effort to do this for yourself. Remember the messages at the start of the book. It is absolutely okay to put yourself first and take the time you need to focus on yourself in terms of diet, physical activity and just generally looking after your body. You have gone through big physical changes – which may have depleted your resources and left you feeling weak in all sorts of places. Helping your body recover is a vital part of not only having the energy to care for your baby, but also to prevent injury and ill-health in the future. Don't see it as a nice optional extra or something that can wait – put it in the same category as brushing your teeth (hopefully an everyday thing!).

It's also about looking at your body in a different way. Ignore the media and articles about getting your pre-baby body back. Your body is still your body and it just grew an entire new human being. Focus on its strengths and your strength. Look at what it can do and give yourself time. Remember that regaining strength and eating and exercising to thrive not only helps you physically, but also supports your mental health and wellbeing. You matter!

Chapter twenty-one

Pains, posture and pelvic floors – recovering physically from your birth

→ Your body spent nine months changing during pregnancy before you had either a vaginal delivery or a caesarean section. Both stress the body in different ways. You're now carrying round a small human being, bending and stooping and tiptoeing about the place trying not to wake them up. Is it any wonder that many women experience aches, pains and weaknesses after birth?

Pain is linked to a number of different elements of your pregnancy and birth. You are more likely to (although not everyone will) experience postnatal pain if you had:

- Symphysis pubis dysfunction (SPD) during pregnancy (also known as pelvic girdle pain or PGP)
- A caesarean section or assisted vaginal delivery
- A long pushing stage
- An epidural

> **" Take time and focus on rest and not feeling pressure to be back out there doing it all. "**

If you are experiencing pain, or even if you aren't, the key to becoming stronger and fitter again after pregnancy is to give it time, go slowly and work on strengthening muscles that may have become weaker during pregnancy and birth. Gentle postnatal exercises focusing on your pelvic floor (more on this in a bit) and stomach muscles should be at the core(!) of this.

Physically recovering from the birth

Whether you've had a vaginal birth or caesarean section things are going to be tender and painful for a while. It takes time for bruising and swelling to go down and stitches to heal. Be kind to yourself and treat yourself like you would any patient after an operation. Take time and focus on rest and not feeling pressure to be back out there doing it all.

Some tips for easing pain from a vaginal birth include:

- Keeping a jug or small bottle of water by the toilet and squirting it over your labia and perineum when you have a wee – it helps stop any stinging from tears, cuts or stitches.
- Try a sitz bath – run a bath just deep enough to cover your hips. Keep the water warm. This can soothe your perineum, help stitches heal and also keep everything clean. It's also great if you have post-pushing haemorrhoids.
- You can buy cooling pads that you put in the freezer and then pop in your pants. Not glamorous but definitely cooling and soothing on your perineum and any stitches.
- You can buy or hire something known as a valley cushion – essentially a supportive cushion that is designed to let you sit comfortably without putting pressure on your perineum. Some local NCT groups have them for hire. These are better than the 'donut' cushions you might see as they help air circulate more freely.
- You can take paracetamol or ibuprofen to help with the pain (if you were able to take these before pregnancy).

'Normal' post-delivery pain should get better gradually, a little more each day or in leaps over a few days. If you are still in pain six weeks after birth speak to your GP.

If you've had a caesarean section the NHS advise:[1]

- Gently clean and dry your wound and don't wear tight clothing around it. Watch closely for any signs of infection such as increased pain, redness, swelling or a nasty smell and contact your midwife or GP immediately.
- It's important to try and remain active and move around – but gently. You should have been supported to get up and move around in the hospital after birth. Ask for support getting up and down from your chair if possible in the early days, or ask your partner to pass your baby to you.
- Don't carry anything heavier than your baby, try and move furniture or lift things.
- In terms of more strenuous things like driving, exercise and sex the advice is that if you feel ready and comfortable then you are probably fine – and vice versa. However, check with your car insurance company as some have different rules. You need to be recovered enough to know you could stop abruptly in an emergency.
- Take painkillers for the pain – there is no need to tough it out! These might be prescribed to you or you can take over-the-counter painkillers.
- Be kind to yourself – remember you have had an operation.

How long am I going to bleed for?

Bleeding after birth – or to give it its technical name of lochia – can come as a shock. It's surprisingly common in a first pregnancy not to know this is going to happen, but it does, even if you've had a caesarean section. The lochia is your body getting rid of all the extra tissue, mucus and blood that lined your enlarged uterus, and the site where your placenta was attached to your womb is healing. Bleeding can last for around six weeks after birth.

At first the flow will be heavy and red and you may have some clots. It will become browner and lighter over time – usually after a couple of weeks or so. Clots are normal, but if you have any large ones or are worried, tell your midwife. You can save them to show them. You'll probably find the bleeding seems heavier in the morning as you've been lying down. Also, exercise (even gentle) can make it heavier. You might find it increases with each breastfeed as breastfeeding gently contracts the uterus. You will probably need super-absorbent maternity pads at first, but can probably move to normal sanitary towels after it slows down. Don't use tampons for lochia as they can increase the risk of infection.

If the bleeding is very heavy after birth tell your midwife – it could be a postpartum haemorrhage. If it becomes very heavy or you start to feel unwell with a fever or feel shaky, have pain in your uterus that isn't like period pain, or your lochia starts to smell, do contact your midwife, health visitor or GP. It could be the sign of an infection or something known as retained placenta – where part of your placenta is stuck inside.

If you do experience a postpartum haemorrhage or retained placenta be aware that it can affect your milk supply if breastfeeding. A lot of blood loss may lead to a lower milk supply initially. Similarly, a retained placenta can lead to a delay in milk production, because it is the removal of the placenta that leads to the drop in progesterone that helps kick-start milk supply. If this happens to you, don't panic: your supply is delayed rather than missing. Speak to your midwife for more support, keep feeding your baby as much as possible and keep an eye on your baby's weight. If it does drop, make sure you get support from a specialist (see Chapter 9).

In terms of when your periods will return, if you're not breastfeeding they'll probably be back at around 6–8 weeks. So remember you need contraception if you don't want to get pregnant again! If you are breastfeeding exclusively – giving your baby only breastmilk and no formula on top – and are feeding them whenever they want, including at night, and are not using a dummy in between feeds, the chances are your periods won't come back until your baby starts solids or starts sleeping all the way through the night, or maybe even later. Breastfeeding in this way has also been shown to have a 98% contraceptive effect (i.e. as high as condoms but less hassle) in the first six months after birth as long as your periods haven't returned. However, some women do find that their period returns sooner, and remember you will ovulate before you see your periods are back. So if you definitely don't want another baby yet, be careful!

Did I just have another contraction?

Afterpains feel like mild (ish) contractions. They happen as your uterus reduces to close to its pre-pregnancy state. You might find they are more common during feeds if you are breastfeeding, as the action of your baby suckling helps stimulate the uterus to contract. A bonus is that breastfeeding helps this happen more quickly and efficiently. You might find afterpains a mild annoyance, or you might benefit from a heat pad and over-the-counter painkillers. They unfortunately appear to get worse with each baby (why does no one tell you this?). But thankfully they don't mean that there's another baby in there trying to get out, even if it feels like it.

Why am I sweating so much?!

Another 'normal' and common experience postnatally is to sweat lots, especially at night as your body gets back to normal. This is thought to be linked to the drop in oestrogen after birth (a bit like hot flushes during the menopause). It also helps you get rid of any excess fluid (your blood and other bodily fluids increase by about 50% during pregnancy) that is no longer needed. On a positive you'll also see a drop on the scales as this happens.

Excess sweating should pass by around six weeks, with a peak at around two weeks postpartum. If it carries on, especially if you're feeling shaky or anxious and losing weight quickly, check with your GP about thyroid issues (more on this later). The usual tips for staying cool apply: try cool clothes in natural fabrics, keeping windows open and air circulating (maybe not in deepest winter), drink lots of cold water, try avoiding foods that can raise your temperature such as alcohol, caffeine and spicy foods, and make liberal use of fans. And remind yourself it will pass!

There is some evidence that hot flushes are more common if you have symptoms of anxiety and depression. Some think that changes in brain physiology during anxiety or depression increase the occurrence of hot flushes. Others think that the experience of hot flushes, if extreme, can increase symptoms of anxiety and depression. In either case do speak to your GP if you are feeling this way.[2]

And my hair's falling out?!
Yes, sorry. Glamourous, isn't it? The drop in hormone levels after the birth means you start to shed some hair. Don't panic – you probably noticed your hair becoming thicker in pregnancy and this is just it returning to normal and starting a new cycle.

Back and pelvic pain
One study found that back pain is very common in postnatal women, with 68% reporting significant back pain at eight weeks postpartum and 60% at eight months. It's unsurprising really given the stresses your body has been under. Taking care of your back is really important. Some ways you can reduce the chances of it hurting are:

- No carrying, lifting or moving heavy stuff in the early days and weeks.
- Make sure you bring your baby to your breast if you're breastfeeding, rather than your breast to the baby – no leaning over or hunching up.
- Change your baby's nappy either on the floor while you sit down or on a higher surface where you're not leaning down to them. Likewise kneel down rather than lean over your baby if you're bathing them.
- Try not to carry your baby on one hip all the time – swap hips or ideally get a comfortable sling.

You might also still be experiencing some pelvic pain if you suffered from SPD or PGP during pregnancy. If you had this painful condition it can take a while for things to return to normal after the birth. You may well feel some relief after giving birth, but it is likely that it will take several weeks for the pain to gradually reduce and you feel close to normal again. Be gentle with yourself and do whatever helps with the pain. If it doesn't get better speak to your GP.

You might also like to think about visiting an osteopath or chiropractor to help you with any aches, pains or posture issues. It can help straighten out any issues (pun intended) which might be putting strain on your joints or muscles.

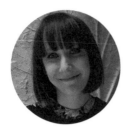

The benefits of osteopathy for new parents

Emma Hayward M.Ost DPO is an osteopath and specialist paediatric osteopath based in Kent and London. She works closely with lactation consultants to help with breastfeeding, infant feeding and supporting mother and baby wellbeing and is also a volunteer breastfeeding peer supporter. Emma is also a trained Pilates teacher and uses movement and osteopathy to support postnatal recovery and women's health throughout a woman and her family's lifetime. You can find her clinic Emma Hayward Osteopathy at www.emmahayward.co.uk.

What is osteopathy?

Osteopathy is a form of manual therapy that endeavours to support the body to maintain health and recover from injury using hands-on treatment – some of this therapeutic touch is very gentle and still (cranial osteopathy) and sometimes it involves stronger massaging, stretching and joint mobilising. All of it is aimed at supporting your body to function well by releasing areas of strain or tension that prevent you from recovering.

Osteopaths train for at least four years at university and are trained to diagnose and triage alongside bespoke treatment. In the UK we are Allied Health Professionals alongside physiotherapists and occupational therapists. Some osteopaths go on to do extensive postgraduate study in the fields of paediatrics and women's health, but all osteopaths are qualified to treat everyone from birth throughout life.

Why see an osteopath if you've had a baby?

There are many reasons a new mother might come to see an osteopath. Supporting your postpartum recovery will help your baby, but that's not why you should see an osteopath. You should see one because you matter. You being comfortable matters right from the start.

How we feel in our bodies matters. It matters to how we relate to the world around us. How easily we can self-regulate. How easily we can relate to others. When we feel comfortable we feel more at ease, are more able to interact externally, more able to manage. Of course this helps you connect with your baby and helps you help them to self-regulate, but regardless of your baby, your feelings and your body matter.

During pregnancy, our bodies undergo huge postural changes. The nine months of pregnancy takes well over a year to 'recover from'. The changes we go through take time to reintegrate, reorganise and heal. We are encouraged to 'bounce back' and 'lose the baby weight' by the media and society. I want to offer a new narrative. Our bodies are incredible, beautiful and powerful and deserve this reverence. Honouring this time of recovery is important, as is seeking out support for pain and dysfunction. There is so much help available and osteopathy can be part of it.

Childbirth is an intensely physical event, however our children are born, whether that be vaginally or abdominally. With a vaginal delivery, the whole of a woman's body works hard to open and move her baby into the outside world. A woman's body and her baby do a beautiful dance together, as her baby navigates its way through her pelvis and pelvic floor.

When I see a woman after a vaginal delivery, there are many things I assess and treat. I will look at how her whole body is integrated together. Strains can occur in the pelvis, particularly with very long or very quick births, and with any injury to the pelvic floor. However, the whole body can be affected and it's not uncommon to see neck and jaw strains after birth too. These can be easily resolved with skilled osteopathic treatment. Treatment of the pelvis and pelvic floor has been shown to be an effective intervention for women with urinary incontinence, and I see postpartum work as an important part of supporting a woman's health right through the rest of her life.

With abdominal birth or c-section, a woman will have also been through major abdominal surgery and perhaps other strain from pregnancy and labour. Many osteopaths are also trained in scar tissue release work and visceral techniques (specific abdominal massage-type techniques). This is such important work to have done after a c-section. It will support tissue healing, but also reduce any pain, and adhesions around the scar that can then go on to cause local pain but can also cause problems elsewhere in the back, hips or even with organ function.

Supporting women after traumatic birth is essential too. Therapeutic touch after trauma can be part of the healing process. Safe touch can be soothing to your nervous system and help you to safely reconnect with your body. This is all part of what women's health osteopaths work with. Whether you are two weeks or 22 years postpartum, your body holds all your experiences. Working with our bodies to release the physical strains can gently allow space for processing our birth experiences.

Can osteopathy support breastfeeding?
Osteopaths often work in breastfeeding. It's not uncommon to be told to take

your baby to see a 'cranial osteopath' by a midwife or lactation consultant. There is much we can do to support a baby to be able to achieve better positioning and attachment in terms of reducing strains through their body, neck and jaw. Osteopathy can be a huge piece of the puzzle when resolving breastfeeding difficulties.

However, breastfeeding isn't just about a baby. It's about the two of you – the dyad. There are many things I look at when working with a breastfeeding mother. 'Breastfeeding neck' anyone? Learning to breastfeed takes time and care and making sure your baby latches well can cause a lot of neck strain. Craning your neck to see their latch, and holding tension in your neck and shoulders if there is any pain or anxiety associated with feeding, all contribute. Neck and mid-back pain are very common postnatally from the increased demands on this part of your body as you feed and care for your baby (on broken sleep). However, common doesn't mean 'put up with it!' This discomfort is very treatable and pain often improves very quickly with hands-on treatment and management advice from your osteopath.

We also can look at treating the chest and breasts themselves. While there are several causes of breast pain when feeding, one cause is due to blood vessel constriction due to chest muscle spasm/contraction. This can be improved with osteopathic treatment, as can recovery from blocked ducts and mastitis. While these are due to the breast not being effectively drained by the baby, an osteopath can support tissue healing and fluid drainage around the chest and breast which can reduce engorgement and speed up recovery by improving lymphatic drainage.

What about osteopathy for partners?
Osteopathy isn't just for the birthing parent. Working with families is wonderful work. Each member influences all the others and helping one will help all. The physicality of caring for a new baby, alongside the huge emotional transition, can influence the health and wellbeing of both parents. It's very common for me to see male or female partners for back pain when their partner is pregnant or postpartum. Caring for your loved one and holding the weight of this transition can be deeply stressful (as well as deeply joyful). Stress absolutely impacts our physical body. Our breathing changes, our muscles are more tense, and we don't sleep as deeply.
All these factors and more can prime us for physical strain or injury. So often in my practice, I see people with back and neck pain or other injury, with a huge life stressor alongside, such as job uncertainty, a home move, or a new baby. So be kind to yourself if you are going through a challenging or transitional time. Self-care can be so important, and beyond that, or perhaps part of it, can be getting support and care from an osteopath.

What happens during a typical session?

In your first session with an osteopath they will chat to you about why you have come in and about your general and historical health. They will want to get a sense of what your body has been through, as often our bodies 'keep the score' of all these accumulative life events, as well as giving us an indication of how quickly your body might recover.

They will then assess you to form a working diagnosis. The assessment will involve watching you do certain movements and then placing their hands on you to assess your joints and muscles and do any neurological testing that is indicated, such as reflex testing.

If it's appropriate (i.e. you don't need a medical referral), and with your consent, they will do hands-on treatment. This may be very gentle holding (which is seen in cranial osteopathy), massage-type techniques, stretching or mobilising joints. Most people need a few appointments to recover from injury, although this can vary depending on the cause and other factors. Your osteopath can discuss your personal case with you in terms of expected management.

Where can I find out more?

In the UK the vast majority of osteopaths work in private practice and you will be able to self-refer directly. A small number work in GP practices within the NHS.

Osteopathy is a registered profession and all osteopaths in the UK are registered with the General Osteopathic Council, which has a list of all osteopaths and their practice locations on its website. Many osteopaths are also members of the Institute of Osteopathy and there is also a list of members on the website. There are also other smaller training organisations such as the Osteopathic Centre for Children. This organisation trains osteopaths in paediatrics and offers a postgraduate Diploma. A list of alumni is on the website.

Your pelvic floor

Pregnancy and birth can cause issues with your pelvic floor either temporarily or longer term. This is caused simply by the growing weight of your baby pushing on your bladder, moving it around and increasing the size of the neck of your bladder opening. Most pregnant women therefore end up needing to urinate more frequently, struggling to urinate fully or in some cases having some urinary incontinence both during pregnancy and in the early months as their body recovers.

However, research shows that for *most* women this goes away by the time their baby is 10 months old. I know, you're asking what you're meant to do for 10 months, but it is at least reassuring that for most women the problem is temporary. Unfortunately, some women are left with longer-term problems, including pain and discomfort, urinary and anal incontinence, an overactive bladder and pelvic organ prolapse.

Some women are at a genetic risk of this becoming a longer-term issue. Some research suggests that these women may be at risk of longer-term changes to the collagen and other connective tissues in the pelvic floor, which mean it doesn't return to normal after your baby is born. Birth can also play a role. Although women who have a caesarean section can also experience pelvic floor issues (due to changes in pregnancy), the process of a vaginal birth does increase the risk of future issues. As your baby was born they would have stretched the muscles, nerves and fascia of your pelvic floor. Any tearing appears to increase the risk. Therefore women who have had a very large baby (particularly a large head), a longer pushing stage or a forceps delivery are more at risk of longer-term issues, alongside birth complications such as significant tearing or shoulder dystocia.[4]

The good news is that for most women, the right support and exercises will improve things. In particular, a systematic review found that pelvic floor exercises do work to reduce urinary incontinence, particularly if you use a vaginal device that provides resistance or feedback against your squeezing.[5]

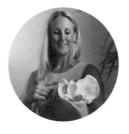

Strengthening your pelvic floor

Jo Perkins is a sports medicine physiotherapist specialising in women's and pelvic health. After her first baby, which was an assisted birth, she was shocked at how little support there seemed to be for regaining strength in the pelvic floor and core system. She now works with women in pregnancy and postnatally to help them restore their bodies. She can be found at www.mummaphysio.co.uk.

After an assisted first birth, I was really shocked at how I felt postnatally, not only in terms of some of the symptoms I experienced, but also because the routine rehabilitation processes that I applied to every other injury in sport seemed not to exist for women postnatally. There was a real culture of 'just get on with it' and I was very naive to think that being a physiotherapist would make me exempt from changes to my body. It was only after a failed return to running that I realised that of course I need to prepare my pelvic floor and core system for returning to impact, just like I would prepare my hamstring if I had torn it.

This sparked a real passion for women's health, and through further training, combined with my sports medicine background, I developed my own rehabilitation strategies, which allowed me to get back into running and complete a marathon without symptoms that had once plagued me. I went on to have my son in 2018 and had an entirely different pre and postnatal experience using my rehabilitation strategies.

What are the pelvic floor muscles?

The pelvic floor can still be a bit of a taboo subject, and many women aren't told about its significance in pregnancy, postpartum and for long-term health. However, it is important to understand that the pelvic floor forms an important part of everyone's core (including women who haven't had children and men!) There is a misconception that our 'core' only refers to our abdominals, but it actually includes the interplay of lots of different muscles.

Think of your core as a cylinder, which has a top (diaphragm muscle), front (deep abdominals), bottom (pelvic floor) and back (back muscles). These muscles work together in a coordinated way with our breathing to not only remain continent, but move efficiently and without pain by managing our intraabdominal pressure. We need our pelvic floor to automatically respond to larger increases in pressure like when we cough, sneeze, lift something heavy, run or jump.

Furthermore, the pelvic floor is just like any other muscle in the body; it has a blood supply and responds to strengthening programmes. It can get weak, injured or stretched, too tight or overused. It is the floor of our pelvis, layered up in deep and superficial muscles to support us. The muscles of the pelvic floor run from our tailbone at the back, to our sitting bones on the side and pubic bone on the front, forming a diamond shape. This is important to know so that you ensure you are recruiting all parts of the pelvic floor when doing strengthening exercises.

How might I know I have a pelvic floor issue?
Signs and symptoms of pelvic floor dysfunction can vary greatly between women and can include, to varying degrees:

- incontinence (faecal or urinary)
- pelvic, low back or hip pain
- heaviness, pressure or dragging in the pelvic area
- pain during sex
- pain inserting tampons
- constipation
- abdominal pain, which often worsens with exertion or exercise
- difficulty fully emptying your bladder or bowel
- the feeling that you need to have several bowel movements during a short period of time
- a frequent need to urinate. When you do go, you may stop and start many times

Some women may only find they leak with a full bladder if they sneeze, for example, whereas for others it can be a regular occurrence throughout the day, which can be hugely upsetting and demoralising.

What can I do about it?
The most important thing is to not suffer in silence. A whole host of people help and support women, and the bridge between rehabilitation concepts applied in sports medicine and those for women postpartum is becoming established. It is something we are talking about more openly, removing the stigma of incontinence and encouraging women to prioritise their own recovery like they would from any other injury or operation. You should never be told 'it's normal to leak' or 'you'll never run again after you've had a baby'.

Incontinence isn't unusual postpartum, particularly in the early days. Unless you have been told otherwise or have a catheter in, you should start doing pelvic floor exercises straight away, aiming for 10-second holds × 10, followed by 10 quick on/off contractions. You should aim to do this three times a day.

The NHS 'squeezy app' is a really useful resource to help guide your pelvic floor exercises. Start lying down, with less weight going through your healing tissues, then progress to more upright postures. This will help get your fundamental strength back. This connection can take a while, so don't worry if initially you don't feel you can get a contraction or you can't hold it for very long. You will have to work up to the 10-second holds but stick with it and you will start to feel a connection and strength return, as well as your continence.

It is always worth getting a women's health physiotherapy assessment to give you a more thorough idea of how your pelvic floor muscles are working and a bespoke rehabilitation plan. Everyone will recover at different rates, and you are not exempt from pelvic floor issues if you had a caesarean, as your pelvic floor still had increasing pressure on it for nine months, as well as the trauma to your abdominals.

When we exhale, our pelvic floor is naturally recruited so try and do your contractions then, rather than holding your breath which can raise your intraabdominal pressure. It is also important to practise something we call 'the knack', which means pre-contracting your pelvic floor prior to a sneeze or cough. This helps train the pelvic floor to respond automatically like it used to.

Also think about exhaling when you lift the buggy and car seat, recruiting your pelvic floor as well. The next stage is to progressively load your core system with movement, or weights, before returning to running or jumping, just as you would if you were returning after a hamstring tear, for example.

If you have symptoms that indicate your pelvic floor is overactive, such as constipation, pain with tampons or sex, or difficulty fully emptying bladder or bowels, it is important to focus on diaphragmatic breathing, allowing the muscles to relax. A women's health physiotherapist can assist with this and give you exercises and treatments.

Chapter twenty-two

Eating for strength, health and wellbeing

→ Eating a well-balanced, nutrient-rich diet is important for anyone's health and wellbeing, but especially so when you're a new parent. Sleep deprivation, stresses and strains and general exhaustion from caring for someone else can all place stress on your body. Therefore, giving it a fighting chance with a good diet really helps. The usual rules apply: eat foods that are going to benefit your body and mood rather than junk and empty calories, lots of fruit and veg, whole grains and seeds, and lean proteins. There is, however, nothing wrong with the occasional cake/burger/wine – whatever takes your fancy. It is about balance and also being kind to yourself.

What about going on a diet?

I'm going to sound really boring here. Yes, absolutely you can lose weight as a new parent, but the key is to go slowly. Crash diets or weird replacement meal substitutes are not a great idea when you're recovering from birth. You need enough energy to see you through everything. However, eating a diet rich in nutrients, cutting back on junk food and making sure you're not eating huge

> **" Crash diets or weird replacement meal substitutes are not a great idea when you're recovering from birth. "**

amounts of food so you lose weight at a safe rate of around 1–2 pounds per week is fine.

You can also lose weight if you are breastfeeding, but again the emphasis is on doing it slowly. How many calories a day you need depends on your height and weight and how active you are, but reducing daily calories below 1,500 per day while exercising is not advised. Focus on eating nutrient-rich foods to keep your energy up.

Breastfeeding uses up around 500 calories per day and it used to be thought that this would automatically help with weight loss, or that you could eat that much more. Newer research suggests that for some breastfeeding women the body slows down the metabolism, meaning they see no real impact of breastfeeding on their weight. It makes sense really – our bodies think that if we reduce our food then there must be a food shortage, so they try to preserve as much energy as possible.

Across the whole population of women, breastfeeding can help you lose weight in the months after birth. However, it doesn't seem to have an even impact. Some women find the pregnancy weight drops off, while others find their body seems to hold onto it until they stop breastfeeding – again most likely to make sure the baby is protected by there being enough energy for milk production. Also, although headlines might like to suggest that breastfeeding leads to amazing weight loss, the actual data shows there is only an average of around 1–2 kilos difference in weight between women who breastfeed or don't at six months postpartum.[1]

There are a number of reasons why restrictive diets are not a great idea, particularly when you've just had a baby:

1. Diet can affect your mood and energy

A very low-calorie diet or one that is missing a lot of nutrients can affect your mood. It has been linked to everything from low energy and feeling down, to mental health difficulties, particularly with anxiety and depression. Diets that are high in sugar and carbohydrates such as white bread and rice are associated with higher levels of low mood, low energy, anxiety and depression.[2] Meanwhile, a diet high in fruit and vegetables, seeds and nuts, eggs and lean meat and fish is linked to better mood and higher energy.[3] Restrictive diets can also lead to or exacerbate nutrient deficiencies, which can give you a whole host of physical and cognitive symptoms. For more details see Chapter 24.

2. Diet can affect aches and pains

Again, foods high in sugar and carbohydrates are associated with increased inflammation and pain in the body.[4] A diet high in saturated fat is associated with increased joint and muscle pain.[5] Meanwhile, a Mediterranean-style diet high in fruit and vegetables, whole grains, fish and olive oils can help with joint pain.[6] Spices such as turmeric and ginger not only taste nice, but help in reducing inflammation in the body, reducing pain and also stress levels.[7] Inflammation in the body can be particularly high in new parents due to sleep deprivation and stress, so eating to reduce this can really help you feel better.

3. You're more likely to break a very restrictive diet

I know it's boring, but losing weight is about doing so steadily and making real lifestyle changes you can stick to once you've lost the weight. Crash diets or ones that eliminate foods make you more likely to snap and binge eat, which leads to increased weight. Typically, the foods you end up craving are the ones that lower your mood and increase pain.[8] Slow and steady really does win the race.

Some ideas for healthy eating

It can be really tough to get the balance right while you have a small baby to care for. Here are some top tips:

- If you're home with the baby all day ask your partner to help prepare some healthy, nutrient-rich snacks you can eat easily throughout the day. Also look at those snack box subscriptions you can get that focus on healthy snacks such as nuts, seeds and fruit. Expensive, but so easy.
- If people ask whether you need anything, or ask what sort of baby gift you would like, you could suggest high-quality healthy snacks (ready-prepared fruits, nuts and seeds, for example), either home-made or bought from upmarket retailers.
- If you are struggling to prepare healthy meals you could focus on nutrient-rich fresh ready meals (they do exist), a meal delivery kit or try to order healthier takeaway options. There are all sorts of great food box delivery services now that have all the ingredients you need ready chopped. They are expensive, but cheaper than takeaways every night.
- Ask friends or family if they can help if you're struggling. Also, batch cooking of healthy easy to heat portions for the freezer really does help even if you don't feel like it.
- Use supplements carefully. A high-quality multivitamin can help plug the gap. It should contain vitamin D3 as lots of people are deficient, especially by March due to a general lack of sun.
- If you have any symptoms such as feeling very sluggish, aches and pains, brain fog and weight gain, it's worth thinking about whether you might have any nutrient deficiency. More details in Chapter 24.

Finally, realise that everything is a spectrum. Diet is not an either/or. It's

> **" Focus on what you can add to your diet in terms of nutrients rather than what you take away. "**

the broader pattern of what you do. Increasing the amount of nutrient-rich foods you eat is better than nothing, even if you can't eat as much as might be recommended. Focus on what you can add to your diet in terms of nutrients rather than what you take away. Eating a healthy takeaway is better than a less healthy takeaway. Mental health also matters – don't make yourself miserable in the name of a supposedly perfect diet.

I'm feeling really miserable about how I look

Pregnancy and birth is a time of huge change for your body, both what you can see on the outside and inside. You're not alone in feeling unhappy about the changes. Body dissatisfaction during pregnancy and after birth is sadly very common and can last long after your baby is born. In some research we did with pregnant women we found that 60% were worried about losing their baby weight, 68% were worried about the effect of pregnancy on their body and 56% frequently compared their body to others.[9]

The media of course play a significant role in whipping all of this up. Almost every day there seems to be a feature about some celebrity or other who is either vowing to lose the baby weight, losing the baby weight, or indeed has just lost the baby weight. Newspapers and websites are full of stories praising women who supposedly look like they've never had a baby. And baby magazine covers portray photos of smiling, rested, sparkly mothers and babies (where the baby is often just draped in a white towel... why?!). Our study found that the more women used social media, the worse they felt about their bodies.

None of this is real. Okay, maybe for a very small percentage of the population it is realistic (with the right lighting and a baby who happens to have slept through miraculously for a few days). But for most women? Far from it. Images on social media are rarely the true picture. We know this, don't we? If you post on social media, do you genuinely just take one photo of yourself and post it regardless? Or do you take several... choose the best... maybe crop them... or even filter them before you post? Yet somehow, despite many of us selecting or altering our own photos, we seem to think others don't do it! It's all a blurred, altered and well-shot version of reality.

Give yourself a break, and know that all this is designed to create unhappiness and anxiety because that's what sells products. The pressure is all part of a huge industry based on making women feel insecure about their bodies in new and ingenious ways. You can buy all sorts of (expensive) treatments for worries you never knew you had. These range from the fairly innocuous 'anti-ageing golden collagen crystal masks for firming, skin nourishing, fine lines and wrinkle removal' for your cleavage, through to the horrendous-sounding nipple-bleaching kits, which recommend you first exfoliate your nipples. And it is gendered. Sure, there are articles about 'dad bods', but on balance they're humorous, accepting and full of stats about how many women apparently prefer them.

Your body just literally created a baby from tiny cells. We should be celebrating this and any changes, seeing it as a sign of power. Eat to nourish yourself and make yourself feel better. Exercise to feel stronger, fitter and happier. But don't starve yourself because society wants to keep women in their place. Know that most women have stretch marks, and most of them on social media have filters.

Focus instead on positive imagery of what bodies look like after having a baby. Check out the following links:

- My Post Baby Body **mypostbabybody.org**
- The Shape of a Mother **theshapeofamother.com**
- The 4th Trimester Bodies Project **www.4thtrimesterbodiesproject.com**
- The Take Back Postpartum Instagram account **www.instagram. comtakebackpostpartum**
- The #celebrating_my_postpartum and #bodyafterbaby hashtags on Instagram

What if I'm breastfeeding?

You might have a lot of questions about whether what you eat and drink affects your milk. The good news is that, in general, eating a well-balanced diet is important for your health and wellbeing, but does not have any real effect on how much milk you produce, its content or its safety.

Does diet affect my milk?

Not really, no. Research shows that as long as you are not very underweight and are not restricting your eating too much with really weird diets, it won't affect how much milk you make. Your diet also doesn't need to be perfect to make nutrient-rich breastmilk. The human body is very adaptable. Bear in mind that many women around the world have nutrient-poor diets or find it hard to get enough energy, yet breastfeed just fine. Research into diet and volume and content of milk finds no real link apart from a small suggestion that consumption of omega-3 might increase the levels of omega-3 in milk, although research is not conclusive. You might like to eat a diet including oily fish or take a supplement for the additional health benefits, but there is no clear evidence it 'improves' your milk.[10]

However, just like in pregnancy your body will take what it needs to prioritise your baby, so if you are not eating a well-balanced diet while breastfeeding you will start to feel run down. So eating a balanced diet helps support your health. Remember you matter too!

There is a lot of debate about whether your baby can react to certain foods you eat. Some women find their baby does seem to react. If your baby seems unsettled you could try to identify what in your diet might be causing it and then eliminate it to see if the symptoms go away. This is really tricky though, especially for things like cows' milk, and the evidence is not clear. I recommend you talk to a breastfeeding specialist before trying it. For more details see Chapter 9.

Can I drink coffee?

Yes! Caffeine does transfer to your breastmilk, but not in huge amounts. Although it can differ slightly between women, only around 1% of what you drink will get into your milk. It is unlikely that your baby will be affected, unless you are consuming over 750mg of caffeine a day. This is equivalent to around five cups of coffee, but that does depend on the size of your cup (1.5 large coffee chain cups can put you at 750mg). Caffeine is also found in other drinks, and indeed in some foods. These include tea (including green tea), sports drinks and even some bottled waters. Also check herbal remedies and medications. Chocolate can have quite a lot of caffeine in it too. Some babies will react to caffeine by becoming more unsettled. If they do you can simply cut back and the caffeine will leave their system too.

Can I drink alcohol?

Yes, if you'd like an alcoholic drink there is no reason why you can't do so if you breastfeed and the NHS agrees that 'an occasional drink is unlikely to harm your baby'. Drinking too much is not advised due to the impact on your health, but is unlikely to affect your baby unless you are consuming very large amounts regularly.[11]

Alcohol does get into your breastmilk, but at very low levels. The level of alcohol in your milk will be the same level that is in your bloodstream. If you have, for example, a 175ml glass of 11% wine, that's roughly two units. Your blood alcohol level will be affected by your gender and weight, but on average that glass of wine would give you a blood alcohol level of 0.04. To put it in perspective, any drink with 0.05% or less alcohol in it is considered 'alcohol free', and anything between 0.5% and 1.2% is considered 'low alcohol'. So a drink or two isn't going to affect your milk.

Although research shows that alcohol in breastmilk can have a small impact on a baby's development, the research is based on much higher levels of drinking – like a bottle of wine every night drinking. When you get into that territory it's really difficult to say that any effect is just due to the alcohol – it's likely that other factors that are causing someone with a young baby to drink a bottle of wine every night are playing a role too.[12]

Really, the main thing to worry about when it comes to alcohol and breastfeeding is whether you are safe to hold your baby. You accidentally dropping or suffocating your baby is more of a risk if you have had several drinks – and you should never co-sleep after drinking alcohol. But if we are talking about an occasional drink and it isn't affecting your behaviour (or you have more but someone else is looking after the baby), then it's fine.

The other thing to remember is that alcohol doesn't stay in your breastmilk, it is metabolised and leaves your milk just like it leaves your blood. Alcohol leaves your bloodstream at the rate of roughly one unit per hour, so once it has left your bloodstream it will have left your milk too. So there is no need to 'pump and dump' (expressing milk and throwing it away), because the alcohol will be broken down over time anyway, and new milk made will continue to contain the same level of alcohol as is in your bloodstream. You might like to pump for comfort, but it isn't about getting the alcohol 'out'.

What about if I smoke?

There are many health reasons (for you and your baby) to cut down on smoking, but if you do smoke the guidance is to continue breastfeeding as it can help protect your baby. This is because the immune properties in breastmilk help decrease the risk of your baby developing an infection. Babies who live in a house with someone who smokes are at increased risk of respiratory infections, but their risk is lower if they are breastfed. Other components in your breastmilk also protect your baby. For example, smoking is associated with reduced iodine levels, but breastmilk contains iodine to support your baby.[13]

You should not smoke around your baby and ideally not in the house. Try not to feed your baby immediately after smoking as smoke will stay on your breath, hair and clothes. Nicotine does pass into your breastmilk and could make your baby unsettled. Smoking also reduces how much prolactin you produce, which can reduce your milk supply. Keep an eye on your baby's weight gain.

Will breastfeeding affect my breast shape?

Despite the rumours, breastfeeding actually has little impact on your breast size and shape long term. Studies led by plastic surgeons suggest that it is in fact pregnancy, plus naturally getting older, that leads to any change in shape. I respect those findings as I think if plastic surgeons could drum up more business, they would![14]

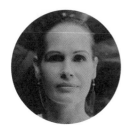

Eating your way to health and wellbeing

Magda Jenkins is a nutritional therapist specialising in all aspects of family health. She has a huge passion for supporting women as they go through pregnancy and the first year of motherhood. Her approach is holistic, drawing on wisdom from all around the world and the science of functional medicine. She works mainly with diet and also uses laboratory testing and supplements to support clients. You can find her at www. magdajenkins.com

The months following a baby's birth are an important adjustment period for everyone in the family. Many non-Western cultures consider the first months to be a special restorative and bonding time. In Ayurvedic medicine, which has its roots in ancient India, mothers are looked after by their female friends and relatives; their food is prepared for them, and any non-helping visitors are kept to a minimum. In China and Japan new mothers practice 'sitting the month' as their female relatives take over the domestic chores and bring in special restorative herbs and foods.

This level of care is rarely possible for most new mothers in the West but we can adapt these traditions and their wisdom to our lives here. I always recommend that my clients ask for as much support as possible: for friends and relatives to bring food, perhaps having a postnatal doula, or a friend to visit regularly for a chat and to hold the baby so that you have the time for something as simple as washing your hair. New mothers should not have to do it all and having this support will make a huge difference to your health and wellbeing at an important time.

For many families in the West, once the baby is born all the attention is on the baby and mothers find themselves exhausted and often with a low mood. My role as a nutritional therapist is to bring attention back to the mother by hearing about her symptoms and offering simple and effective nutritional and lifestyle tips which are relevant to her individual situation.

Good nutrition is not just about bouncing back and getting into pre-pregnancy clothes. I always remind my clients that it took nine months to grow the baby and it will take nine months – if not longer – for the body to fully readjust to life with a baby. It takes time and patience, which can be difficult with the unrealistic expectations set by the media's obsession with celebrity body shapes.

The food you eat is your medicine. It has the power to help rebuild your energy and give you the resilience you need even if you wake up several times at night to feed the baby. This will help avoid long-term postnatal depletion, which is now an officially recognised syndrome. In my practice I often see women with this syndrome: exhausted mothers whose children are already 5 or 10 because they have never had a chance to recover after giving birth.

Nutrition can help cleanse the uterus after birth and heal the tissues that have been stretched or torn during pregnancy and birth. It is needed to support breastfeeding and to optimise your and your baby's microbiomes, the microbial species in our guts which are responsible for most of our immunity, mood, hormone balance and almost every aspect of our health.

My nutritional recommendations for new families are:

- Make time to eat and listen to your body's hunger cues. Always have healthy snacks at hand with a focus on real food : granola bars and flapjacks (without refined sugars), fruit, carrot with hummus, or a soup – so you don't end up feeling exhausted and then grazing on foods which are not healthy.
- Sit down when you eat and chew your food thoroughly until it is more like a smoothie in your mouth. Digestion really begins in the mouth as it stimulates the release of digestive juices and enzymes to enable you assimilate all the nutrients.
- Always have breakfast. This will help lower stress hormones which can inhibit milk ejection reflex, and also lead to low mood and fatigue. My go-to breakfast for mums is porridge, to which you can add seeds, nuts, coconut, grated apple and berries. If you don't have time to cook breakfast, smoothies are another great option – they only take minutes to make and are an effective way of getting nutrients into your body.
  Healthy smoothie recipe, serves 1:
  ½ cup blueberries or raspberries, ½ avocado, ½ banana, handful broccoli florets, small bunch of parsley, 1 tbsp chia seeds, five Brazil nuts, a cup of water or plant milk. Blend all ingredients together in a high-speed blender, pour into a tall glass and enjoy.
- Focus on warm dishes as cooking helps assimilate nutrients especially in the first three months following the birth when your body needs to heal and during colder winter months when our digestive enzymes are naturally lower. Batchcook and freeze meals as much as you can to minimise cooking time and to maximise the time you spend with your baby. Eat stews, cooked greens, soups, slow-cooked chicken bone broths.

which are delicious as a stand-alone snack or as a base for your stews and soups, eggs and fish. Avoid large fish such as tuna and swordfish as these may have a high level of toxic metals.

- Use warming herbs such as black pepper, ginger and cinnamon which will support your blood sugar levels and eliminate any sugar cravings. If you are anaemic, and if you eat meat, I recommend consuming organ meat such as liver, which is full of iron and also B12, which is needed for your baby's brain development. If you are not too keen on the taste of liver, it can easily be 'hidden' in meatballs, shepherd's pie and chilli.

- Always have some good quality protein and fat with your main meals as this will help you stay full for longer and will balance your energy levels for the entire day. I have found that this helps many mums who are experiencing low mood, irritability and even postnatal depression. Protein is not just meat. Good sources of protein include eggs, beans, nuts, seeds, and even vegetables and legumes.

   Because life with a new baby is busy, it can be a good idea to have some hemp or pea protein to add to your drinks, smoothies and even soups. Healthy fats include butter, ghee, coconut oil and oily fish such as wild salmon and mackerel. I also recommend supplementing with good quality omega-3 as most people do not get enough from their diets; this will also help with your mood and your baby's brain health. Research shows that fatty acids in breastmilk help prevent eczema, asthma and also allergies in babies, and I always prescribe omega-3 to clients who are experiencing postnatal depression.

- Many sure you aren't drinking too much. If you are, the colour of your urine will become very pale, and when you are dehydrated your urine will become dark and have a stronger odour. I recommend drinking to thirst, avoiding cold drinks and instead sipping herbal teas and warm water throughout the day. Many women find it easier to make a large jug of herbal tea in the morning and then keep it warm in an insulated flask. The best teas for new mothers are:

  - Dandelion leaf tea, which also contains iron and is gently detoxifying. You could also pick fresh dandelion leaves and add them to salads or sauté in oil.

  - Fennel tea helps digestion and eliminates bloating and gas. I recommend steeping a tablespoon of fennel seeds in a cup of boiling water for 10 minutes to drink between meals.

  - Red clover blossom tea is useful if you are experiencing anxiety.

Most mothers I test are deficient in many micronutrients despite taking a daily multivitamin. I often see low levels of both zinc and iron, which are the main cause of dramatic hair loss and restless leg syndrome. Many of these symptoms start showing at around six months postpartum when there is a change in hormones.

Other symptoms of nutritional deficiencies include brain fog. I truly believe that nature would not willingly design mothers, the very people whose responsibility it is to raise the next generation, to have brain fog. As mothers we are meant to be growing new neurons and connections in the emotional centre of the brain, which increases our IQ! Brain fog is a symptom of not getting enough real nutrients, such as B12, either from a vegan diet without appropriate supplementation, from having low stomach acid levels, or from having an intestinal bacterial overgrowth which would need to be professionally addressed.

I recommend also checking your vitamin D levels, as it's such an important nutrient to support your immunity and healthy bones. Depending on their test results, breastfeeding mums often need to take as much as 6,000IU D3 per day.

Another important nutrient is iodine, which is essential for your baby's brain development and also protects your thyroid from postpartum thyroiditis, which affects 1 in 12 women and is the main reason why some mothers start feeling sluggish and unable to lose weight. I always test the thyroid, especially if there is an additional history of preeclampsia, postnatal depression and constipation. In my practice I see women who are unable to get up in the mornings and they have been told that this will pass. This is unacceptable, and these women are not getting the right treatment for a potentially serious condition.

It is important to test the full range of thyroid hormones – TSH, Free T4, Free T3, Reverse T3, and also TPO and TG antibodies – to help identify and navigate appropriate treatment. Seaweed is a good source of iodine – I recommend using sushi nori as wraps for your salads, laverbread if you are in Wales and real sea salt instead of refined table salt. I also recommend eating a handful of Brazil nuts daily, as these are filled with selenium, which can support thyroid health and also reduce anxiety. Other selenium-rich foods include salmon, mushrooms, eggs and sunflower seeds.

Simple lifestyle tweaks can also help rebuild your energy levels – choose a peaceful environment, restrict non-essential visitors, go to bed early with your baby and be gentle with yourself. Adaptogenic herbs such as Tulsi and Siberian Ginseng can be very helpful, along with balancing blood sugar by eating a palm-sized portion of protein with every meal. If you make this your new healthy motherhood lifestyle, it will stay with you for life and support your health.

Pay attention to your digestion. As your baby inherits the maternal microbiome, any issues with your own gut are likely to show up in your baby.

Conditions such as cradle cap, colic and reflux are usually an expression of your and your baby's gut health. Because these conditions occur so often, they have been accepted as normal. If your baby is experiencing reflux or colic, I recommend treating yourself and your baby together. Probiotics should not be given to babies under six months of age, so treating through the mother is helpful as probiotic species will transfer to the baby via her breastmilk.

Colic may be a reflection of potential food sensitivities in the mother. In my practice, I often see dairy, wheat, corn, soy, and sugar as the main culprits. To determine which foods your baby is reacting to it is helpful to create a food/symptom journal with a section for your baby's poo and any other details such as a red bottom or insomnia. As a nutritional therapist I ask about poo all the time as it gives me so much information about the inner workings of the body!

Sometimes colic can be caused by low digestive function in mothers – in such cases I sometimes prescribe digestive support supplements to optimise digestion and absorption of foods and remind my clients of the need to eat mindfully. Reflux has been discussed a lot in recent years, but it's important to remember that everyone has some reflux, even adults. We just see it more in babies because their stomach sphincter is immature and they are on a liquid diet. We need to be cautious with treatments as these can interfere with mineral uptake and lead to deficiencies in magnesium and zinc, and contribute to other digestive issues.

Many babies who do not have at least one bowel movement per day have skin issues as their bodies struggle to detoxify. Quite often, mum is constipated too and it is important to keep elimination going by addressing the root cause. Stool testing can reveal so much about the microbiome and the entire digestive function, which is often essential to determine treatment. It may help to eat more fruit and vegetables (having a kiwi fruit per day is particularly helpful because it contains pectin, which can stimulate the movement of the digestive tract) and to soak up magnesium in a relaxing Epsom salt-filled bath.

Nutritional research shows that people with the most diverse microbiomes are healthier, more resilient and less prone to depression. We need a diverse diet of real unprocessed food to feed the thousands of different species which live in our guts. Aim to eat 40 or more different real (not processed) foods every week and make your dishes as colourful as possible. Colour is not just pleasing to the eye, but is also the language of the plant kingdom informing us which nutrients are present. By eating the rainbow, we also include many diverse nutrients.

Eating together as a family will teach your baby about a healthy approach to food and will also boost the hormone of love and calm – oxytocin. This is a very valuable learning from within our kitchens and dining rooms which stays with us for life.

Chapter twenty-three

Exercising again (or just exercising)

$\rightarrow$ If you were active during pregnancy or before you got pregnant, you might be chomping at the bit to know more about when and how you can start exercising again. If you weren't, you might be more reluctantly thinking about exercise to strengthen your body after your birth. Exercise has so many benefits after having a baby (as it does at any time), but you have to find something that suits you, fits with your family's patterns and benefits your lifestyle. This is not about losing baby weight because you need to 'get your body back' or society has told you that you should look a certain way. It's about working the benefits of exercise slowly back into your life.

After having a baby things are going to have changed. You will most likely feel more stretched or weaker than before, coupled with a nice dose of sleep deprivation. This isn't the time to suddenly run marathons if you haven't before. It's about looking at what exercise can bring to you and how that can benefit your new life as a parent. And being active can benefit you in a lot of ways. Aside from feeling physically fitter and every health benefit we know that can bring, exercising can improve mental health, sleep and be a positive source of social interaction with others.

311

When can I start?

There are two main rules about starting to exercise again after the birth.

1. Start when you feel ready, are physically healed and want to, rather than feeling any pressure that you 'should' be exercising.

2. Start gently and build up from there. Remember, you have just grown, birthed and are now caring for a whole new tiny human being. It's okay to be gentle and give yourself some time.

In terms of how long it is best to wait to start exercising again (or indeed just start), there are a number of things to take into consideration.

1. What you're going to be doing

It's best to wait until around six weeks after the birth and your postnatal check to do anything that would be considered strenuous – both in terms of high-impact exercise or lifting heavy weights. You're going to want to check that any stitches are healed, and anything too strenuous too soon can put you at risk of uterine prolapse. If you had a particularly difficult birth or were unwell, you might need to wait longer. Six weeks is just a guideline, not a target, and certainly not a time point by which you *must* start exercising. Talk to your midwife, health visitor or GP.

In terms of exercises to start gently strengthening your core (the key word being gentle) or a stroll with your baby in the park, then it is more of a case of when you feel ready. However, if you do experience any pain or your lochia starts getting heavier again, slow down! This is about making you feel better, not meeting some imagined standard.

2. What type of pregnancy and birth did you have?

If your birth was straightforward and you have little residual pain, then you're probably going to feel ready sooner (at least to think about the possibility of exercising) than if you had a more complicated delivery. If you had a caesarean section remember it is abdominal surgery and be kind to yourself. If you had significant tearing or stitching, again be kind to yourself and give yourself time to heal. Likewise, if you had joint problems during pregnancy such as SPD/PGP you may need to be careful after birth. Although the pain may be receding, your joints may still be loose for a while yet. Be careful and don't push yourself.

3. How fit were you beforehand?

You may have felt fit and well enough to exercise through pregnancy and didn't really stop. But maybe you weren't very active in pregnancy due to pelvic pain, a giant bump or general exhaustion, or are new to the idea of exercise. Go slowly and be realistic rather than throwing yourself in at the deep end (either literally, if swimming, or metaphorically).

What exercise can I do?

Anything goes really, with the proviso that you feel comfortable, are not in pain and it works for your body (more on exercising with a physical disability coming up). You might have preferred classes or activities, or you may be fairly new to exercise. The main thing is to choose something that makes you feel good. Postnatal exercise isn't about exercising to within an inch of your life. It should be about getting stronger again, feeling more confident in your body and improving your wellbeing. And there is no set activity, intensity or duration of exercise that will do that for everyone. The key is to find something that makes you happy – whether that's intense gym sessions with a scary instructor or long strolls in the park that end with an ice-cream. If you're looking for inspiration or just want to mix things up check out the BBC Get Inspired web page **www.bbc. co.uk/sport/get-inspired**.

Strengthening your stomach muscles

One thing that every postnatal woman should think about is how to gently work to strengthen the core muscles after they have been stretched during pregnancy. This isn't about getting yourself a six pack (though if you want to work towards that, crack on) but more about regaining strength and stability. These muscles around our stomach, back and pelvis play an important role in our posture, stability and keeping us pain free.

Your stomach muscles come in two sets, one each side of your belly button. During pregnancy these become separated to allow for your growing baby. In the weeks after birth they should return to normal again by the time your baby is about eight weeks old. Some women find they do not and this is known as diastasis recti. If you think you have it, talk to your GP about a physiotherapy referral. It's important to help the muscles get back to where they should be as otherwise you are more at risk of weak stomach muscles, back pain, poor posture and even constipation and bloating, as everything has a knock-on effect down there.

To test whether your stomach muscles have gone back to normal or not, lie down with your legs bent and with your feet flat on the floor. Raise your head and shoulders as if you were doing half a sit-up. Feel with your hand above and below your belly button. Press your fingers down gently and slowly. If your muscles are still separated, you will feel a gap there. If it is more than about one or two finger widths, you may need more support. Your physiotherapist or GP can recommend some exercises and they will advise you to avoid heavy lifting.

Even if you don't have separated muscles, take your time in recovering.

> **"Anything goes really, with the proviso that you feel comfortable, are not in pain and it works for your body."**

They will have been weakened and strengthening them is important for regaining good posture and reducing the chances of back pain. Go gently – now is not the time to start with major ab sessions. Also, forget everything you might have been taught in school gym class about tightening stomach muscles. Do not do traditional sit-ups – they can actually separate the muscles. You want to focus on a motion that draws your muscles closely together and that you have control over so you can stop if it hurts.

Find a position you are comfortable in, either sitting cross-legged, lying comfortably or standing. Draw your stomach muscles in towards your spine. Gradually draw them closer and closer in and hold. You can increase the amount of time you hold this for as you get stronger. You can then do this multiple times a day, wherever you like – cooking dinner, in the supermarket queue or waiting to pick up your takeaway. This method has been shown to significantly tighten your stomach muscles, reduce diastasis recti and generally help you tone up.[1] You can find out more on the website of one of the personal trainers who studied the impact of this move here on the Every Mother website **every-mother.com.**

Be gentle with your joints

During pregnancy you produced lots of a hormone known as relaxin. This had the effect of loosening your ligaments and muscles so that your pelvis could open up during birth. Unfortunately it also has the effect of loosening other muscles, like knee and ankle joints. Relaxin doesn't disappear after the birth – it can stay in your system for up to six months. So it might be best to avoid twisty type movements like football or basketball until you feel more stable again.

For inspiration for gentle postnatal exercises that support your joints while also healing and strengthening your body, check out the Strong Mums Northern Ireland Facebook page – not just for those in Northern Ireland! **www. facebook.com/strongmumsni.**

With or without your baby?

This may or may not be an option for you, but one thing to think about is whether you will exercise with or without your baby. There are lots of fitness classes that you can take your baby to, or you might choose to run or walk with your baby in a pram. However, research has shown that if you have the opportunity to exercise without your baby (some or all of the time) it might have added benefits for you. Workouts tend to be more intensive, but also one study showed that solo (or non-baby) exercise was better at reducing symptoms of anxiety and increasing wellbeing. It makes sense: exercise isn't just about the physical activity, it's about the head space and time to invest in yourself.[2] So if you have the chance to take that time alone, even if it's the only alone time you have all day, it can give you a much-needed psychological boost.

Walking

Walking is a really effective way to build your strength and fitness, especially if there are some hills involved. And you don't need any 'equipment' or to pay expensive class fees (bar a comfortable pair of shoes). You can pop your baby in a sling and get an even better workout.

There are a number of 'buggy fit' style classes around, where new parents meet with their baby in a buggy and do walks and sometimes strengthening exercises. These work really well both in terms of improving fitness, and also in increasing feelings of wellbeing and reducing symptoms of depression.[3] Importantly they can also be a great source of social support and offer the chance to develop friendships that last much longer than pushing your baby around a lake.[4] The only downside is that in the UK these things tend to be a bit weather dependent. There's nothing wrong with a bit of rain, but a howling gale is probably not conducive to improving wellbeing.

Swimming

Swimming is a brilliant postnatal activity as the water takes your weight and it's gentle on your joints. It's advised that you wait until around seven days after your lochia has stopped to start swimming again. This is because you're more at risk of infection while you are still bleeding. If you still have stitches in, check with your health visitor or GP.

One stroke you might like to avoid if you had SPD during pregnancy or have any residual pain or weakness in your pelvis is breast stroke (well, the legs – you could do the arms and simply kick your legs front-crawl style). For more ideas about how to build your strength with swimming (and indeed with any postnatal exercise), fitness coach Vanessa Barker has a great website www.vanessabarker.com.

Yoga

Yoga can heal your body and bring brilliant core strength after having a baby. But it's about more than that – it's about reconnecting with your body, slowing down and making peace. You don't need to be lithe, bendy, and permanently zen to do it – exercises will range from the very gentle to the more advanced.

You might like to join a postnatal yoga class. Again, research into the benefits of such classes shows it's not just about the physical benefits, but the connection and being part of a group. One study showed how stories shared during classes about birth, caring for babies and motherhood instilled connections between participants that lasted long after classes ended.

Classes brought a feeling of wellbeing and belonging alongside perfecting the downward dog.[5]

There are also parent and baby yoga classes. Not only do these mean that you can exercise and connect with others while also caring for your baby, but gentle baby yoga moves also help them. Although nothing is a miracle cure, there is some evidence that the touch, ritual and connection can help reduce symptoms of colic and improve sleep for babies.[6]

Social media appears to be the place to go to follow all sorts of great yoga accounts. You might find your own favourites (and other accounts are available!), but a quick poll of my yoga enthusiast friends suggested these to start with:

- Lush Tums www.instagram.com/lushtums
- PAH Pregnancy Yoga www.instagram.com/PAHPregnancyYoga
- Stretch London www.instagram.com/stretch_london
- Black Girl Yoga www.instagram.com/blackgirlyoga
- This is Nave www.instagram.com/_thisisnave
- Veronique Denise www.facebook.com/VeroniqueDeniseYoga
- Happy Yoga Newcastle www.facebook.com/happyyoganewcastle
- Birthlight www.facebook.com/birthlight

Another really inspirational account for doing yoga with your baby is MummyYoga – handy if you don't want to or can't leave your baby but still want to get involved www.instagram.com/mummyyoga. Pregnancy yoga also do online parent and baby sessions www.pregnancyyogabristol.co.uk/online-pregnancy-yoga-classes.

While you're limbering up, for sheer yoga inspiration check out Erika Harper's Insta page www.instagram.com/harpererika7/ – I'm so going to master that headstand one day... On another note, many yoga accounts are run by women, but of course men can do yoga too. For some male yoga inspiration a great account is dade2shelby www.instagram.com/dade2shelby/. I also really like the Instagram account Afro Yogi for showing body positivity outside the typical thinner body found on many Insta accounts www.instagram.com/afro_yogi.

Finally, yoga isn't just for the very bendy. Check out the Accessible Yoga page if you have issues with mobility – and more on exercising with a disability later. www.instagram.com/accessibleyoga

Becoming a running evangelist

Really? Yes, really. If you haven't run before, give it some serious thought. After you've had the serious thought you can go back to ignoring me if you like. But it seems that the time after having a baby is actually when a lot of people get into running. Now of course, this will totally depend on your recovery from birth and any physical challenges you might have, but if you're looking to get more active and have never considered running, read on.

Why running? Well, it's a brilliant way to get fit, but the impact on well-being can be huge. It's not just about all those lovely endorphins that are released, but more the sense of strength and freedom it can bring. It is also the perfect thing to get some time alone, or with the option of placing your baby or even baby and older child in a running buggy and just going for it (a definite workout).

With the caveats that it displays a lot of privilege (health, living in an area that's safe, supporters to care for my children): running. I only took it up after some sort of existential crisis when my oldest was three months old and I suddenly had a panic that now I had a baby I had to be as healthy as possible (side portion of anxiety about being the unfit embarrassing mum who couldn't kick a ball around with him). I'd tried taking up running a couple of times but it never really 'took' – I'd get tired, hot and have sore knees. But then I did Couch to 5k. I think that the combination of breastfeeding and running has been synergistic in teaching me new things about my body: that it's not just decorative, that what it does is more important than how it looks, that at very nearly 40 I can go out and run in shorts, something I wouldn't have even imagined doing 10–15 years ago. Pregnancy, birth, breastfeeding and then running taught me lessons I hadn't learned before about the power and strength of my body. <u>Vicky</u>

Top tip – you don't actually need to run the whole way, you can walk in places too, just keep moving! It's a myth that you have to run flat out to be a 'runner'. If you are running, you are a runner and actually the act of combining running and walking in places (known as 'jeffing') can help you become fitter and run further. It's about building up slowly and enjoying the experience rather than immediately trying to do a half marathon. The Couch to 5K programme is amazing in helping you start slowly and build up your endurance. It's got an amazing reputation for getting people who can barely run to the end of the street to run 5km in one go! It's hosted on the NHS website where you can find the app to download **www.nhs.uk/live-well/exercise/couch-to-5k-week-by-week**.

Running can be done any place, any time as long as you have the right shoes (these are really important). Pick the time and location and it can be really relaxing too (yes, honestly!). This is a great video on the BBC website from endurance athlete Sophie Radcliffe, showing her running at sunset. **www.bbc.co.uk/sport/av/get-inspired/47772119**

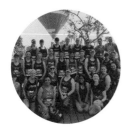

The Run Mummy Run Facebook group

Leanne Davies is founder and owner of Run Mummy Run – a supportive online community for female runners. You can find out more about them and join at www.facebook.com/groups/runmummyrun, www.instagram.com/run_mummy_run or www.runmummyrun.co.uk.

I have always loved running, but after having my children (two boys) I found it much harder to keep to a regular running routine. I just didn't seem to be able to plan ahead, go to structured club sessions or commit to runs – no week is ever the same with young babies and children. I really missed the interaction with other runners, so in December 2012 I decided that I needed to create a network of like-minded women who loved running as much as I did, but understood the challenges of juggling running around children. I sat in my kitchen and set up a small Facebook group of just three people. Other ladies joined in my local area, then from further afield and it just kept growing! We now have over 64,000 ladies in our community, talking about everything to do with running and parenthood (though any lady can join, not just mums).

We are mainly on Facebook, as that's where the majority of our community are. We have a closed Facebook group that is the main hub of our activity. We also have social network channels on Facebook and Instagram, and a website, which has a shop for running kit and expert blogs on all sorts of topics that are relevant to running mums, supporting them through their journey. Finally, we have a sub-group called The Healthier Balance, which covers more than just running, including self-care, nutrition, family meals, cross-training and much more.

I know, from experience, that running after having a baby can be a whole different ballgame. Even though I ran before I was a mum, it was still very different. We always advise ladies to listen to their bodies and start slowly. The majority of problems and injuries are caused by doing too much too soon. Be kind to yourself – your body has been through a lot! You can start with regular walks in your local area, and build that up to include short running intervals. Programmes like the NHS Couch to 5K are perfect – even if you have run before, this helps you build up slowly and sensibly. Take it one run at a time, and it will get easier and you will get stronger. Running can give you so much more than fitness – it gives you a mental break and time out, which is so important when you have a young baby. Plus, being active helps set a good example for your child as they get older. One day, they might even come running with you and that's a great feeling!

What if I have a chronic illness or physical disability?

Physical activity can benefit almost everyone, but making sure it fits your own needs and scope is really important. Far too often chronic illness or physical disability is overlooked in 'getting fit after pregnancy' articles, but there is certainly support out there. Yet obviously you still benefit from the benefits of activity for physical health, wellbeing and a sense of achievement.

What exercise you can do will of course be based on your personal physical health and preferences. Be especially careful about not overexerting yourself if you have an autoimmune chronic illness such as rheumatoid arthritis or multiple sclerosis, as some women find that their symptoms, while reduced during pregnancy, flare in the postnatal period. This might increase joint pain, muscle pain or feelings of exhaustion so please, please listen to your body.

The most important thing is to choose an activity that suits your physical health and wellbeing. It might be that your disability allows you to swim, walk, do yoga or weight lifting with the right support. Or it might be that you have to look for classes and activities that have made the effort to be inclusive and supportive. Finding these can be challenging, so here are some ideas to start with if you are unsure:

- Check out the Activity Alliance website. It gives a list of leisure and activity centres around the UK that have adapted facilities to be more inclusive. They also have lists of sporting and active events in your local area. Pop in your postcode to find out more. **www.activityalliance.org.uk/get-active/inclusive-gyms** Similarly the Parasport website has great ideas and links to local activities **parasport.org.uk**.
- Check out this HuffPost article with advice from Dom Thorpe, founder of Disability Training, with ideas for exercises depending on your physical range **www.huffingtonpost.co.uk/entry/exercises-to-do-at-home-if-you-have-a-disability_uk_5878b3bfe4b0f3b82a37408e**. Dom's website is also full of ideas for those wanting to be more physically active with a chronic illness or disability **dt-training.co.uk**.
- Also, follow KymNonStop on YouTube. Not only does she have the most amazing abs, but she has a great set of workouts for those in a wheelchair or with limited mobility **www.youtube.com/watch?v=d6zHyxXd1Dk**. Jessica Smith is another amazing follow **www.youtube.com/watch?v=1xC9khisFPA**.

Finally, for inspiration for anyone, the BBC has some great videos:
- 'I'm just living' – triple amputee Mark Ormrod's inspirational journey **www.bbc.co.uk/sport/av/get-inspired/45967595**
- 'We're coaching deaf ladies, not deaf disabled ladies' **www.bbc.co.uk/sport/av/get-inspired/47886506**
- The female boxer with cerebral palsy **www.bbc.co.uk/news/av/uk-england-dorset-43843170/the-female-boxer-with-cerebral-palsy**

Can I exercise if I'm breastfeeding?

Yes, you can breastfeed and exercise – maybe not literally simultaneously, although I breastfed a number of times while out walking... There are some things to think about though.

1. Invest in a good sports bra (or two)

Larger breasts give greater potential for bounce and you'll want to keep things secure. If one doesn't keep them under control, some women find wearing two works. The most important thing is to make sure the bra is well fitting so the breasts aren't compressed. Also, take it off as soon as you have finished exercising, as too much compression could increase the risk of mastitis.

2. Feed before you exercise

If you are still in the earlier stages of breastfeeding and you feel engorged before a feed, it's probably a good idea to try and time exercising around feeding. Give a feed before you go so things are more comfortable. This probably also gives you more time to exercise.

3. Shower if you need to before you feed your baby

The taste of sweat and salt on your skin might put some babies off, so factor in having a shower if you have sweated a lot. There is no need to if your baby doesn't mind – it's not as if your nipples themselves will be coated in salt.

4. Build up gently

This applies in general, but you might find that your baby reacts differently to your milk if you exercise very hard. Lactic acid, if produced at high levels, can get into your breastmilk in small amounts, possibly enough to make it slightly more bitter-tasting. Many babies are just fine with this, but it's best to build up gradually rather than do a really hard session and find out your baby has decided to be one of the discerning ones.

There is no real evidence that by doing too much exercise you'll affect your milk supply – after all, our ancestors would have been much more active day-to-day. But again, it's best to build up gradually, mainly to make sure you don't feel too exhausted. Saying that, there are many stories of women running marathons while breastfeeding, or even the inspirational case of Sophie Power who, on breaks during running a 103-mile race, breastfed her three-month-old son while also expressing some milk for him. You can hear her story on BBC Radio 5 Live **www.bbc.co.uk/ news/av/uk-45560184/ultra-runner-sophie-power-on-breastfeeding-during-a-103-mile-race**.

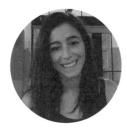

Recovering your postnatal strength – a whole-body focus

Betsan de Renesse is an NASM certified personal trainer and pre and postnatal exercise specialist. After having her first baby she wanted to regain her pre-baby strength and fitness, but couldn't find any programme that met her needs, so she founded her own system – the GLOW method.

What is the GLOW method?

The GLOW method is more than just postnatal exercise or trying to lose weight. It is a whole body approach that focuses on your posture, alignment and breathing. It focuses on a functional fitness approach, helping you rebuild strength in a way that benefits you every day as a mother, with all the lifting, carrying, pushing and pulling you do. It takes a whole body approach, looking at muscles that are under and over used, aligning our bodies to be as strong as they can be. Importantly though, the approach doesn't just focus on your physical wellbeing, but your emotional wellbeing too. Classes give you space and me time, with chance to repair the everyday stresses and strains. It empowers you as a mother and a woman, allowing you to return to or become whatever you want to be.

You can find out more about the approach and articles to help you thrive on the Glow Method website **www.theglowmethod.co.uk**.

We also have an online class, which is great if you can't come in person. It's a full core and pelvic floor rehab and fitness programme for women to access no matter where they live. You can find it at **www.theglowmethodathome.com**.

What are some of the most common concerns you see in women postnatally about getting back into exercise?

I think some of the most common concerns come from the mixed messages women receive from the media, friends, medical professionals and even family. This is tricky to counteract, although there's definitely a much more forward-thinking movement of medics and fit pros making huge changes in the UK. It's increasingly easier to find consistent and accurate return to exercise information, and even media messaging about postnatal bodies is changing.

Despite a slow but steady rebellion against the idea of 'bouncing back to your old body post-baby', women are often concerned about losing baby weight. I completely support and empathise with this feeling, but I'd always advise working on the functionality of your body as well as aesthetics. Ideally, and with the correct support, both come hand in hand.

Ladies are also often concerned about when to start. Advice varies from 'return to normal after six weeks, even running is fine!' to 'postpartum is forever and you'll never do a sit-up or plank again'. It's no wonder women feel confused. My advice would be to find a knowledgeable and forward-thinking fitness professional (or programme) to help you achieve your goals safely and progressively. It can help to think about your return to exercise post-baby in the same way as you'd think about a return to exercise post-injury. Progressive overload and a core and pelvic floor focus is key. There have recently been some excellent guidelines published to help guide women's return to movement and running.

Mums are also often concerned about pelvic floor function and abdominal wall separation or weakness (this can also sometimes present in lower back pain, or what's described as a 'mummy tummy'). I'd always advise an appointment with a specialist women's health physio before starting any exercise programme post-birth. Or if you start to experience any symptoms like leaking, heaviness in the pelvic area, or pain during exercise. The women's health physio can do a full internal exam, which really isn't as scary as it sounds. They even check you're doing your pelvic floor exercises correctly.

What would be your advice to someone who is worried about getting started or taking the time for them?
I think my best bit of advice would be to adjust your mindset around taking care of yourself. When you become a mum you quickly relegate yourself to the bottom of the importance list, when in fact your physical and mental wellness is actually as important to you as your whole family. If you try to think that you have a responsibility to take care of your body and mind so that you can care for and really enjoy your baby, it can really help to rebalance the urge to look after everyone except yourself. The old saying 'you can't pour from an empty cup' becomes so true and if you see your exercise time as essential self-care, as opposed to a selfish or superficial pastime, it can really help give movement the importance it deserves. I don't personally find self-care like a long bubble bath, or a manicure fills my emotional cup, or gives me the physical and emotional resilience I need for motherhood as effectively as drinking enough water, eating well and moving my body.

Apart from the importance of regaining strength after having a baby, what are the benefits of taking time out to be active once you've had a baby?
Taking time out to be active once you've had your baby can have huge benefits

for both body and mind. Something as simple as getting out into the fresh air for short (to begin with) and progressively longer walks can increase feelings of wellbeing and decrease cortisol levels. It will also help you get some essential vitamin D.

If your mood is low and you're feeling sluggish, even a short burst of movement can flood blood to your muscles and your brain causing a release of endorphins. These endorphins will help you feel more cheerful and energised. Evidence suggests that regular exercise can act as a mild antidepressant. Powerful stuff.

If you're feeling stressed and anxious, multiple studies have shown that even a short yoga practice can decrease the secretion of cortisol, the primary stress hormone, and this can in turn ease stress and lower anxiety.

I also believe exercising with your baby helps to entertain both of you. It can become a fun activity in what can occasionally feel like a long day. It also helps to demonstrate self-care and the importance of movement to your little one. I'd always advise working out while your baby is awake. If you wait for nap time it might never happen because naps are notoriously inconsistent. If you schedule exercise as part of your day you're more likely to stay motivated and consistent. It will also mean you can save nap time for a cup of tea or a much-needed rest.

Chapter twenty-four

Postnatal deficiencies and disorders

→ Pregnancy, birth and breastfeeding (and let's face it, just looking after a baby) can be a drain on your system, especially if your diet was affected by things like prolonged morning sickness. There are some common symptoms that can be a sign of nutritional deficiencies or other health disorders that can be brushed aside by you (or sadly sometimes medical professionals) as 'just' being because you're tired and not sleeping well as you care for your baby. These include:

- Overwhelming fatigue that doesn't go away after a good night's sleep
- Aching joints or bones
- Feeling fuzzy headed or like you have brain fog
- Changes to weight and appetite
- Changes in mood including feeling down or anxious
- Migraines or headaches

If you are experiencing any or a mix of these issues and it's possible to try and get a few nights of good sleep, then try that first. Otherwise, or if you try that and they don't go away, it's worth making a visit to the GP to talk about how you feel. There are a few things that they might be able to test for with a simple blood test. Some of the more common issues could be:

Vitamin D deficiency

Vitamin D is a really important vitamin and one that we seem to be finding out more about all the time. It is important in the development and maintenance of healthy bones, but also seems to play a role in autoimmune disorders, cardiovascular disease and musculoskeletal health problems. There are even suggestions it may play a role in dementia, depression and other cognitive disorders. The problem is that many of us do not get enough of it.[1]

The main way we get vitamin D is from the body creating it by sunlight shining on our skin. Vitamin D is found in some foods but in very small amounts. These include oily fish, red meat, liver, egg yolks and some fortified cereals and spreads. But really, our main source is the sun. If you live in the Northern hemisphere, the chances are you are at risk of vitamin D deficiency, particularly during the winter months. Even if you live in sunnier climes, if you work indoors and use sun protection when you are out, the chances of you being deficient are high.

If you are pregnant or breastfeeding, the evidence suggests that you need more vitamin D. One study in Germany found that around half of breastfeeding women and nearly all pregnant women had low vitamin D levels during the winter.[2] Others have found that this also applies to new mothers who aren't breastfeeding, which makes sense as demands on the body from pregnancy still take time to put themselves right.[3]

This is particularly true if you have darker skin, as vitamin D doesn't seem to be produced at such high levels due to sunlight in darker skins. It is thought that higher levels of melanin reduce the body's ability to react to sunlight. Also, if you have a BMI over 30, you may need a higher intake to achieve the same levels.[4]

If you have low levels of vitamin D, some of the symptoms you might experience include:

- Feeling very tired
- Bones and joints aching
- Muscle weakness
- Feeling depressed or anxious
- Getting a lot of infections
- Slow wound healing
- Hair loss

Again, lots of those symptoms could be attributed to not sleeping properly and carrying an increasingly heavy baby around.

There are two main ways to increase your vitamin D. The first is more time in the sunshine. This is more of an option if you live somewhere where it's sunny (or perhaps if you happen to have the money and time, you could disappear for some medicinal weeks in the sun – for your health, obviously). For this to work in the UK and the rest of northern Europe it a) needs to be sunny, b) needs to be roughly between 11am and 3pm, c) needs to be between March and September and d) you need your arms or legs uncovered. You also need to be outside – it doesn't work sitting in a sunny window, for example, as the UVB rays need to reach you.

The important part is that you need to expose your skin without sunscreen, as it blocks the UVB rays from reaching your skin. Herein lies the problem for many pale people. You don't want to go out in the midday sun to get your vitamin D but burn and put yourself at risk of skin cancer. It will take roughly 15 minutes in the midday sun for a person with pale skin to get enough vitamin D... but how long to burn? For those with darker skin, you need an increasingly long time to make enough vitamin D – up to two hours for those with the darkest skin. You might find yourself at less risk of burning (but remember you can still burn, no matter how dark your skin, if you're out too long without protection), but how many new mothers (unfortunately) have two hours to sit in the sun each day – if it's even sunny?[5]

For this reason, it is recommended that most people would benefit from vitamin D supplements (look out particularly for vitamin D3). This includes breastfed babies (because they already add the vitamin to formula) and children. There is some evidence that if mothers are well supplemented with vitamin D their breastmilk will have enough for their baby, but given there is not lots of evidence for this, and vitamin D is easy to take, it is recommended that all pregnant and breastfeeding women take a vitamin D supplement too. You can get them free if you quality for the Healthy Start scheme in the UK. If you still don't feel better, visit your GP.[6]

Vitamin B12 or folate deficiency anaemia

This happens when a lack of B12 or folate (B9) means you produce red blood cells that are too large and can't carry oxygen around your body properly. This affects the functioning of your nervous system and gives you a whole host of generalised symptoms that could be brushed off. Signs of not having enough B12 include:[7]

- Exhaustion
- Breathlessness or dizziness
- Pale skin
- Feeling fuzzy headed or not being able to concentrate

- Sore tongue or mouth ulcers
- Pins and needles or restless legs
- Difficulty falling asleep
- Fuzzy vision
- Headaches
- Depression or anxiety

It's possible that you have a B12 deficiency because of following a very restricted diet, particularly one that is vegan. Some of the best dietary sources of B12 are fish, eggs, milk and meat – obviously putting vegans at risk, but also vegetarians. You can get some B12 from fortified cereals. If you are feeling this way and think your diet is low in sources of B12, consider taking a B-complex multivitamin.

If that doesn't work, or you think your diet is fine, see your GP because there are a number of other conditions that can mean you don't absorb the B12 you do eat. These include the autoimmune disorder pernicious anaemia, in which your body decides to attack the cells in your stomach, meaning it's really difficult to absorb B12. There are also certain medications that might affect how much you absorb. If your low B12 is caused by either of these, you should be offered regular B12 injections to help bring your levels back up.

Iron deficiency anaemia

Anaemia is another common postnatal deficiency affecting up to around a third of women. It occurs when we have too little haemoglobin in our blood, meaning our red blood cells can't effectively distribute oxygen. Anaemia is common in pregnancy and can continue postnatally, further increased by any postpartum haemorrhage. Again the symptoms are similar to other deficiencies – tiredness, low mood, brain fog. You may also look pale.[8]

If you are feeling this way, especially if you had low iron levels in pregnancy, try a multivitamin supplement alongside eating iron-rich foods. There are two sources of dietary iron: haem iron and non-haem iron. Haem iron is in meat and oil-rich fish and non-haem iron is found in leafy vegetables, cereals, beans and lentils. The iron from haem sources is better absorbed than that from non-haem sources. However, consuming these two types together increases how much iron is absorbed from non-haem sources. The amount of non-haem iron absorbed by the body also depends on the body's stores. If you are iron deficient you will absorb more of it than if you are not. It also depends on what you eat with it – vitamin C may help absorption, while foods such as unleavened bread, whole grains, cheese and green leafy veg can reduce it. Tea reduces iron absorption by nearly two-thirds, which is one reason why it is not recommended as a drink for young children.

If your GP recommends treatment as your red blood cell count is low they might prescribe you stronger iron supplements. Some people find these difficult to handle, with symptoms of constipation or diarrhoea (or both), heartburn, stomach pain and nausea and black poo. You might find you manage better on liquid sources of iron such as Spatone, which you add to water or orange juice. If you are prescribed tablets make sure you keep them away from any children as they are toxic if ingested in large amounts.[9]

> **" Anaemia is common in pregnancy and can continue postnatally. "**

Postpartum thyroid issues

Your thyroid is a small gland in your neck that produces hormones that play an important role in a whole range of bodily functions particularly around growth and metabolism. Unfortunately, it can sometimes go a bit haywire, producing too much or too little thyroid hormone, and this is particularly common in women – around 15% will develop an issue during their lifetime compared to less than 3% of men. One of the most common times for it to go wrong, temporarily or triggering a longer-term change, is after pregnancy, so it's important to keep an eye on any symptoms. Again, you've guessed it... these symptoms can often be written off as part of being a new parent.

There are a number of different thyroid disorders. Many are a type of autoimmune disorder, where the body's immune system goes into overdrive and starts attacking the healthy tissue. Hashimoto's disease (or hypothyroidism) occurs when the thyroid produces too low a level of thyroid hormones and Graves' disease (or hyperthyroidism) occurs when the thyroid produces too much. Unfortunately, it appears that pregnancy can either increase the risk of an autoimmune disorder developing, or accelerate one that was already developing or present at a very low level.[10] And post-pregnancy is one of the most common times for a woman to develop an autoimmune thyroid disorder.[11]

Broadly, two of the most common patterns in thyroid dysfunction after pregnancy are for either a temporary issue to occur lasting just a few months or so (postpartum thyroiditis) or for a lifelong disorder such as Graves' or Hashimoto's disease to develop.

Postpartum thyroiditis

This disorder typically develops within a few months of birth and disappears after about a year. A pattern is often seen. First, the body starts to attack the thyroid (often in the months after birth) meaning thyroid levels go too high, causing the symptoms of hyperthyroidism. You might have symptoms such as:

- Losing weight quickly
- Feeling shaky
- Not being able to sleep
- Feeling anxious
- Sensitivity to heat and feeling hot
- Irritation and anger

Then, after a few weeks of this, the thyroid gland becomes unable to keep up, and thyroid hormone levels drop really low, causing the signs of hypothyroidism. Symptoms of an underactive thyroid include basically the opposite:

- Gaining weight quickly
- Feeling sluggish
- Feeling exhausted – like you are dragging something around
- Constipation
- Muscle aches and feeling weak
- Dry skin and brittle nails
- Feeling cold

Treatment

If you are experiencing the symptoms of an under or overactive thyroid, it's important to make an appointment with your GP for tests. Unfortunately, it seems that a number of women in the UK struggle to get tested correctly for thyroid disorders and receive sufficient treatment. It's a bit strange given how common the disorders are, how simple it is to test and how relatively easy it is to fix with the right medication. My suspicions are that it is not taken seriously enough because it affects mainly women, post-pregnancy and at menopause. These factors appear to play a role in how easily women get diagnosed and treated.

Taking a positive stance and assuming you have access to a GP who is switched on and aware of the importance of diagnosing and recognising thyroid disorders, your symptoms should mean you are offered a blood test. Some GPs will offer only a simple test. They will ask for the level of the thyroid hormone T4 to be measured, alongside something called TSH (thyroid stimulating hormone). TSH rises when you do not have enough thyroid hormones circulating in your body, so the higher this hormone is, the more your body is struggling to produce sufficient thyroid hormones. The problem with this test is that it misses some other important markers and also does not necessarily identify whether your thyroid is operating optimally for a number of reasons:

1. The T4 test only measures levels of the hormone T4 in your body. Your thyroid gland, if working correctly, produces two hormones known as T4 and T3. In terms of overall levels, roughly 80% is T4 and 20% T3. In simple terms T3 is the active version of the thyroid hormone that helps all your metabolic processes. When your body is working correctly it will convert T4 to T3. However, some people have a problem converting T4 to T3, so if the blood test only measures T4, it would not pick up that you do not have enough circulating T3. Therefore, ideally your T3 levels should be measured too.

2. Your body might be making just about enough T4, but be under autoimmune attack making it really difficult. Autoimmune disorders attack healthy parts of the body. Thyroid antibodies attack the thyroid, meaning it has to work really hard to carry on sending out enough thyroid hormones. Therefore, ideally your antibody levels should be measured too. Medication would mean that your body didn't have to put up the fight to make it.

When you get your blood tests back, the GP will typically tell you whether your thyroid levels are 'within range' or not. The problem with this is that sometimes people can have a level within range but it has dropped *for them* – and without earlier levels you wouldn't be able to tell if it's normal for you or not. The whole point of a range is to show a level of normal across a population, but just like many things, being at the top or bottom of a scale might or might not be normal for you.

Sometimes you might be within range but very close to either edge – known as borderline. There is some evidence that treating you if you are borderline can help either slow down any development of an illness or simply help with your symptoms. This is especially important in the UK, because our cut-off levels for determining whether TSH is raised, are higher than in the USA or Australia.

If you are diagnosed with a thyroid issue you will most likely be prescribed medication. For those with an overactive thyroid you will be given treatment that aims to reduce the amount of thyroid hormone your body is making. The most common medications prescribed are carbimazole and propylthiouracil, and you may also be given a beta-blocker to help reduce symptoms such as anxiety and a fast heart rate. In more severe and long lasting cases you may also be offered radiotherapy to kill off some of your thyroid cells and therefore reduce how many hormones it makes. This obviously has long-term implications and is not suitable for short-term cases or if you tend to bounce between hyper and hypo thyroid as some people do. In the most severe cases you may have surgery to remove your thyroid and be given thyroid replacement medication for life.

If you have an underactive thyroid you will be given medication to increase it. This is usually Levothyroxine, which is based on the thyroid hormone T4.

Some people do well on this medication, but others struggle. They might have problems digesting it or in some cases they might be struggling to convert T4 into T3. Guidance is to take it on an empty stomach, at least an hour away from coffee as it can interfere with its absorption (tricky in the mornings!). Some people have luck with vitamin supplements such as selenium which are thought to help with absorption (although pro tip – two Brazil nuts have all the selenium you need and yes, it works if they are chocolate-covered).

Again, if you are struggling go back to your GP. If you haven't had your T3 levels checked then this might be the time to see whether the medication is actually helping raise your levels. Also, you could ask to trial a different type of medication – a combination of T3 and T4, or T3 alone. Unfortunately this is no longer a recommended first port of call treatment in the UK and is much more expensive than plain old T4, so a lot of GPs are reluctant to try it. There are many anecdotal cases of symptoms improving after a trial and guidelines do say that if you are not improving with T4 alone that you should be referred to an endocrinologist for a trial of T3.

The good news about postpartum thyroiditis is that often things return to normal by around 12 months after your birth.

What if I can't get treatment?

Unfortunately there is a tendency for some GPs to dismiss or not treat thyroid issues, especially underactive thyroid. Symptoms are brushed off as being due to the exhaustion of new motherhood or – ironically given an underactive thyroid will most likely make you gain weight – some women are told their symptoms are due to them being overweight. Sometimes you might only be able to get a basic T4 or TSH test, which as explained above doesn't always give you the full picture.

Not being listened to, at a time when you are already run down and exhausted, is soul-destroying. If this happens to you there are a number of options:

1. Get a new GP or ask to see someone else
2. Push to be referred to an endocrinologist
3. Make an appointment to see a private doctor specialising in thyroid disorders
4. Order private blood tests and take the results to your GP

Obviously, numbers three and four are only available if you have the money. You should not need to do this, but if you are convinced your symptoms are due to a thyroid issue, especially if you have any kind of family history of thyroid difficulties, it can be worth the investment.

- A good source of information for support with thyroid issues is Thyroid UK **thyroiduk.org**
- The British Thyroid Foundation is also great. It publishes a small book with lots of further information which is a great read **www.btf-thyroid.org**.

"

Part five

Let's talk about relationships

"

As we've already seen, becoming a new parent is a time of change.

You've got a new identity and a relationship with a whole new person and it may have changed your career and friendships (for better or for worse). But a big part of becoming a parent is how your relationship with your partner changes, if indeed you have a partner.

Your relationship is all part of being a new parent and how you experience it. Maybe you have a good relationship, maybe you don't. Maybe you don't have a partner or have split up with your partner. Maybe you are experiencing different challenges as an LGBTQ parent.

This section is going to explore the different challenges you might face – the most common arguments that couples have and how to work towards solving them, how to spot the signs of domestic abuse, and dealing with people's stupid questions as an LGBTQ parent. It also explores your feelings if you're a single parent, looking at the challenges of maintenance, contact and communicating with an ex-partner and offers real-life expertise on how to manage alone.

We look at topics such as the mental load of motherhood and how we can tackle the increasing burden of women taking on more at work and at home. There are ideas for how partners can support each other, tips on how to have a good argument and ways of working out what is fair in your relationship.

Advice from relationship experts will help you nurture positive relationships and deal with challenges, while making sure you get the support you need.

Chapter twenty-five

Your new relationship with your partner – what's normal?

→ The period after having a baby is not only a transition to becoming parents, but it's also a big transition in your relationship. You both now have additional roles and connections with each other, not just as partners or lovers, but as co-parents. You are both learning the ropes of caring for your baby, and in relation to supporting each other. It can be a big change: suddenly one of you may be not working, and the dynamics of your days can be very different.

It's normal for this time to feel really challenging. A lot of adaptation is going on and the dust needs to settle on your new normal. Although not all couples feel this way, it is normal for relationship satisfaction to decline after having a baby, although part of that is just relationships naturally declining over time – it happens to couples without a baby too. It's normal to feel more comfortable and less ecstatic over time. However, this decline in satisfaction is stronger for women than it is men.[1] This is unsurprising, because a common source of dissatisfaction is feeling like your life has changed and your partner's life has not.

337

We're arguing more – is something wrong?

Most new parents find that they argue more with their partner after having a baby.[2] It's unsurprising really: everyone feels more on edge and things seem much worse when you haven't had much sleep. Research by the counselling organisation Relate found the most common arguments among new parents were based around money, sleep, task sharing and sex,[3] although other hot topics included differences of opinion on how to raise your baby and interference from family and friends. This article on Fatherly has 22 ideas for possible fights to have if you are looking for some inspiration: **www.fatherly. com/love-money/new-parent-arguments-first-baby**. Let's look at some of those sources of conflict in more detail:

1. Money

Let's face it, this is one of the biggest things couples argue about outside of having a baby.[4] But money arguments are increasingly common in the first year after birth. There is likely a lot of change going on. One of you is on maternity leave and probably receiving less pay, so there's less money all round. You might be thinking about when to return to work and disagreeing about that. Maybe one of you has more opportunity to spend money on leisure and it feels unfair. And maybe one of you has a middle-of-the-night Amazon habit during night feeds. No comment.

Having a baby is a time when financial and power inequalities in your relationship can arise if you're not careful. It's a common pattern, after a first baby in particular, for women to reduce their paid employment and increase how much housework and childcare they do, while men do the opposite.[5] This can be the start of imbalance in your relationship, and contributes to widening financial inequalities between men and women later in life.[6]

It's a source of many arguments. As a society we tend to value paid work and status and undervalue unpaid work, when actually it is all interlinked and part of the wider jigsaw of supporting a family. This can mean, however, that one partner is in a place where they get a lot of clear rewards – a wage, feedback at work, promotions, status, a feeling they are financially supporting their partner and a feeling of value within society. The other partner can feel that their life is full of thankless tasks that have no clearly defined reward. You might also feel like you are slipping away from each other in terms of shared experiences and goals.

This can lead to conscious or unconscious imbalance in financial control in couples. The partner who is working can sometimes see their wages as theirs alone, or believe they should have more control over the money. They may accuse the non-working partner of not bringing any money in, ignoring the fact that it is very much because their partner is not working, and is taking the childcare and household load, that they can work without paying for childcare and work longer and more flexible hours. The partner who isn't working may feel uneasy or guilty about spending money that they didn't earn.

Some ideas for reducing arguments:

- Value each other's contribution and recognise that you are both supporting the family in different but interconnected ways. Try to make sure you both have equal amounts of time to relax rather than thinking about who brings what to the partnership.
- Listen to each other about what has been stressful in your days. Don't try to compare it or get into the 'I wish I had your stress' type arguments.
- Support each other in whatever you are both working towards. For one that might be a promotion. For the other it might be simply getting your baby to nap for longer. Be each other's cheerleader.
- Try to find some shared goals that you can both look forward to and build towards.

2. Sleep

Let's face it, no one is getting much sleep as a new parent. Sleep satisfaction and duration declines for both parents, but mothers are more affected.[7] Especially if breastfeeding, mothers are more likely to lose more sleep at night, but on average make up for it slightly with daytime naps.

Sleep deprivation is awful. It affects your mood, your immune system and your physical wellbeing.[8] It's linked to feeling more stressed as a parent and feeling like you can't cope during the day.[9] If you're exhausted by the end of the day you're less likely to be able to positively engage with anyone and are going to fall into bed. Is it any wonder this can lead to relationship issues?

Competitive tiredness is a common trap to fall into, and a common source of seeing red when you haven't slept properly for what feels like forever. To be fair, you're probably both tired, just in different ways. Caring for a baby is exhausting. Working is exhausting. You might get breaks at work, but you probably don't get naps. You might get naps at home, but the relentless tasks and night feeds mean it's not exactly like being on a spa break.

Some ideas for reducing arguments:

- Recognise that each of you is tired but perhaps in different ways.
- Look after each other. What do you both need most? Can one of you support the other to have 30 minutes' peace when they come in from work, and then they support the other to have 30 minutes all on their own? Do

what you can to give the other more time to relax and rest. Make each other cups of tea.

- Realise that the grass likely isn't greener. Working is hard. Looking after a baby is hard. Different types of hard, but still both hard.
- Tag team your sleep and lie-ins. Maybe you will decide to protect the working partner's sleep during the week, as long as they in turn give you chance to go to bed earlier or at least rest in the evenings. Maybe each of you gets a lie-in on one day at the weekend. If this is difficult with breastfeeding, maybe one does the night feeds and after the first morning feed the other takes the baby for a bit.

3. Task share

Another common source of arguments is who is doing more in the relationship. It's too easy to fall into a pattern where somehow the partner at home is taking care of the baby and doing all the housework, meaning their working 'day' never ends, especially if you add night feeds in. This can be a particular issue if the working partner is working long and irregular hours.[10]

Ideally, couples would come to a balance where each is putting equal amounts of hours into the needs of the family, whether that be through working, housework or childcare. Both of you should have equal opportunity for time to yourself and rest. It's highly unlikely that just because 'work outside the home' and 'work inside the home' falls into two neat categories that they are equal in load. Housework and childcare are not a 9-5 job, but couples can easily fall into a pattern where a partner at home is continuing to do more in the evenings and on weekends, meaning they have less downtime overall.

It's also not just a simple case of how many hours you are both putting in. Thinking back to the section on money and how we value making money, equal hours of housework and childcare versus working can feel very different. One can feel thankless and repetitive and lonely. The other can be linked to rewards, the chance to socialise and identity. Saying that, it all depends how much the working parent likes their job. If they hate it, they have a nasty manager or they have little control then they may envy the parent at home who isn't getting shouted at or criticised. Additionally, if they have a tiring, physical job they may be too exhausted to do much on getting home.

This perceived unfairness is often at the heart of arguments around who does what, with the partner who is at home often feeling much more dissatisfaction.[11] It also becomes a particular issue when maternity leave ends and both partners are working. It is easy to have fallen into patterns that don't change as much as they should, especially when it comes to household chores.

The not-so-small issue of household chores

Research consistently shows what many couples already know: housework is a huge source of contention, particularly when both partners are working. Data shows that women do more housework than men – even when they are the main breadwinners, they are still more likely to do more household chores.[12]

For example, in one analysis of how much paid work, childcare and household chores each partner in a couple does, women were found to do the majority of housework and childcare even when they were the main earner. Men were very rarely both the main wage earner and did more childcare and housework.[13] The researchers found that:

- In dual-earner families, 60.5% of women report doing over 10 hours of housework per week compared to 22.9% of men.
- When women were the main wage earner 58% still did more than 10 hours a week, with 49% of men doing more than 10 hours.
- When men were the main wage earner 87% of women reported doing more than 10 hours a week, while 14% of men did.

In terms of who does the childcare:
- When both are earning, roughly two-thirds of couples say they share child care equally, while a third of women do more, with men doing more about 2% of the time.
- When women are the main wage earner childcare is still shared equally about 60% of the time, done mainly by the father about 25% of the time and mainly by the mother 15% of the time.
- When the father is the main wage earner, childcare is shared equally about 14% of the time and done mainly by the mother 85% of the time. Men take the lead just 1% of the time.

Similarly, in research from the USA, a pattern was observed that when a male partner earned more than a female partner, she took on more chores. When a female partner earned more than a male partner, he did proportionately less.[14]

- When a father stayed home while the mother worked, he did on average 18 hours of housework and 11 hours of childcare, while she did 14 hours of housework and nine hours of childcare per week.
- When a mother stayed home while the father worked she did 26 hours of housework and 20 hours of childcare while he did seven hours of housework and six hours of childcare.
- Notably, stay-at-home dads had on average 20 hours more leisure time than their working partners, while stay-at-home mums only had on average four hours more leisure time than their working partners.

"Housework is a huge source of contention, particularly when both partners are working."

Why does this pattern consistently happen, even when women earn and work more? One reason is a tendency for couples to subconsciously conform to gender expectations. Men feel challenged by not meeting the societal expectation to be the main wage earner, so do not want to 'feminise' themselves by doing more housework. Women worry about not being good enough mothers or partners (according to societal expectations), so do more housework. This fits with research that shows that when individuals go against the societal gender norm at work, they try to balance it out at home. So men who are nurses are more likely to spend leisure time doing 'manly' stuff like putting up shelves, while women who are police officers do more baking.[15]

Oddly there also sometimes seems to be some kind of cognitive dissonance about who is bringing what to the family. In one strange study, where women contributed at least 80-100% of the family income, just a third of women and their partners actually considered the woman to be in the main provider or breadwinner role. This was despite inclusion in the study being based on women earning more. So couples knew the woman earned more, but didn't want to see her in, or her to be seen in, a provider identity. Why? Most likely the explanation is those strange social expectations about what makes a 'good' partner – women are not viewed as good mothers unless they give up everything to be with their child, and men aren't men unless they're the breadwinners.[16]

The role of the mental load

This double burden of tasks has been referred to as a 'second shift' for working mothers. Researchers in the 1980s found that as the number of women in the workforce increased, there was little change in who completed household chores. Women carried on doing the bulk of chores and childcare, effectively working a 'second shift'.

What is interesting about research that looks at the impact of this second shift is that quite understandably, women aren't very happy about it. But what is intriguing is that men often don't understand what their partner is unhappy about. They think that they are sharing responsibilities equally. Indeed, in one study of couples, 40% of men felt things were equal, but only 20% of women did.[17] Likewise, in a poll in the *New York Times* about who was taking most responsibility for home schooling during the COVID-19 pandemic, 45% of men thought they were, but just 3% of women agreed.[18] Research shows that men consistently overestimate how much time they spend on household tasks and underestimate how much time their female partner spends. Women are more accurate.[19]

Why is this? It's probably the effect of the mental load.

The mental load – or emotional load – is a common reason for arguments, especially when you've just added a new baby to the mix. This term refers to all the stuff that needs thinking about and planning rather than just the everyday things. Like remembering you need to buy more nappies, or thinking about what you'll need to pack to take out with you, or remembering to have bottle sanitising fluid in, and so on and so on. Some people have described it as like being a project manager or wedding planner or personal assistant... or someone who organises a lot of stuff behind the scenes to make things happen. So when you open a changing bag to change your baby's nappy when you're out and about, all the stuff you need is in there. It is very eloquently summed up by French columnist Emma in her cartoon about the mental load: www.theguardian.com/world/2017/may/26/gender-wars-household-chores-comic.

The mental load grows exponentially when you have a baby as suddenly there is a whole new person to be organised who can't do stuff for themselves, exacerbated by the fact that until recently you never knew half of this stuff needed doing anyway. The core issue is that it is kind of invisible, and therefore not 'counted' in tasks or associated with any gratitude. It's not about giving the baby a bottle, which you can see happening in front of you. It's the making sure there was a clean bottle – or a bottle in the first place – and that it was filled with breastmilk that you expressed (and bought the pump to do so and cleaned the pump and stored the milk...) or bought the right stage formula (as you'd researched it) and stored it correctly and made it up correctly. This invisible stuff often takes far more time and effort than the visible act of actually giving the bottle.

The idea of the baby-related mental load has been around for a while. In 1996 Professor Susan Walzer published a research paper entitled 'Thinking about the Baby: Gender and Divisions of Infant Care' which presented her findings from interviewing 25 couples about how they cared for their baby. Walzer identified that not only did mothers do more of the planning and organising, they also did much more worrying and delegating of tasks, meaning their overall time spent thinking about 'stuff' was far longer.[20]

Worrying

Mothers worried more about their babies than fathers did, and then worried more about them precisely because the father was not doing much worrying. Many women described simply 'worrying about everything', which was attributed to society holding women more to account for their baby's health and wellbeing than men. A common way of describing the worry was that their baby was just 'continuously at the back of their mind' even when they weren't with them.

Somehow worrying was seen as synonymous with good motherhood – some mothers even worried that if they stopped worrying about stuff, it was a sign they were not a good mother. Notably fathers in the study exacerbated this issue, with one describing his wife as a good mother because 'she worries a lot'. Another mother talked about how she worried that if she wasn't the main one doing things for her baby, then she wasn't a good enough mother – doing half was too little in her view; it had to be most, even though she was also earning a very high salary. Guilt and anxiety drove her to need to be there as much as possible.

Notably no father in the survey expressed a similar feeling – when they were away from their baby, they were away from their baby. Instead fathers worried about how much time they spent with their baby when they weren't doing something else – attributed to pressures to provide and do well at work. Men often said that they felt their partner worried too much, notably without seeing all the things that needed worrying about. One described his partner as worrying too much about things like making sure their baby got all their immunisations, doctors' appointments and vitamin drops, noting that he didn't bother worrying about those things.

Delegating

Another common finding in the study was that even when tasks were split equally, it was the mother who was in charge of thinking about what needed doing and asking for it to be done. Many fathers talked about how they did an equal share of things *when they were asked* rather than identifying that something needed to be done. Insightfully, Walzer notes: *While on one level it appears that women are 'in charge' of the division of labor, the assumption of female responsibility means that, on another level, men are in charge — because it is only with their permission and cooperation that mothers can relinquish their duties.*

This continues to be a source of contention in 2020. When it comes to the mental load, it is not necessarily that male partners are less willing to do the tasks, it's that they don't see that they need to be done in the first place. A common response to you losing your rag and yelling 'Why are there plates all over the kitchen?' is 'You should have asked me to wash them'. This immediately throws responsibility back to the woman – she is 'in charge' of managing the household and noticing things and delegating things as well as often doing more of the things.

One of the clever things about the mental load is that it often isn't categorised as 'work'. So going back to the example of giving the baby a bottle, we might recognise and see the work of feeding the baby, as it's physically there in front of us, but we don't see the thinking and the planning. But thinking and planning is exhausting and means we never switch off. I bet when you're thinking about buying or organising *all the stuff*, you don't formally sit down and think. You're thinking while stuck at traffic lights/bathing the baby/cooking the dinner/having mediocre sex.

You would think this imbalance would make women feel angry. And indeed, it does. But the study also talked about how this unseen labour and responsibility led to women feeling another emotion – loneliness. They felt unseen in their relationship and unseen in their role. Unappreciated. And this led into another idea – that they were missing out on gratitude and recognition – known as the 'economy of gratitude'. Think of everything a couple brings to a relationship. They might bring money or completion of chores. These are visible things. Things we see happening and are grateful to each other for. But the planning and the worrying of emotional labour often goes unseen and therefore doesn't count in the labour of the household. This is exacerbated even more if fathers are seen to be 'doing a favour' to the mother if they do the things she asks.

Finally, this all gets further ingrained by society's views on good mothers and fathers. Society still seems to excuse or forgive men who don't do things for their children in a way it never would for women. Women are judged more harshly for forgetting small things – things that men wouldn't even be expected to remember. So when women push back against the emotional load by simply refusing to do things, they pay a higher price – both through society's judgement and their own increased worry for their baby.

Some ideas for reducing arguments:
- A starting place is talking to your partner about what really needs to be done now you have a baby. Talk about everything you do, how relentless it can feel and how it could be more equally shared.
- Make a list of everything that needs to be done – both visible and invisible tasks.
- Divide up the tasks so you have equal responsibility – earning money, caring for your baby and housework. This isn't necessarily straightforward, nor will there necessarily be balance every single day.
- Look at your own pattern of functioning, no matter how hard this is. Have you fallen into a traditional pattern, perhaps observed in your own parents, of you taking on more or less or doing only certain things – and then feeling bitter or helpless about it?

Ideas for dividing up tasks

You could start by working out what practically needs to be done by one of you. Perhaps you are the one breastfeeding and your partner is the one working outside the home – and it's not like you can just rock up at their workplace and they take over feeding the baby (though never say never!). Then perhaps there are things that make more sense for one of you to do – so it's easier for you to pop washing on because you're at home, and it's easier for them to drag the bins out as they're not recovering from a c-section. Or maybe there are things you are 'better at' and they are 'better at'. By this I mean stuff like maybe one of you is more interested/has more access to financial deals or whatever, *not* somehow being more skilled at the washing up. Or maybe there are things you would prefer to do over others and so on.

Compromising on some things is a good idea. Maybe one of you really cares about dust on the top of the fridge and the other one couldn't care less and can't see it anyway. If it's not life-threatening, let it go. It also needs to be fluid. Some days you might be more knackered than others, or the baby screams all day or your partner has to stay late at work. Don't hold each other strictly to account or time each other or whatever. Some weeks some stuff won't get done.

It can really help to approach this task from this perspective because it involves sitting down and discussing who will take responsibility for what (well, in theory). After you have had this discussion, you have moved responsibility from you to both of you – you have shared the responsibility. You are no longer in charge of noticing and delegating.

Roughly speaking, three main things need attention: your baby, your home and your finances. You're aiming for roughly equal amounts of free time each, but again preference and compromise will help you sort it fairly.

4. Sex

Arguments about sex are also really common. Sometimes it's actually about the sex and sometimes it's really just about the connection and intimacy. Most couples find they have less sex after having a baby, but with communication and understanding this doesn't have to be an issue. A really good read on this topic is the book *Mind the Gap: the truth about desire and how to futureproof your sex life* by Dr Karen Gurney.

Some ideas for improving communication and intimacy

Talk to each other
Don't try and avoid talking about the fact that you are having less sex. Talk about how you are feeling and what might be affecting your lack of interest. It might be a simple case of both going '*Wow, we're exhausted, aren't we?*' or it could run much deeper than that. Memories of birth, fear of it hurting or worries about feeling different as a parent can all play a role. Tell your partner how you feel without accusing them. Listen to your partner when they do the same.

Go slowly
Research has shown that in the first few months after giving birth 83% of women experience some sort of physical issue, including pain from tearing or stitches, vaginal dryness, thin vaginal tissue, pain or soreness. Many of

these are exacerbated by fatigue and unsurprisingly are linked to low libido.[21] Go gently and talk to your partner if it hurts. Remember sex doesn't have to mean penetration – there are many different ways and stages of being intimate! Always remember you can stop at any time. Talk to your partner about this. You might be wary but willing to give things a go on the understanding that they will stop if you ask them to.

If you experienced a very difficult birth and are feeling a lot of trauma about that, you might be finding the idea of sex very difficult. It could bring back memories of the birth, consciously or subconsciously, and you might find yourself recoiling or panicking. Do talk to someone. Look at the chapter on birth trauma and find someone who can support you. You might also find that postnatal depression is making you feel unlike sex. Again, there is support. Treat both of these as if they were physical health issues, even if you are physically healed. You might also find this article from *Elle* magazine useful: **www.elle.com/uk/life-and-culture/culture/articles/a38516/sex-after-trauma-giving-birth-postnatal-depression**.

Recognise the role that hormones play

It's easy to fall into the trap of arguing when one of you doesn't want sex, thinking that it's about attraction. It's not. It's about hormones, how they change after the birth and how exhaustion affects them. Sleep deprivation and tiredness lower libido.[22] It's likely that on an evolutionary level we are designed not to risk pregnancy soon after having a baby, or expend energy away from caring for them.

After birth women's oestrogen levels fall quickly and may stay low, possibly even lower than pre-pregnancy levels if you are breastfeeding. Oestrogen plays a role not only in libido, but also in vaginal lubrication, meaning you might be at increased risk of dryness, irritation or bleeding during sex. You might also be worried about leaking breastmilk during sex. Talk to your partner – it's all normal.

Men also experience a drop in testosterone which can reduce sex drive – fathers with the largest drop in testosterone report the largest drop in sexual activity.[23] Always talk to your GP if you have any physical concerns.

Check your health is okay

Depression, anxiety and nutritional deficiencies can all affect sexual desire. If you're avoiding sex, is it just exhaustion or could it be something else? Make an appointment with your GP if you are concerned.

Focus on intimacy not sex

If you feel unable to have sex due to pain, or simply feel exhausted, focusing on intimacy instead in your relationship can really help. Talk to each other, hug, sit together on the sofa. Make time for each other and to be together. As intimacy and affection builds, your libido may too.

Also, ask yourself how much it really is about sex. Is it the physical act? Or is it actually the intimacy, connection and simply time spent together one on one? These can be worked on outside of actually having sex if you are feeling unable to for whatever reason.

Think about whether you're feeling touched out

I had this really strong feeling of all my senses being overwhelmed. I didn't want anyone to touch me or sit too close or speak to me. Sometimes even strong smells would annoy me. It was like being touched hurt, like an electric shock. I hated it and obviously my partner took it personally but he hadn't had a small person glued to him, pawing at his breasts all day. Kellie

Feeling touched out – not wanting anyone to touch you or even be near you – is a common feeling among breastfeeding mothers, although anyone can feel this way. You may feel intensely irritated by the thought of your baby touching you, and want desperately to put them down and escape... and then feel guilty for feeling like that. It extends to everyone else too – once you've put that baby down you don't want someone else making demands on you.

This is such a natural feeling. Your baby has perhaps been glued to you all day or will only stop crying if you hold them while standing up. Then just as you get them down your partner comes home and tries to hug you and bang... you recoil. But obviously it can have the effect of making them feel rejected or unloved.

It might seem odd, but the solution might actually be to spend time being more physically intimate with your partner. Feeling touched out is often blamed on having a baby pawing at you all day long or needing to be held. But it's not always about the touch, it's about the neediness. In fact, being touched in a nice way – a massage, a hug or whatever you fancy – can help as long as it is focused on what *you* need. It can help to explain this to your partner, talking about how you need touch to be about shared intimacy rather than a demand.

It can also help if your partner gives you time to have physical and emotional space – chance to be alone and no one to need anything from you. This can act as a reset, making you more open to feeling intimate later.

Recognise things will likely change in the future
Most couples find they start having more sex once they are less tired. It's not exactly rocket science, is it?! And you will feel less tired one day. Look at all the second and third and subsequent babies out there – living proof it happens!

Public service announcement: if you don't want another baby, use contraception!

Know the difference between a good and a bad argument

Disagreements between couples are absolutely normal. It's not so much about how often you disagree, but how you communicate those disagreements and how you deal with them and make things better.

- Do talk about how you feel – arguments have a short-term negative impact on relationship intimacy, but in the longer-term lead to more satisfaction. Conversely, suppressing your emotions can lead to resentment.[24]
- Stay calm if possible – and never try and hurt your partner to win an argument.
- Recognise your partner's fighting style (and your own). Do you yell? Run away? How does that make your partner react? Is it constructive? If you both tend to yell and then forget all about it, it's less of an issue than if one of you is a yeller and one of you panics at a raised voice. It's also worth taking some time to think about where your argument style comes from. How did your parents deal with disagreements? How did they communicate with you? Thinking back may give you a number of clues about why you react in a certain way. Remember, your partner is not your parent!
- Try not to accuse the other of '*always* acting in a certain way'. They most likely don't.
- Describe how an action makes you feel, rather than how the person makes you feel. For example, 'I feel frustrated when you don't do the dishes' rather than 'You are frustrating'. This is also a great tip for talking to your child when they are older.
- Try and discuss what you are really upset about. Maybe they haven't been loading the dishwasher. Is it really about the few minutes that takes, or is it actually about how that makes you feel?
- Try and keep arguments concise and to the point – and therefore possibly more frequent – rather than letting things build up and you having a long list of things to say. Try to not drag up absolutely everything from the past while you're at it.
- Try to make requests rather than complaints: 'I need you to do the dishes more often' rather than 'You never do the dishes'.
- Recognise your own patterns. Do you always have a certain fight at a certain time? Are you trying to avoid something? Is it because you're frazzled about other things at a certain time? Are you just hungry?
- If possible, try not to discuss things when you're exhausted, have no time or the baby is crying. Ask if you can discuss it later, or choose your moment to bring things up.

- Know when to apologise and how to do it. How do you like to be apologised to? How does your partner? Is it about a show of affection? Or about reassuring them about certain things?

Some more ideas for strengthening your relationship

- Be kind to each other – realise you are both on a huge learning curve. Remember you love each other and are both trying to do the best you can in the situation. Also remind yourself it is the situation not each other – things will change and pass.
- Do try and prioritise time together. You might want to make this a regular 'date night' or you might cringe at the term or feel exhausted just thinking about it. But regular time is important. Maybe it's sitting down at the end of the day together or declaring nap time when you're both home as time to forget everything else and be together.
- Present a united front against interfering family and friends. Don't let them interfere. And certainly don't pass on messages that they think your partner is doing things wrong.
- Read about love languages. Although this can be overly simplistic, think about how you feel loved and express love – and how your partner does too. The love languages idea is based on the concept of five ways of expressing love – through words, gifts, acts of service, physical touch or quality time. We each see different options as being a sign we are loved or a way of showing love. Talk to your partner – what makes them feel most loved? Words about what a good job they are doing? A surprise gift? Time focusing on you? Responding with what they feel shows love has a higher chance of making them feel important.[25]
- Find a shared goal you can both work towards in the future even if your current days are exhausting. This especially works well if you feel your daily lives are now very different. It might be a plan to move to another house or area, train, pick up a new hobby or simply a holiday or night out once your baby is sleeping more. See yourself as a team with shared goals.
- Just keep talking. Talk and try and understand your partner's view and experience. How are they feeling? What are they stressed about? What do they hope for? How do they see the future? Really listen and be supportive (where possible!).
- Do consider external relationship counselling as an option if you are struggling. Relate provides counselling **www.relate.org.uk,** as do private counsellors. Try the British Association for Counsellors and Psychotherapists to find support local to you **www.bacp.co.uk**.

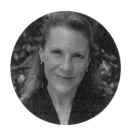

Five tips for staying connected to your partner

Interview with Elly Taylor, a perinatal relationship specialist based in Australia. Her website 'Becoming Us' has resources and courses for parents and professionals to support them in navigating the journey to becoming new parents. You can find it at www.becomingusfamily.com. Her book *Becoming Us: The Couple's Guide to Surviving Parenthood and Growing a Family that Thrives* is available now.

1. Know that most couples have relationship struggles in early parenthood. In fact a whopping 92% of couples report increased conflict during this time. More arguments don't mean there's anything wrong with you, your partner or your relationship, so don't panic, it's normal.

2. When we're having problems, we tend to look for someone to blame. Don't blame your partner. It's likely that you both could have done with more preparation and support for your new life with a baby so you could be there for each other. Unfair blame leads to resentment and you don't want that to get in the way of your connection.

3. Make it safe to talk about anything and everything. There are so many changes going on inside new mothers and new fathers, that it can be easy to start drifting apart when you're not sharing them with each other. Check in with your partner every day to see how they're doing. This could be the beginning of deeper conversations that connect you on an emotional level.

4. Staying connected as partners needs to be a priority when most of your time and attention is likely to be going to the baby. Connection doesn't have to be a night out or a weekend away. Small things that only take a moment can be more than enough! A loving look, a kind word, an affectionate gesture or a thoughtful gift all keep you connected on a daily basis.

5. Couples' sex lives usually change when they become parents. Even when your doctor gives you the six-week OK, most parents, mothers and fathers both, still aren't ready. Stay connected in other ways and your new normal sex life will return more naturally sooner rather than later.

Chapter twenty-six

When things can't be fixed – spotting the signs of relationship breakdown and domestic abuse

$\rightarrow$ Sadly, sometimes relationships cannot be fixed. The previous chapter was all about strategies for working together to improve your relationship and be a team. But it all relies on you both wanting to be in that team, and a willingness to put in the energy and effort to help each other. Sometimes relationships simply break down. You realise you have grown apart or want separate things. But sometimes there are deeper issues around control, coercion and violence that you might need support in escaping from.

Both men and women can be victims of domestic abuse. However, women experience higher rates and more serious injuries. They are also more likely to experience coercive control.[1] On top of that, the most common time for a woman to experience domestic abuse is when she becomes pregnant, and the majority of women who are victims of abuse are either pregnant or have dependent children.[2] Data from 2018 collated by Women's Aid from domestic

> **Many women will not ever report abuse, or will wait to experience multiple occurrences before they contact anyone.**

abuse organisations in England found 6% of women who accessed help were currently pregnant (compared to a figure of roughly 2% across a population), with 58% having dependent children.[3]

However, it is likely that the numbers of women actually experiencing abuse are much higher. It is extremely difficult to accurately report how many women experience domestic abuse each year. Many women will not report it, either from fear of further consequences, fear of not being believed or sometimes not even realising that what is happening to them is abuse. To show the scale of it, data shows that every hour the police across England and Wales receive over 100 phone calls relating to domestic abuse, yet other surveys have shown only around one in five women will ever report an incidence.[4]

There is a difference between reporting domestic violence in a survey or to a health professional and making an official report to the police. In research that tries to estimate the number of women who experience domestic violence in pregnancy, figures suggest much higher rates than 6%. For example, one study in Ireland that examined antenatal records found that 12.9% of women reported a history of abuse, while a survey in northern England found 17% of pregnant women reported a history of physical, emotional or sexual abuse. Many women will not ever report abuse, or will wait to experience multiple occurrences before they contact anyone. On average this figure is 35 times.[5]

Why does domestic violence increase in pregnancy?

Lots of reasons have been considered to explain why violence may increase during pregnancy - none of which are your fault. Research has shown that for some men sexual jealousy increases alongside what they perceive to be a limitation on your sexual availability. Some are jealous of your relationship with the baby. Others are worried about the changing status of your relationship or financial concerns. Some seize upon a woman's increased physical and potentially economic vulnerability during pregnancy, or conversely are jealous of her perceived sexual and reproductive power.[6]

Some doubt they are the father of the baby or want to end the pregnancy, particularly if it was unplanned. A study from the World Health Organization found that 90% of women who were physically attacked during pregnancy were attacked by the father of their baby. Up to half experienced direct trauma to their abdomen.[7]

Domestic abuse is not just about physical violence. The charity Women's Aid lists seven different main forms of domestic abuse, including:

- Coercive control
- Psychological and/or emotional abuse
- Physical or sexual abuse
- Financial or economic abuse
- Harassment and stalking
- Online or digital abuse

At the heart of any of these is often an attempt to control. A partner can be controlled through fear of what will happen if they trigger the abuse, or fear may be used as a form of abuse itself.

Signs you might be experiencing domestic abuse

Some aspects of abuse might be easier to spot than others. If someone physically hits you this is a clear marker. But remember, physical abuse doesn't just involve physically hurting you. It might also include:

- Threats to hurt you such as pretending to punch you, squaring up to you
- Punching a wall or a sofa or throwing things
- Hurting a pet
- Threatening to hurt your children
- Breaking your possessions
- Driving too quickly with you or your children in the car
- Restraining you and preventing you from leaving

Other forms of abuse may feel more subtle, which is most likely the aim of the abuser. Recently, 'coercive control' has been made a criminal offence. This type of abuse is based around control, limiting your ability to live a confident and 'free' life. Abusers use tactics such as slowly isolating their victim from other forms of support, making them financially dependent and undermining their confidence through humiliation, insults and intimidation.

Often from the outside these individuals look like great partners. They might be in good jobs, have lots of friends and be very sociable. In fact they thrive by presenting as one person to the outside world and then treating you very differently in private. You might have a night out with friends and think that the evening was great, but once you get home your partner starts telling you that you made a fool of yourself or them. Maybe they take you aside at a quiet moment and tell you this in public, or give you a private look to let you know they are not happy. They control you by making you doubt yourself and feel embarrassed or ashamed, while giving the impression that everyone else thinks they are wonderful.

Some signs you might be experiencing coercive control:

- You are not allowed (or are strongly discouraged) to see family or friends
- You get regular put-downs or attempts to embarrass or humiliate you
- Your time is not your own; you have to ask to go out, rest or do hobbies
- Your finances are strictly controlled
- You are told, directly or subtly, what to wear
- Your partner threatens to leave, telling you your life would be worthless without them
- Sulking or silence when you don't 'behave' or disappearing to punish you
- Removing access to your things or hiding them
- Preventing you from doing your work
- Criticising you in front of others
- Taking money from your purse or asking to borrow your card and spending money you didn't say they could
- Invading your privacy, e.g. hacking your email or looking at your phone

Spotting the abuse–forgiveness cycle

A key trick of abusers is to repeat a cycle in which they are abusive and then beg for your forgiveness. Many try to persuade you that it's not really their fault: you pushed them into it, or other stressors in their life are so great that they just couldn't help themselves. They might try to persuade you this is normal and happens in all relationships. Or suggest that you are overreacting and they didn't do anything that bad.

They may also engage in 'love bombing', where they shower you with love, affection and gifts for a period of time until you forgive them. This then ebbs away, before they restart the abuse. This is a really common trick in cults, because it increases feelings of connection and obedience, meaning you are more likely to forgive and follow orders. It can be used positively with children when you spend lots of time concentrating on them – obviously without then pulling all affection away and abusing them.

I'm really not sure if this applies to me

If you recognise things in this chapter as applying to you and your relationship you might be worrying that you are overreacting or doubting whether they are occurring or not. This is really common and something that abusers will deliberately encourage you to feel so that you don't leave. They may also try to whittle down your confidence – again so you don't leave. Or limit your access to
money – so you don't leave.

The Freedom Programme is a brilliant online course that you can access for around £12. It talks through what a good relationship looks like, different signs of abuse and supports you in working out whether you are in an abusive relationship. You can find more about it here – there are different versions for men and women: **freedomprogramme.co.uk/online.php**.

Practical steps to change your situation

If you recognise the signs of abuse and make the decision to leave then Women's Aid has lots of information on how to access support on its website **www.womensaid.org.uk/information-support**. The charity also has an excellent handbook on how to spot abuse and what to do next, including guidance for seeking alternative accommodation, your legal rights and money **www.womensaid.org.uk/the-survivors-handbook**. These guides include information on helping you think through things like:

- Finances
- Housing
- Supporting your children
- Making an escape plan
- Packing your belongings to leave
- Your legal rights
- Protecting yourself

You do not need to fear that your children will be taken away because you re-port being abused. In fact, one of the best things you can do for your children is to remove yourself from the situation. One of the most common risk factors for someone experiencing abuse is having seen their own father physically attack their mother. It becomes 'normal'. Removing yourself from the situation and saying enough is enough sends an incredibly strong message to your children.[8] All the evidence around the impact of separation on children's wellbeing points to the fact that it is usually not the separation itself that causes any issues, but having to live in difficult or abusive circumstances. Again, removing yourself from the situation is one of the best things you can do for them.

Your next steps will be specific to you. If you have a job and income or family and friends who can help you then it may be easier than if you are more dependent on your partner. Do read through the guides – they have supported many people to leave abusive relationships and start again. A newer, more positive life is possible.

Chapter twenty-seven

Thriving as an LGBTQ parent

→ The number of same-sex-couple families is increasing rapidly in the UK, supported by changes to same-sex marriage in 2014. In 2015 there were 152,000 same-sex-couple marriages in the UK compared to 232,000 in 2018.[1] Many of the relationship difficulties you might face as a new parent will be the same as any couple. However, you may find you experience some additional challenges. Although attitudes have hugely improved in the UK over the last three decades,[2] LGBTQ couples still face ridiculous questions and reactions, particularly when it comes to having a baby. This chapter is going to look at some of those and ways to get support.

The good news – *better* relationship satisfaction

To start with the good news, research has consistently shown that same-sex couples have much better relationship satisfaction on becoming and being parents than heterosexual couples. A number of studies show that lesbian couples in particular are far better at sharing childcare and household chores than heterosexual couples,[3] meaning they experience much less couple dissatisfaction upon becoming parents.[4] Research has also rated communication, co-operation and intimacy between same-sex parents as much stronger.[5]

The challenges

Unfortunately, becoming a new parent as a same-sex couple can throw up a number of unique difficulties. On top of all the day-to-day stresses new parents face in adapting to parenthood, you are possibly dealing with additional pressures on top. These might include:

- Subtle or more overt prejudice from others. Gay fathers in particular can face stigma. Some people with very traditional views seem to believe there is only one way to be a family, which of course causes a lot of grief for perfectly happy couples falling outside their imposed rules. A common prejudiced opinion is that somehow children of same-sex parents have worse outcomes than those with heterosexual parents. Quite simply this is nonsense and lots of science backs this up - outcomes are no different across educational, social and emotional measures. The main predictor of secure children is having consistent and loving relationships with parents, whoever they are. One study even showed better health and family cohesion in same-sex-couple families.[6]

- Having to spend time explaining things repeatedly or even reassuring the health professionals who are meant to be supporting you. Some couples have talked about health professionals getting confused and asking daft questions about 'Who is the mother?' or 'Where is the father?', despite it being explained. These everyday micro-aggressions can feel really challenging, especially as they increase and become repetitive during pregnancy and birth.

- Dealing with the ridiculous questions people ask you that they wouldn't ask a heterosexual couple, like 'How did you get pregnant?' or 'Who is really the mum?' You might find this video relatable - heterosexual parents are asked the same questions same-sex parents often get. It shows just how intrusive and ridiculous this can be **www.youtube.com/watch?v=4RH7zX6QSUM**. There are also some great responses in this article: **metro.co.uk/2017/03/09/8-things-you-should-never-say-to-same-sex-parents-6491323**.

- A chance that you will fall into typical traditional heterosexual roles if one partner stays home with the baby and one becomes the main wage earner - and feeling really uncomfortable with that.

- Challenging emotions around who will carry a baby or who will feed the baby. Even if one of you didn't actually want to do either, it's still normal to feel jealousy. Or perhaps if you are both women, the partner who didn't give birth might induce lactation to be able to feed the baby too. This can be challenging, but many couples feel it's something worthwhile. Of course, you can then get stupid questions from people who are very confused and feel it's their right to pry in a way they wouldn't with a heterosexual couple. For more support on inducing lactation, La Leche League has great information here: www.laleche.org.uk/relactation-induced-lactation, or check out my own *The Positive Breastfeeding Book* for tips and stories from those who have induced lactation.

- A larger social burden than heterosexual couples. Research has shown that for same-sex female couples, the social burden typically placed on women within family structures can be really high. Often, in heterosexual couples, women report having to do all the 'wife work' for the family, including things like remembering relatives' birthdays, organising socialising or taking care of other family members. They are expected to be nurturing, thoughtful and caring for others. Research has shown that when two women form a relationship and have a baby, their families often, subconsciously or otherwise, really ramp up expectations of *both* women, expecting them to be the couple who supports everyone else. This is obviously stressful and extremely frustrating and can leave you feeling that you have little time for each other between juggling everything.[7]
- Stress involved in proceeding with legal changes such as adoption for non-biological parents. For legal information, Stonewall has great resources to support you through the process www.stonewall.org.uk/help-advice/parenting-rights.
- Potential discrimination from employers who may not be up to speed or make insensitive comments. Same-sex parents have the same rights as heterosexual parents – the partner who gives birth can take maternity leave, and the partner who does not can take paternity leave, or you can take shared parental leave. For more information on leave see Chapter 29. The Maternity Action website is a great source of information maternityaction.org.uk/advice/same-sex-partner.

Ideas for support

- Recognise the additional stresses you experience and that they are coming from outside your partnership, not within. Be kind to yourself and each other and seek as much support as possible, whether that is from friends, allies and family or more formal support from relationship counsellors. Never underestimate the power of support from other LGBTQ parents who understand what you are experiencing.
- Check out the website and blog of Amber Wildes about her experiences of same-sex parenting meetthewildes.com.

- Send family and friends who want (or you think need) to learn more to the Families and Friends of Lesbians and Gays website which has great resources **www.fflag.org.uk**.
- B.J. Epstein Woodstein has written a great piece for the Association of Breastfeeding Mothers on supporting LGBTQ parents with breastfeeding. A number of the points might resonate with you and it could be a useful starting piece to refer health professionals to **abm.me.uk/breastfeeding-information/tips-for-supporting-lgbtq-families**.
- The Australian Psychological Society has a great review bringing together all the evidence supporting same-sex parents, should you ever need such references **www.psychology.org.au/getmedia/47196902-158d-4cbb-86e6-2f3f1c71ffd1/LGBT-families-literature-review.pdf**.
- Books that are worth a read include:
  - *Pride and Joy: A Guide for Lesbian, Gay, Bisexual and Trans Parents* – Sarah and Rachel Hagger-Holt
  - *Gay Parenting: Complete Guide for Same-sex Families* – Shana Priwer and Cynthia Phillips.

Chapter twenty-eight

Thriving as a single parent

→ Almost a quarter of families in the UK are now headed up by a single parent, with the majority of single parents being female. Being a single parent can be as brilliant as it can be challenging. This chapter is going to look at some of the challenges you might encounter and where to get support.

Your experience of being a single parent is going to be affected by who you are or are not parenting with. Your partner may have left but still be engaged as a good co-parent, they may have left and you are fighting while trying to co-parent, they may have left and are nowhere to be seen, they may have died or you may not actually know them at all. You may also have chosen single parenthood deliberately – by adopting or having IVF. Maybe you've now got a new partner yourself or maybe you haven't.

Sometimes being a single parent, especially if you have an okay relationship with a co-parent and a new relationship yourself, can actually be a positive experience. Whatever your situation you might find it much more positive than still being in a relationship with them. Or maybe you're really struggling. Have a look through the sections in this chapter and pick which may or may not be helpful to you.

Financial support

Women who are single parents are one of the population groups most likely to live in poverty. You only have one adult to bear the brunt of the living costs and may find it difficult to work, especially irregular hours or if your child's other parent is not on the scene.

Make sure you are claiming everything that you are entitled to. The Entitled To website has a calculator that will identify everything you might be able to claim. It can be found here: **www.entitledto.co.uk**. You may be entitled to benefits including help with childcare costs and housing. If you are on a low income you may also be entitled to Healthy Start vouchers which can be used to buy cows' milk, fruit and vegetables and first-stage infant formula. Check your eligibility here: **www.healthystart.nhs.uk**. If you are ever struggling to buy food speak to your health visitor. They may be able to refer you to a food bank. You can find more information on the Trussell Trust website **www. trusselltrust.org/get-help**.

What you are entitled to will depend on whether you have a new partner that you move in with. Unfortunately, it will take their income into account even if they do not pay towards your child (who they have no legal responsibility for). Think carefully and discuss how finances would be shared before moving in with someone.

Child maintenance

Child maintenance is paid by one parent to the other who has more responsibility for the child. It is based on how many children you have with that parent, their income and how many nights they have them in a typical year. If you share care equally they do not have to pay. There is a calculator here where you can estimate what they should pay: **www.gov.uk/calculate-child-maintenance**.

This figure is meant to be the minimum figure for contributing to supporting a child. It could be suggested that the parent should pay half the costs of raising a child, which of course will be much more if you take into account things like childcare. Many parents agree to a regular amount plus half of all big costs. Try to open the discussion with the other parent, perhaps with a list and evidence of the actual costs. Unfortunately, there is nothing you can do to actually make them pay half costs if they decide not to.

The Child Maintenance Service prefers co-parents to discuss and arrange payments between themselves. If this is impossible you can use the service to collect money, but it will charge you both a fee. Again this is obviously unfair if the other parent is choosing not to co-operate. Unfortunately, there are a lot of gaps in this service, including:

- Parents who are full-time students or in prison do not have to pay maintenance. It is easier to understand why someone in prison cannot pay maintenance than that a parent can give up a job and become a full-time student and therefore no longer have financial responsibility for their child.
- You may also face problems with some self-employed co-parents arranging their accounts so they have to pay less money. This is a common area of concern and again unfortunately one that a lot of co-parents experience. You can try to collect evidence that they are likely being paid more. And you can challenge their accounts through the Child Maintenance Service by raising a complaint.
- Maintenance also reduces if the other parent moves in with someone else who has children and claims they are paying towards their costs, or has another baby with them. Again this can feel very unfair as of course it does not reduce costs for your child.
- Finally, maintenance is based on the co-parent's salary only. If they move in with someone who earns more money it does not take this into account (yes I know, even though if *you* move in with someone the benefits system will take your partner's income into account). If the co-parent gives up work and has no income, yet is being fully supported, they will have no legal requirement to pay.

The system is deeply frustrating and causes a lot of pain to the parent doing most of the care and paying most of the costs. I should also stress that you are not allowed to prevent the other parent from seeing their child if they refuse to pay maintenance. The government suggests getting a mediator involved but that obviously requires the other party to agree to meet a mediator. They recommend using this website: **www.familymediationcouncil.org.uk/find-local-mediator**.

The system is deeply unfair and I wish I had a loophole that I could point you towards. In terms of protecting your own mental health, look after yourself as much as possible. Talk – to friends, family and in particular other single parents. Focus on what *you* are doing – stepping up and caring for and supporting your child and feel a lot of pride in that. You might also want to get some legal advice on whether it is worth you pursuing any claim.

If your co-parent is avoiding paying by trying to trick the service and repeatedly changing jobs, or just refusing to pay, then you can take action. The government has put together a document here that has lots of information: **assets.publishing.service.gov.uk/government/uploads/system/uploads/attachment_data/file/325186/if-child-maintenance-isnt-paid.pdf**.

Contact with the other parent

How often your child sees the other parent will depend on a number of factors. What any legal expert will tell you is that any decision should be made in the best interests of the child. Your child has the right to build a relationship with their other parent even if you hate them – unless it is established that they are a threat to the child in terms of violence or lack of care. I won't pretend this is easy, especially when they are tiny. On the flip side, there is actually no law that says they must see them and share the parental load if they don't want to. Yes, again this is deeply frustrating and shows the real inequity and lack of support for single parents who are mainly women.

How often the other parent sees your child will depend on how old they are. With older children a typical pattern is every other weekend and a night in the week. This seems to work well in making sure children aren't moved around too much but do see their other parent. It will of course depend on things like where any childcare, work or school is and if the other parent lives close to you.

- With a young baby though, this might be very different, especially if you are breastfeeding. I'm going to use the most common descriptors of mother and father here because it becomes confusing otherwise. When babies are young most are cared for by their mother (and this is the biological norm), with their father having contact. It is unlikely that a judge would rule that a young baby should have overnight stays with the father unless this was something you both wanted. Remember the key phrase – in the best interests of the child.
- If you are separated from the other parent from before birth or in the early weeks a more typical pattern would be for regular short visits, usually in the company of the mother too or even in your home if that is okay with you. Contact is important to build a bond, but it should not be at the expense of a baby who needs to form a core attachment relationship with a primary caregiver. This can change slowly over time. As your baby grows their other parent may take them out for the day, for example. You could work towards overnights by the end of the first year or so, dependent on whether your child is still breastfeeding.
- If you do have a good relationship with your co-parent things might be different, especially if you haven't started new relationships. Some former couples might consider having an overnight at each other's house – in a separate bedroom – so that the baby has contact with the other parent but is not away from their mother. This also helps if your baby is breastfed.
- You might find yourself in a situation where the other parent demands that breastfeeding stops so that visits are easier, or they think the baby is too old or it doesn't matter. Breastfeeding is in the best interest of the child and

therefore this is not something the other parent can ask. They can ask for more access, and you should give genuine consideration to how that could be managed, but they cannot prevent you from breastfeeding. La Leche League

" You might find yourself in a situation where the other parent demands that breastfeeding stops. "

has a great information sheet here: www.laleche.org.uk/breastfeeding-contact-cases.

- You might want to consider drawing this all up in a parenting plan between you and your co-parent. You could agree things like pattern of contact, drop-offs, rules for caring for your child (e.g. they are vegetarian, religion, screen time or whatever you like). CAFCASS has a great document here: www.helpguide.org/articles/parenting-family/co-parenting-tips-for-divorced-parents.htm.
- If you are struggling to agree on a contact plan, the government has advice on getting mediation or legal support. If you cannot agree, a legal order can be made setting out minimum contact arrangements www.gov.uk/looking-after-children-divorce/types-of-court-order.

Coping when your baby is away from you

The first times your baby is away from you can be really difficult. Try and keep yourself as busy as possible when they are away. Plan work or meet-ups with friends. Do all the things you can't do when your baby is with you. Sleep. Lean on family and friends.

Dealing with a difficult relationship with your co-parent

It may be that you have a very difficult relationship with your co-parent. They do still have a right to have contact with their child unless they are violent or neglectful towards them. How you interact with them will depend in part on how they engage with you, but the following ideas may help.

- Ask for communication to be in writing, maybe via an email address that you don't have message alerts on so you can check at a regular time suitable for you.
- Try to communicate calmly with them and don't put any rants or threats in writing. Text as if your messages could be read out in court – calmly and politely. What you mutter while writing them is up to you.
- Involve your co-parent in decisions if possible. Try and ask their opinion and take it into account rather than just making big decisions for your child.
- CAFCASS has some great ideas for communicating with your co-parent here: www.helpguide.org/articles/parenting-family/co-parenting-tips-for-divorced-parents.htm.

- You might want to try keeping a diary between you where you record useful information on your baby and their care. This saves you having long conversations but keeps you both updated and helps you share stuff you'd like them to do.
- Meet on neutral ground for handovers so they do not need to come to your house.
- Try to stick to a regular pattern of contact so you don't have to keep making arrangements.
- Try to remain calm in front of your baby and as they grow older not to complain about the other parent in front of them. When children feel that their separated parents have a civil relationship they feel more secure. Yes, this does take intense gritting of teeth. Again lean on friends and family and consider counselling if you're really struggling.
- Choose your battles. Your ex is going to really frustrate you at times (remember that's probably why they're an ex). But try and let the little things go. Don't let them goad you. Focus on the important stuff. This is a great skill to practise for when your baby is a teenager.
- Finally, if you are worried about your child's safety or your ex-partner is making threats towards you, you can contact CAFCASS for advice on whether a court could be involved in reducing contact or preventing them from coming near your home www.cafcass.gov.uk/grown-ups/parents-and-carers/divorce-and-separation/harmful-conflict.

For more support and information on thriving as a single parent:

- CAFCASS has lots of information about managing a separation and co-parenting here: www.cafcass.gov.uk/grown-ups/parents-and-carers/divorce-and-separation.
- Gingerbread is a charity that supports single parents and has lots of information www.gingerbread.org.uk.
- You might wish to consider counselling or mediation with an organisation such as Relate www.relate.org.uk.
- If you are really struggling to communicate with the other parent you might like to consider the CAFCASS-run Separate Parents Information Programme, which covers different challenges you can face www.cafcass.gov.uk/grown-ups/parents-and-carers/divorce-and-separation/separated-parents-information-programme.

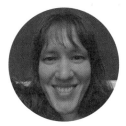

Thriving and surviving as a single parent

Jennie was a single mum to Emily who is now 18. She stayed at home with her for a year, supported by benefits before starting university when Emily was 12 months old. Jennie is now married, a step mum to two more daughters and works full time.

I was a single parent from when I was a couple of months pregnant – I think it's important to recognise it from that point, as the fact that you are single at that point can be really relevant, aside from the fact that even being pregnant makes you a parent.

To give a bit of background on me, I had always wanted to be a mother, more than anything else. It was my biggest dream growing up. I didn't get particularly worried about how I would look after a baby, I used to put that down to being quite a practical and logical-minded person, but looking back on it, I think quite a bit of it was actually because I got pregnant at 19, had my baby at 20 and so was young enough to not have some of the worries and overthinking many of us develop as we get older! As well as much less knowledge of what could go wrong!

Pregnancy as a single parent starts from the scans, the blood tests, the midwife appointments. I had some very supportive friends, but I was also very determined to be independent, so I did a lot of things alone. This was a challenge, as I didn't drive, so I had to either get a lift from friends or use public transport, which at the time wasn't straightforward from where I lived – the hospital was out of town in a different area to where I lived, so it was a bus into the centre and a bus out again. I didn't drive until she was about three, so I travelled on buses, just the two of us, a lot!

I was living in a room in a shared house when I became pregnant, which was certainly not suitable for a baby, so I had to register as homeless and was living in a mother and baby unit when my daughter was born. This was both a Social Services assessment house and supported flats (where I lived), which were mainly populated with people who had come out of the Social Services house. I think watching how many parents never made it out of the Social Services house into the flats (their children were removed) made me appreciate my daughter even more; it was a very sad place to live from that point of view. I lived there until she was about four months old, when I got a council flat.

A few thoughts about being a single parent:

People assume it will be hard

One of the things I found really fascinating about being a single parent is that everyone assumes it will be hard, and that you would be better with someone else. I dispute this, and if I could give one message to 'other people' about single parents, I would ask them to stop assuming it's a problem to be a single parent, that it's going to be hard, that you should feel sorry for us. In fact, I know friends of mine who have struggled much more who are not single parents. There are different challenges, of course, and for some people it will be really hard and for some much less so, but I do think it's important to recognise that for every parent, not assume the single ones should struggle.

Personally I honestly started to question what I was doing wrong because I wasn't really finding it particularly hard, but so many people were saying, 'I don't know how you do it, it must be so hard'. They meant well, of course, and I appreciate that they cared, but it wasn't particularly helpful! I think other people's use of language really makes a difference. If only people would ask about how parents feel, rather than assume based on their circumstances. A parent with a baby whose partner is working, not helping and expecting them to continue to cook meals, clean and so on is in a much harder situation than I was. And believe me, it can be very much easier to be the only one making the rules and not have to try and compromise on how you look after and parent a child with a partner!

Be prepared

As a single parent there isn't anyone else who can just pop out when you need something. You do need to be well prepared! Have an emergency stash of everything you can and keep it somewhere separate so you don't use it by mistake when you are tired and not thinking straight! A few spare nappies (clean ones if they are reusable), spare wipes, spare milk if you are bottle-feeding, spare food – all the things you might need for baby. But also things you might need for yourself - spare breast pads, spare tinned or frozen food, sanitary pads, toothpaste, clean clothes! And an emergency kit for a hard day – chocolate, bath bomb, whatever will help you feel a bit human. Obviously this is difficult if you are short of extra money, as I was, but even doing a little bit of this can be really helpful. When you wake up feeling ill and can't go out, the last thing you want is to find you have run out of nappies. This is also great advice for friends and family who want to help - make up an emergency kit as a gift.

Keep money available if you can, both in the house but also when you are out, and keep it separate from the rest of your money as emergency cash. Again, you never know when you might need a last-minute taxi or some supplies for your baby that you are not prepared for. With card payments these days this is much less of an issue than it was when I had a baby, but it's still good advice.

Keep a bag packed for going out – it's good to get into the habit of replacing everything in the bag as soon as you get home so that it is immediately ready. Obviously that's good if you have to go out in an emergency, but also when going out with a small baby anything can happen. Once I was about to go for an evening out, all dressed up and doing a last-minute nappy change, and my daughter peed all over me! You never know how long it will take to get out of the door so the more prepared you can be, the better.

This applies when you are pregnant too. I once had to go into hospital as I fell down some stairs. I ended up staying for three days, firstly for observation and then waiting for a doctor to be available to discharge me. I was fine but I had nothing with me, I was in shorts and t-shirt and flip flops, I had no money, no credit on my phone, no change of clothes and nothing to do – it was extremely boring. A 'just in case' bag would have made all the difference.

No, everyone doesn't really want to babysit – identify who is really there for you

This was a real eye-opener. When I first got pregnant so many people were excited and I had endless offers of babysitters, people who couldn't wait to come round and play with baby, or people who wanted to help out. Hardly any of them saw it through. Obviously there were some who were great, but very few. It's worth realising this and identifying the people who really are committed. Recognise that many people do mean what they say, but when it comes to it they don't have time, it's not their top priority and so on.

Find someone who will go through the whole process with you – not just a birthing partner for when baby is born, but a pregnancy partner who will come with you to scans and blood tests. Fortunately I didn't get any bad news at any of these, but I am not sure how I would have coped if I had done and been on my own, getting the bus back home alone after that.

It's definitely worth having friends who also have children if you can – get to know others through antenatal classes or online local groups before birth and through local groups afterwards. I did find that generally speaking it was the people with children who were there for each other, as we really understood the challenges each other was going through. Especially those who were single parents as we all appreciated each other's adult company! When other friends were having adult-only nights out, we single parents would get together with the children and have sleepovers all together. Which leads on nicely to...

YOU are important – don't feel guilty

So many parents recognise that once you have a child you become their 'mum' almost in place of your actual name. (If you are a single parent with a child who has their father's name, you also often become 'Mrs father's surname'. Always ask what a parent's name is or what they would like to be called.) Obviously, as a good parent you are prioritising your child and your role as parent, but that shouldn't mean you lose yourself. You are a person as well as a parent.

This can be hard as a single parent. When you feel like all of your day and night is taken up with looking after your baby, the last thing you want is something else to do. But it does help to hang on to your own identity. It doesn't have to be anything huge and it will be easier for some people than others, but:

- Take up the offer of someone coming to sit with the baby even for half an hour and do something you enjoy. (Note to friends and family: half an hour sitting with baby is not too small an offer. Don't feel that just because you don't have much time to give that it will not be valuable. That could be the thing that makes the whole day manageable.)
- Don't feel that every spare moment not looking after baby has to be filled with housework. Your house does not have to be perfectly clean and tidy. Your mental health needs to be cared for just as much as your house. Do things that make you happy, make you feel more like you, remind you what you enjoy (or just sleep).
- Sleep when baby sleeps – good advice for anyone, but even more essential when you are the only one who is looking after the baby. Again, don't feel that when baby is asleep you have to do all the housework. You are the most important thing for the baby and you need to take care of yourself.

Train them early

Invest in equipment that will help you take baby safely with you around the house so you can start training them in housework from a very early age... I jest, but it's a serious point. It can seem like you need to be doing things for your baby and concentrating on your baby when they are awake and then rush around doing everything while they sleep. As a single parent that just won't work. Invest in a good baby carrier or sling that you find comfortable and can move around in easily. Also get a very portable chair for your baby – I had a really simple bouncer that I could take from room to room and she was very happy in – nothing heavy that will be difficult for you to transport. Set them up so they can see you and get on with the cooking or washing or cleaning. Keep talking to them – this can take a bit of getting used to, especially when they are tiny, but your baby will love hearing your voice.

Again, don't feel guilty: your baby doesn't know you are doing a boring job, as far as they know you are dancing with the clothes while hanging them out or doing a little wiggle dance as you clean the oven.

Push for useful information and support
It can be really difficult to get the information you need when you are a parent and especially when you are a single parent and you need to plan even more carefully. There are often schemes available that can help and support you but they are not well advertised. Find out about local support groups by asking your medical professionals or local community groups. And don't give up when you need things to support you – for example, I really struggled when back at work with the fact that teacher-training days were always announced last minute, leaving very little time to arrange care for my daughter. I went to the school and talked to them about this and managed to get much more information on when most of them were planned for, so I could make better arrangements. Some swimming pools will have special sessions for single parents with more than one child to enable them to attend (as the usual adult to child ratios can prohibit this). I wish these things were better advertised but don't give up, you have the right to equal opportunities as a single parent, so keeping pushing for the support you need to get that.

All in all I think I would say, 'You can do it alone but you don't have to'. Never feel that as a single parent you are inadequate or not good enough, rejoice in the positives and recognise that everyone has negatives, whether they are single or not. Know who you can rely on and never be afraid to ask for help – and also be honest about how people can really help. Try to always be prepared and don't lose yourself. You are by far the most important treasure in the world to your baby, so treat yourself with the attention that you need and deserve.

"

Part six

Let's talk about going back to work (or not)

"

At some point the question of returning to work or not will come up.

Maybe you already had plans when you became pregnant, or looked into options before your baby was born. Possibly you have now changed your mind, or are looking at ways of being more flexible. It's a big decision. Finances are likely to play a role, both in terms of how long you can stay at home or affording childcare on return. There might be many, many questions going around your mind.

This section will look at some of the options available to you in terms of policy, rights and plain facts. But it's going to do more than that, by exploring how you feel and why you might want to consider different options. It will challenge gender stereotypes, looking at issues such as fathers choosing to stay home and breadwinning mothers. It will tackle the stupid things people will suggest, such as you returning to work will harm your baby (nope), childcare harms your baby (nope) or that stay-at-home mothers have it easy (err, nope again). It will also look at the practicalities of combining work and parenting, including things like getting organised, planning childcare locations and continuing to breastfeed on return to work. Hopefully it will help you think through different options and feel a whole lot more organised and confident.

Knowing your rights as a new parent on return to work is useful in ensuring that you can have the adaptations in place that you are entitled to. Unfortunately, not all workplaces will be up to speed on the necessity or value of these, for you and them. This isn't necessarily deliberate – it might be that in a smaller organisation they haven't had many women return to work. Although it shouldn't have to be this way, knowing your rights can help you broach potentially difficult situations.

One of the best websites to refer to if you have any difficulties is the Maternity Action website https://maternityaction.org.uk. This provides all sorts of information on your rights during pregnancy, maternity leave and return to work, including specialist help on benefits and immigration questions.

Will I harm my child by working or staying home?

Of course not. What is best for your child is what works best for your family, practically, emotionally and financially. Men and women have social pressures in different directions - men are generally more likely to feel the pressure to work, while women feel the pressure to stay home. In reality, many families muddle through doing a balance of the two based on what works best for them. Do not let society dictate to you what you 'should' be doing or feeling.

There are so many articles about whether mothers affect their children by working or staying home, but unsurprisingly there are very few about fathers. You can find articles on your child's social development, cognitive skills, friendships... just about anything being affected positively or negatively by either option if you look hard enough. However, the consensus is that basically, if your child is loved, well cared for and secure then they will have the best outcomes. Do what is right for you and your family. That will be based on things like:

- How much you like your job
- What your income after childcare might be
- Your long-term earning potential
- Whether you are single or in a partnership
- Whether you are married (from a legal protection perspective)
- What childcare options are in your local area
- Your personal values and beliefs
- Your child's needs
- Your own health

All of these are important elements in your decision and it's a good idea to take your time and think through what the pros and cons might be. You might also decide to think outside the box by both cutting down your hours and sharing care, or working alternate hours so your baby is cared for at home. There is no one option that is right for every family - and never let anyone tell you otherwise.

Chapter twenty-nine

Understanding maternity, paternity and shared parental leave

→ This chapter explores your rights when it comes to your entitlement to maternity/paternity pay and leave and the potential option of shared parental leave. It would be most useful in pregnancy but also is relevant once your baby is here – you have the right (within certain regulations) to change how long a leave you will take and who takes it.

Understanding your rights when it comes to work and having a baby can be a bit confusing. The best places to look for up-to-date information are the Maternity Action website **maternityaction.org.uk** and ACAS **www.acas.org. ukmaternity-paternity-and-adoption-leave-and-pay**. These pages include information on maternity, paternity, shared parental and adoption leave. As these things have a tendency to change over the years, you should check there for the most recent information, but below is an overview. There is also a useful calculator on the HMRC website **www.gov.uk/pay-leave-for-parents**. Please bear in mind that if you're not in the UK, the specifics in this chapter might not apply to you.

Maternity leave rights

Maternity leave is for those physically giving birth to a baby. There is a difference between the right to maternity leave and maternity pay. If you are an employee of a company, i.e. have a contract with whoever is paying you, be that a business, organisation or family as a nanny for example, you have the right to up to 52 weeks' maternity leave. You may also be entitled to maternity pay. Maternity pay is split into:

- **Statutory Maternity Pay (SMP)**
  If you're employed and you've been working continuously for your employer for 26 weeks or more by the 'qualifying week' of your pregnancy. This is the week 15 weeks before your due date. You also need to have earned at least £120 a week on average for the eight weeks before your qualifying week. SMP is paid for 39 weeks from the date your baby is born. For the first six weeks you will receive 90% of your pay. For the next 33 weeks you will get either £151.20 a week or 90% of your average weekly earnings (whichever is lower). You can take a final 13 weeks on top of that but it is unpaid. If you have more than one employer you can only claim SMP once.

- **Enhanced maternity pay**
  Your employer may have a scheme where they add money– typically a percentage of your salary – on top of SMP. Ask your Human Resources department. Sometimes you need to return to work for a certain period after having a baby or repay some or all of the extra money. If you have more than one employer you might get enhanced pay from each.

- **Maternity Allowance**
  If you are employed but not eligible for SMP or are self-employed and paying Class 2 National Insurance contributions you may be entitled to Maternity Allowance instead. It is also paid for up to 39 weeks. You can't claim Maternity Allowance and SMP. You need to have been employed or self-employed for at least 26 weeks in the 66 weeks before your baby was born (known as the test period). Your earnings are calculated from 13 weeks over this period. You can choose these and they don't have to be in a row. You need to average at least £30. Unfortunately student bursaries do not count. The standard rate is £139.58 or 90% of average earnings (whichever is lower).

HMRC has a more detailed guide. It also has guidance on what you can apply for if you do not qualify for any form of maternity pay or allowance, including Jobseeker's Allowance, Income Support and other benefits. More details here: **www.gov.uk/government/publications/maternity-benefits-technical-guidance**.

Paternity leave rights

You qualify for paternity leave if you are the biological father or your partner is having a baby, adopting a child or having a child through surrogacy. If you're a same-sex female partner it's still called paternity leave. You can also receive paternity leave if you are adopting (see more details below). You can still get this leave if you are separated from your partner (as long as you haven't signed away parental responsibility). You might be asked to sign a declaration that you will be using the time to care for your child. To qualify you need to be employed and have worked for the same employer for at least 26 weeks before the qualifying week (15 weeks before your baby's due date).

For paternity pay, the rules above apply. You need to earn at least £120 a week on average over the eight weeks before your qualifying week. It's currently £151.20 a week or 90% of your average weekly earnings (whichever is lower).

Adoption leave rights

If you are in a couple only one person can get adoption leave. The other may qualify for paternity leave (regardless of their sex). Adoption leave for the parent who applies follows the same rules as maternity leave. You need proof you are adopting. You will need to tell your employer within seven days of being matched with your child and the date they will be placed with you. The earliest it can start is when you've been matched with your child, although if it's an overseas adoption it must be when the child arrives in the UK (or within 28 days of this).

You can also receive paternity leave and pay for adopting a child. You have to have worked for the same employer for 26 weeks by the date you are told you've been matched with a child or the date the child enters the UK for overseas adoption. It can continue even if your child is not placed with you.

Shared parental leave

Another thing you might like to think about is how you might share any leave with your partner. You have the right for the mother to go back to work while the father (or the mother's partner) takes over. You also have the right to both take shared parental leave together. In the UK you and your partner may be eligible for shared parental leave after your baby is born (or you adopt). The partner who has given birth must take two weeks' leave after birth (four if they work in a factory), but then you can share up to 50 weeks' leave, 37 of which will be paid. You can take it alone or you can both be off at the same time and you can have more than one period of leave each: so you can have three months off, then your partner has three months off, then you have three months off again.

Shared Parental Leave Statutory Pay is the same as Statutory Maternity Pay - currently £151.20 per week or 90% of your average weekly earnings

" Understanding your rights when it comes to work and having a baby can be a bit confusing. "

(although Statutory Maternity Pay is paid at 90% of whatever you earn for the first six weeks. This doesn't apply to Shared Parental Leave pay). If one of you is on maternity pay and you decide to take shared leave at the same time together, both of you will go on to the shared parental leave package.

However, just like with maternity pay, your employer might offer an enhanced package above the standard rate, although they might have rules. If they do, they must offer the same amount of shared parental leave pay to both men and women (i.e. they can't pay women on an enhanced maternity rate and their partner on a lower rate).

To be eligible

- You are your baby's mother, father or a partner to a mother who has just given birth
- You must be using the period of leave to care for the baby (shouldn't have to be said but...)
- You must both have been employed continuously for at least 26 weeks by the end of the 15th week before your baby's due date
- You must earn on average at least £118 per week (correct as per rates in 2020)
- You must stay employed by the same employer through the period of SPL

The rules are a little more complex than this and it's best to check out your individual circumstances online. If you earn less or are not an employee you might be eligible for just Shared Parental Leave or Shared Parental Pay and not both. Likewise, if one of you does not regularly work, or earns less, you might not be eligible. So your best bet is to look up more details at **www.gov.uk/shared-parental-leave-and-pay** and Maternity Action also has a great factsheet **maternityaction.org.uk/advice/shared-parental-leave-and-pay**.

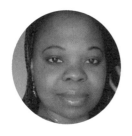

The benefits and challenges of shared parental leave

An interview with Dr Ernestine Gheyoh Ndzi, Course Lead for Law, York St John University. Her research explores the topic of Shared Parental Leave (SPL) and its challenges. More on her work on SPL can be found on www.sharedparentalleave.org and Facebook where she provides free information and advice to parents.

What is Shared Parental Leave?

SPL is a policy put in place by the government to allow mothers to share their maternity leave with their partners, giving mothers the opportunity to return to work early after birth if they so desire, and for fathers to spend more time bonding with the child. Before this policy came into being, mothers could take only maternity leave and fathers paternity leave. The introduction of SPL means that mothers do not necessarily have to take their full maternity leave (which is 52 weeks) alone but can share with their partners. For the fathers (or partners in the case of gay couples), in addition to paternity leave they can take SPL, which gives them more time to spend with the family.

SPL is applicable to parents of babies born on or after 5 April 2015 and is available to biological parents and social parents (including same-sex partners and those adopting children). Biological parents do not have to live together to qualify for SPL. The father and mother (or parent of the newborn) are able to share 50 weeks of SPL after the mother has taken the initial two weeks after birth. This leave must be taken in the first year following the birth of the child.

To be eligible for SPL, both father and mother (or parent) must be employees and have been employed for at least 26 weeks by the 15th week before the expected week of the child's birth. Both parents would have to remain in employment until the week before SPL. The mother must be entitled to take maternity leave or maternity allowance (in the case of self-employed) and has either given notice to their employer that their leave will end or have returned to work. A self-employed mother who is eligible for maternity allowance can still take SPL so long as the partner is in regular employment. If the partner of a mother is self-employed, they will not be eligible for SPL.

Both parents are expected to give their employers at least eight weeks' notice of their intention to take SPL. Furthermore, fathers' notice must be accompanied by the mother/spouse/partner's consent to father taking the leave. Mothers are expected to declare their interest in opting to take SPL and the amount of leave each parent would want to take. SPL can be taken in continuous or discontinuous periods, but the employer has the right to refuse discontinuous leave requests with no obligation to justify why.

However, SPL can only be taken in blocks of weeks and can be taken concurrently or otherwise. This provision gives the mother and father the opportunity and flexibility to share the leave however they want depending on their caring needs. It is worth noting that SPL does not replace paternity leave. SPL and paternity leave are two separate rights for a father.

What are the benefits of SPL?

The aim of SPL is to allow the mother to return to work early if she chooses to and to allow the father of the baby to be more involved in the baby's life. SPL provides greater paternal involvement in childcare, which could have a positive impact on child development and establish long-term happiness and marital stability in the home. Nikki Slowey, Joint Programme Director of Family Friendly Working Scotland, summed it up by saying: *'Creating more options for fathers means mothers benefit from greater choice in how to balance their own work and home life – mothers don't have to be the only parent to take time out. This, in turn, is good for businesses because happier employees are more engaged and productive. Shared Parental Leave is definitely something employers should embrace and encourage.'*

Furthermore, everybody's situation tends to be different when they have a child. Some people require more support than others and/or need their partners around longer than the two weeks' paternity leave. SPL allows parents to be together longer if required or if they decide to, supporting each other and bonding with the baby. A good use of SPL has the potential to improve on maternal mental health after childbirth.

There are numerous reports on how women have been/are being discriminated against in the workplace because of pregnancy and maternity leave. Some have lost their jobs, some miss out on promotion and some have been demoted from their roles. With fathers taking SPL and spending more time with the family, discrimination against mothers in the workplace could be minimised.

What are the challenges of SPL?

The first challenge is to know and understand what shared parental leave is all about. Find out if your workplace has a policy on shared parental leave and what the policy says. The policy on shared parental leave on the government website is difficult to understand and some employers still do not understand either and are therefore unable to advise employees. If this is your situation you may have to contact an expert who can explain or give you advice.

As a mother, you will have to decide to cut short your maternity leave by taking SPL. This might potentially be a difficult decision to make, given maternal bonding and other factors such as breastfeeding. Making this decision also depends on how comfortable your partner is with taking SPL. SPL is still a new concept and both parents might still find it a little odd that mothers can share their maternity leave. However, a good conversation between both parents on what SPL is, how it could benefit them and the impact it could have on their family will make it easier for the mother to reach a decision. Some mothers do find it a little difficult to start such a conversation with their partners and may assume their partners' reaction or response. Fathers may also be a little nervous, because just like mothers they think the mother needs all that time and that they earned it. Either way, the right thing to do is to have that all-important conversation and make a decision together.

SPL is paid at the statutory rate, which might prevent people from taking it if they are not financially able to cover the period. Some employers enhance SPL pay and others do not. Some employers enhance maternity leave and pay, but not SPL pay. Mothers need to be aware of this, because if they take SPL and share part of the leave that would have had enhanced maternity pay, the enhanced maternity pay will stop and revert to statutory pay.

SPL could potentially be challenging if you are breastfeeding and intend to return to work early. You need to know your workplace policy on breastfeeding and the resources available to support breastfeeding mothers returning to work. Where the workplace is not very supportive or doesn't have the facilities that a breastfeeding mother needs (such as private room with sockets, fridge, etc.) taking shared parental leave could have a significant impact on your ability to continue breastfeeding.

How can parents make breastfeeding work if they are using SPL?

It is crucial for breastfeeding mothers to feel comfortable and supported. The benefits of breastfeeding are many and can be described simply as the ideal nutrition for infants with many advantages for both child and mother. Therefore, knowing how to combine SPL and breastfeeding is important for mothers returning to work.

There are several ways in which you can take shared parental leave, go back to work and continue breastfeeding. The first thing to do is to check out your workplace policies and see what support there is for returning breastfeeding mothers. This will include checking if there is a workplace nursery on site, which may allow you to visit your baby and breastfeed during your working day. Check if there are private rooms designated for breastfeeding which you can use to express milk while at work, or to breastfeed your baby if someone can bring them to you at certain times in your normal working day. Even if you do not want to breastfeed at work, the private room should have sockets and a fridge to enable you to express at work. It is always helpful to check if there are other mothers in your workplace who have been in a similar situation, who may have some useful tips to share with you.

Requesting flexible working could also be an option for you. Obviously, flexible working is not an automatic right, and it will be down to your employer to grant or reject it. But flexible working can allow you to change your times of work, or place of work, or days of work (all depending on the nature of your work) to accommodate your breastfeeding plans.

What is your advice for parents thinking about SPL?
If you are considering taking shared parental leave, take some time to find out as much as you can about how it would work in your particular circumstances. Once you have made an initial decision to take shared parental leave, check whether there is a policy on shared parental leave in your workplace and how it might affect you. Check if your employer is enhancing shared parental leave pay and what impact that may have on maternity leave pay if maternity leave pay is enhanced. Find out what support is available in your workplace for breastfeeding mothers. It is crucial that you find out all of this information early to enable you to make informed decisions and give your employer adequate (at least eight weeks') notice.

Chapter thirty

Deciding to be a stay-at-home parent

The decision not to return to work is a very personal one. Around a third of mothers and 2% of fathers in the UK with a preschool child are not currently in paid employment.[1] There are many reasons you might make this decision, including the financial impact of childcare, the logistics of juggling a job and your children, not particularly liking your job or simply a desire to be home when your children are small.

The transition to being a stay-at-home parent is going to be different depending on what you did before. If you had a hectic job with long hours, things might feel very different than if you were already working fewer hours or perhaps had a job you didn't particularly like. It can feel stressful, all-consuming and you might doubt whether you've done the right thing or not. It's normal to spend time missing your job and old role.[2] Give yourself time to get used to it though – it really is a transition in itself.

You might face a number of different challenges depending on what life was like before, what your friends do and what sex you are. As above, just 2% of men are the primary stay-at-home carer for their children, meaning they can face all sorts of weird reactions. More on this later. These challenges might include things like changed relationships, money worries and missing having an identity outside of the home. Here are some ideas for coping with the biggest challenges:

1. Keep the discussion going about what your new roles will look like

Getting used to a new role of not working outside the home can be tough sometimes. Your partner, if they are working, might feel that they're the one out all day working and come home stressed. You've been with the baby all day and haven't had a second's peace. It's easy to get frustrated with each other. Talk and keep talking. Talk about how you feel and explain what is involved in your day. If they don't understand, try to go out for a full day (or more) and leave them with the baby.

Realistic divisions of labour are also important so you don't become the person who does everything at home. You're caring for a baby and may well still be up in the night with them. Yes, you can sort out some stuff as part of your day-to-day life, but sometimes your partner is going to come home and find everything a state. And that's okay. It's normal. You can't do everything at once and they need to understand that. Again, talk about what is realistic.

Another conversation on the tricky list is to make sure you discuss finances, ideally before you actually give up your job. Couples work this out in different ways, but you should have access to money. Withholding it from you, only giving you small amounts when there is plenty and hiding facts from you are financial abuse. Big decisions should be joint. You are saving the family a lot of money. Remember you are much better protected financially if you are married.

2. Try and make time for yourself

It's really easy to get into a pattern where there is little focus on you and everything you do is for your family. All the little moments go – the tea breaks, the five minutes talking to a colleague, even the commute. You might feel you don't have the excuse of 'give me 10 minutes while I get in' or 'I'm really stressed from work so need to do x to relax'.

You might be in your home, but you are working and saving the family a lot of money in childcare and everything else. Remember that (and see the next section on never underestimating your worth). You deserve a break too. Look back at Chapter 3 on self-care and reread all the ideas there, including the importance of making sure both you and your partner have time. Your baby might be a bit older but it still very much applies. It can help to have something structured if possible. So, a set class, activity or coffee with a friend. Make the appointment and put it in your diary so it can't just be forgotten and pushed back.

Some people find that doing something creative or 'constructive' helps, so you feel you have something to 'show for it' at the end. Sometimes, when you are home day after day with children, it feels like nothing gets done and you have no identity apart from serving others. But research shows that if you are doing something artistic or creative, or that requires a skill, it can help with these feelings.[3] Other people are horrified at the idea and feel it's just one more thing on their never-ending to-do list. Volunteering, especially for things that can be done with your baby, also gives some people a sense of purpose or identity. Likewise for small businesses selling things from home. Others feel far too exhausted. The main message is to do whatever makes you happy.

3. Make new connections

If you're new to being a stay-at-home parent it can feel really isolating, particularly if friends are going back to work. You might miss the social side of work, or simply the connection and being around people. It can be a source of frustration with your partner, especially if they come home at the end of the day exhausted and peopled out and not wanting to talk, when you've not seen an adult all day long.[4]

Have a look back at Chapter 1 on finding support – there are some ideas there for finding support and connections within your community. Taking a slightly practical perspective on things, getting involved in your community and meeting other friends with babies also helps your baby as they get older. It helps them make friends and it means you have a support system if one of you needs a favour such as picking up children after school.

4. Never let anyone underestimate your worth

Sadly, we probably all know someone who thinks that a stay-at-home parent is somehow not pulling their weight. Let's imagine for a second that caring for a baby was the easiest thing on earth. Somehow, they just lie there or happily play all day long, occasionally needing a feed or nappy change while you sit on the sofa watching daytime TV. Back in reality we know that couldn't be further from the truth, but even so there are many, many other ways a stay-at-home parent is a huge asset to the working parent and the family in general. Here are a few:

You are saving the cost of childcare fees. Let's say you have two children of pre-school age. Average childcare costs in 2017 were £4.54 an hour per child (some areas might be a bit lower, some much higher). If you were back in work full-time, that's roughly £45 per child per day. So £90 per day, or £350 a week or £1,600 a month. Although most people will qualify for tax-free childcare, that's still roughly the equivalent of the take-home pay of someone earning £27,000 after tax, student loan and pension deductions. And that's before you think of the hidden costs of working – commuting, clothing, inevitable shop-bought lunches.[5]

You are making the other parent's day much, much easier. In a scenario where everything was split equally and one parent did drop-off and the other the pick-up from nursery, you are freeing the other parent from this load. They don't have to worry about getting to work on time because they have to wait for the nursery to open, or getting up an hour earlier to get the kids ready and to take them to nursery. That's potentially 250 hours of sleep a year you're saving them. They don't have to leave work at 5pm on the dot to make sure they can get to childcare to do the evening pick-up.

Do not underestimate the impact of this on their day-to-day life. A recent study found that getting the kids out the door to nursery or school was the equivalent of an additional day's work per week.[6] The absolute luxury of simply leaving the house without children and commuting to work is worth roughly a billion pounds (I may have just made this statistic up, but it certainly feels like an accurate figure). I remember when my own children were old enough to start walking home from school. The sheer relief at not having to go and pick them up felt like some sort of holiday. And we live on the same road as the school.

You are enabling the other parent to work longer, more unsociable or irregular hours – or travel... without needing to worry about childcare pick-up times or additional costs. Linked to point two is the immeasurable benefit of freedom. If they're in the middle of something they don't have to rush off. They can have that after-work company dinner or travel overnight. If they work irregular shifts, say as a health professional, they can do so without worrying about nurseries that open 8–6pm.

And then there's the other huge benefit of not having to make frantic plans when a child is sick. Working parents know the fear that strikes your heart when your phone starts flashing and it's nursery or school. You stare at it for a few moments hoping it's an error (or that they'll give up and ring the other parent). Or your baby wakes up and vomits everywhere and you know that's at least two or three days that one of you isn't going to be able to work.

This really is one of the biggest benefits a working parent can have – a stay-at-home partner. The pattern of women being more likely to stay home and benefit a male partner is one reason for the gender pay gap between men and women and the higher number of men in top management positions.

You are easing other loads on them. Now, I don't think that a stay-at-home parent automatically becomes the cook/cleaner/slave – far from it. But when you're at home during the day you do end up doing all manner of small things that just make life easier. You can put a load of washing on. You're there for a home delivery. You can chuck some food in a slow cooker. Anyone who occasionally works from home knows how much simpler it is to spend a few seconds doing these things during the day than having to juggle them when everyone comes home, fraught and tired. In fact the concept of a stay-at-home partner has been described very much as a luxury.[7]

5. Remember things can change if you want them to

If you are really struggling with being a stay-at-home parent, remember that nothing is set in stone. If the feelings of missing work and your role don't go away there is the option to explore part- or full-time work. Sometimes we get into all-or-nothing thinking and feel the years stretching out ahead of us. Set yourself smaller goals and tell yourself you can reconsider then.

Stay-at-home dads

All of the previous section applies to both men and women. Many of the challenges of being the one at home, caring for your baby, are the same. Your sex doesn't matter when it comes to the frustrations of a baby who doesn't want to be put down, multiple messy mealtimes or trying to persuade the baby that they would like a nap right now. A really long nap.

However, we all know that our society still has a long way to go before it makes no assumptions about who might not be going back to work or who is at home with the baby all day long. Most people still know more women who stay at home than men who do, which results in a number of different challenges that should not exist but sadly sometimes do. So this section looks at why men might choose to stay at home, how they might feel about that and some of the issues they may need to think about.

Challenges of being a stay-at-home dad

Ideally there should be no additional challenges for a man who chooses to stop work and stay at home with the baby he co-created. Unfortunately, our society is far from equal, and continues to judge women who go back to work quickly and men who choose not to. Talking about these challenges helps not only highlight them to others, but also helps you realise that you are not alone.

Why would you stay home?

Well, why wouldn't you at least consider it if it is a serious option? Apart from the fact that you helped create the baby, there are many positives to being a stay-at-home dad that most men do not get the opportunity to experience (due to income imbalances, hang-ups and just an inability to think outside the traditional box).

Staying home you get more of your child's time, especially if until this point it's been your partner off on maternity leave for many months. You have more time to experience firsts, the challenges of caring for a baby (yes, that can be a positive too) and just generally get to be around and witness stuff. All the things in the previous section apply too – more time as a family, more balance for everyone and so on.

There have been a handful of studies in the last few years that address the concerns and issues stay-at-home fathers might face, alongside how they coped with these thoughts.[8,9]

1. Worries about money

We live in a world where on average men earn more money than women for many subtle and not-so-subtle reasons, which lead to men's careers often advancing faster than women's or them simply getting more money for the same work. This is firstly obviously overtly unfair to women, but also places a lot of expectation and pressure on men if their female partner earns more than they do – or indeed is the sole breadwinner.

It's common for stay-at-home fathers to feel tense about not earning money or not contributing as much to the family pot. Men have years and years of being conditioned to be the main earner and to step up to provide for their family once a baby arrives. Maybe you grew up seeing your father and all the fathers around you working more and earning more, with few if any men taking the role of caring for their children.

This can be particularly difficult if as a family you needed to make the decision for the father to stay home, perhaps because of a job loss or job insecurity or simply a major difference in earning potential.

Remember this is all cultural nonsense. Why would having a Y chromosome automatically mean you should earn more money? Why are you not allowed to be the one caring for the baby?

The reactions of those around you can be unhelpful. Some may make fun, in the dubious guise of 'banter'. Why? Realise that this is more about them than you. Maybe they are jealous, having no choice to take this option for themselves. Maybe they think it's the easy job and you're a slacker (ha!). Maybe they simply know no different and are uncomfortable. All their issues, not yours.

2. Worries about your longer-term career

Anyone who takes a career break might worry about what happens in the long term, and this is one of the most common concerns of women who stay at home too. Skills change and workplaces move on and you are not moving with them. People might also be (wrongly, obviously) suspicious of men with career gaps.

There are numerous ways around this, all of which also apply to women. You might want to have some kind of sideline, a few hours out doing a job in the evening or at the weekend, further study or simply keeping your training and skills up to date in other ways. You might, however, be far too knackered and content to not do anything else.

If you are worried about this the Belgian dads suggested reframing things.

Some dads found it useful to refer to themselves as having a career break, sabbatical or being retired rather than being a 'stay-at-home dad'. Whatever works.

> **"It's common for stay-at-home fathers to feel tense about not earning money or not contributing as much to the family pot."**

3. You might feel like you're not contributing your share

She grew the baby and pushed it out after all, didn't she? And what if she's breastfeeding? She's the one feeding it and up in the night with it. What are you doing?

Again nonsense. Reread (or read for the first time) the section on staying at home. You are playing a major role by supporting her in her career. Believe me, when two parents work part-time, the pressure is intense in a different way. Who will take the kids to school? Who will do sick days? Who will leave work to pick them up? By staying at home you are enabling her to focus on work. It really is invaluable and will help her develop and progress in her career. It really is a joint effort.

4. Feeling out of place in the community

Let's face it, stay-at-home dads are still in the minority. You might well be the only man at baby group, or feel you can't go at all. Things are thankfully changing and the world is opening up to be a more accepting place for dads, but sometimes you still can't shake that feeling.

You might also have to put up with other people's prejudiced nonsense, thinking you are odd staying at home.

5. Strange beliefs about your relationship

There are some very odd people out there who can't seem to open their minds to anything being different. Again, this may well simply be their own insecurities, or they might just be plain weird. In the research with fathers two reactions specific to relationships were brought up – either that somehow you can't be bothered to work and are making your partner do everything... or the opposite and that you are being controlled by your partner and made to hide away at home. Stop laughing now. Unless this is actually true – in which case see the section on relationships.

6. Worries about your identity

A common moment of panic for women who stay at home is meeting new people and being asked 'So what do you do?' and not knowing what to say. There is a real social pressure to have an identity linked to your work, with a subtle hierarchy in some circles of whether that is good enough.

If this freaks you out, the Belgian dads have a number of solutions. The first is to remind yourself that this is what you wanted. You made the decision as a family and there are many benefits. It works for you. Don't let some idiot tell you otherwise.

Another idea the Belgian dads had was to pride yourself in stepping away from societal pressure to conform. Society telling you that you must be pigeon-holed? Sod that. You're doing what's best for your family and have the confidence and self-assurance to know that's a good thing.

Also, it's absolutely fine to think about what you like doing and make time for it, so you have some time to just be yourself rather than dad. Some men find it helps for this hobby to be something 'useful', like repairing old cars, photography, or community work. Or indeed a small sideline that brings in a bit of money. Whatever works for you. Equally you might just like one evening a week to meet up with your mates for a pint or to watch the football (or perhaps something less stereotypical).

Finally, if you're feeling really frustrated here's a great video on YouTube to laugh or cry at **www.youtube.com/watch?v=mpsngs9nlW4.**

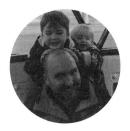

Being a stay-at-home father

Steve Smith is a stay-at-home dad to Tom and Rose, after he and his wife Vicky made the decision for her to return to work as the main earner after their second child was born.

When did you make the decision to be a SAHD?

When did I make the decision? I suppose the answer is over a number of years. We have traditionally atypical financial dynamics in our household, in that my wife earns more than me and always has. I'm sure this is more and more common nowadays, but still not the norm. Following the birth of our first child we needed my wife to return to work after six months in order to keep on top of the bills, as my salary would not cover the monthly outgoings. Therefore I took six months' paternity leave to look after our son, while my wife returned to work full-time as an intensive care doctor. By the time our second child was born my wife had finished her training and had been appointed as a consultant at our local hospital. She had chosen to work part-time to manage the work-life balance, which worked out as approximately four days a week. I was working Monday to Friday, regular working hours. Our son was in nursery, or looked after by grandparents on my wife's working days.

My wife took nine months of maternity leave with our second child, and I took the remaining three months as (unpaid) paternity leave. During this time, and for some months before, we had discussed the financial and other practicalities of how we would manage after this period. We took the decision that I would apply for a 12-month unpaid sabbatical to look after the children and see how this worked. It was a reduction in family income, but one that we decided was worthwhile, as a large proportion of my income would have been paid in nursery fees for both children had I remained in my paid employment. It seemed to us that we would rather not go to work just to pay for someone else to look after our children. The sabbatical worked for us, and towards the end of the 12 months I resigned from my employment to become a stay-at-home dad until the children both went to school.

What's the thing you find best about it?

This is difficult to answer. In the years to come, once I am back in employment and the children are at school, I'm sure I will look back and say the chance to spend so much time with my children was the best part. Right now, it is very easy to feel under-appreciated by the children. I also don't really have a benchmark to say whether my relationship with the children has improved, as I have fortunately always spent a lot of time with them. That said, during lockdown I feel as though my relationships with both of my children have improved. My wife is an excellent parent and has a huge knowledge bank on children and their behaviours (from both her professional career and lots of reading about parenting techniques), she has also been hugely determined to succeed with breastfeeding our children, and to do this for as long as benefits them. There are many, many benefits both for her and the children that most people are not aware of, and it also creates a very strong bond with the children. In earlier years I sometimes felt invisible to the kids as they would instinctively go to her when there was a problem (not all bad by any means as I wasn't the one who was disturbed in the night) but recently I feel that both have formed stronger relationships with me. Especially my daughter, who won't be aware of a time when I wasn't around for her all of the time.

I suppose the best thing currently is always being able to be there for our children. They never need after-school clubs, breakfast clubs, childminders etc. They have a number of after-school activities that are more easily facilitated by me being around and not being tied by work commitments.

My wife has a number of work commitments and does not work regular hours. I think it helps her to know that I am always available and there for the kids, so that if she gets stuck at work (sometimes until after midnight) then it isn't a problem.

What are the things that are more challenging?
I'm sure I experience the same challenges that most parents do, but thinking back to when I started paternity leave for my first child I definitely did feel like an outsider when I went to the baby groups/classes etc. I'm not always the most confident person in new situations and I did find these tricky. The only man in a room full of women, trying to strike up conversations with mothers who had breasts out so that they could feed their babies was not somewhere I felt confident at first, and to be honest I didn't succeed at these classes where my wife had thrived. Over six years down the line this is no longer an issue for me. I have a weekly routine of daytime activities with my daughter and we are both very comfortable with these.

Ongoing things that I do find challenging are that my school-age child has the impression that school teachers know everything and are to be obeyed at all times, whereas he doesn't seem to take my word for it, or believe that I can know things too as I'm just dad, and not a teacher, or anything else in his eyes. Just a dad. Lockdown has seen this get a bit better, but I still feel that we have room for improvement.

At the beginning I did find it difficult at times being a 'kept man' and not having my own money. I would feel like I had to ask if it was okay to buy things, or would feel guilty if I spent money just on me and not the family. And it can feel strange buying someone a present with their own money, if that makes sense. How generous should one be spending someone else's money on them? Different couples find different ways to deal with this I'm sure. I think I am fairly considerate and don't spend money on many luxury items. For example I don't spend loads on fancy clothes, I don't go out spending lots drinking with friends.

What's the most stupid thing someone has said to you about being a SAHD or the most annoying assumption?
The most annoying assumption is that it's easy. It isn't. It can be wonderful and incredibly rewarding, but then it can also be really hard some days. And on those days, when my wife comes home late from work after a tough day, I have the feeling of guilt. I may need a break, but so does she. She needs to unwind from work and be able to look forward to 'mummy time' with the kids rather than coming in through the door to pandemonium and me needing to get a breather. These days are rare, but they exist.

To be honest I don't get many negative things said to me about it. I'm sure there were a couple of comments at my old work but they were very few and far between, and also from people with very different life experiences and backgrounds. None of these affected me or made me reconsider the choice.

What have you learned along the way?
Some days you will be pissed off. Apologies for the language, but when it happens that is how you will describe it. Learn to accept that this is part of it, and take the rough with the smooth.

Say sorry when you are wrong. And sometimes when you're not. It is important for the children to see this.

Do yoga, and meditate. To quote *South Park* it sounds like 'tree hugging hippy crap' but it really worked wonders for me. It just helps, especially if you've never done it.

Do yoga with the children – there are parent and child yoga classes and I think it benefits my children to see that looking after the body helps look after the mind.

Read books to them from a young age, and keep books wherever they can reach them for themselves.

Expose them to music and rhythm from a young age. It may take a while before you see the benefits but they are there, and you get used to the weirdness of sitting around with a group of strangers singing children's songs. Some of my best friendships have been formed at these classes.

Find something for you to do, just for you. In my case I took up a musical instrument and meet up every week with a group of others to learn, play, sing and socialise. Ukulele is fun and a great 'group' instrument to take up if you can. I have no musical background and couldn't read music beforehand. I'm now playing to Grade 3 standard in little over a year.

My wife works unpredictable hours. I used to find it frustrating if she was 'late' for tea or just not knowing when she would be home. While I am sad that she has to work so hard I now just accept that that is the way it is some days, and just get on with the evening without putting any pressure on her to make a time frame. This helps both of us.

Bedtime for two children of different ages when there is only one parent at home can be a challenge. Just roll with it and go with what works. Ideally I would want both kids to just lie in bed and go to sleep. In reality I will often end up snuggling one or both in my bed and then carrying them through to their beds when they are asleep, and this is perfectly fine. We are seeing improvements in their sleep and have never 'sleep trained' as it just strikes us as cruelty by not responding to your children when they are sad and want company/security.

What would you say to a friend who is considering being a SAHD?
If it is something that you can afford, and want to do, then do it. Don't go into it thinking that you're perfect, this is very much learning on the job and you will make mistakes. Learning from these is important, and ongoing. I will never stop wanting to be a better dad. Whether I will achieve it is a different matter, and I am certainly never going to try to be the best dad in the world. The best one I can be is all I can aim for.

Chapter thirty-one

Returning to work

$\rightarrow$ Making the decision to go back to work is a big one. You might have all sorts of emotions including sadness at leaving your baby, guilt at going back, worries about juggling it all, or just be really excited about the idea of lunch breaks. Maybe you need to go back for financial reasons or maybe you simply want to go back. And that's fine – your needs are important.

Full-time, part-time or flexible working?

One thing to think about is the hours you are going to work and whether it's possible to do your job part-time or differently. If you went part-time, would it be easy to increase your hours again in the future if you needed to? Part-time or flexible hours can look very different. You might want set days off, or an earlier or later finish or to condense hours. Childcare costs might play a role – it may be a balance between continuing to work and also not paying more out in childcare costs than you earn.

Asking for child-friendly working hours – aka flexible working
Everyone has the right to ask to change how much, where or when they work as long as you have been employed for at least 26 weeks by that organisation. You can ask for changes to hours, days that you work or even to work from

home. Remember, if you are on maternity or paternity leave you are counted as employed. Both parents can ask for this – flexible working isn't limited to women or indeed the birth mother. In fact, grandparents could also ask for it if they are considering doing some childcare.

You can only ask for flexible working if you haven't made a request within the last 12 months. However, if you are a parent to a child and have a change in circumstances that means you cannot follow your usual working pattern because of childcare issues, such as a nursery closing down or grandparents suddenly pulling out of childcare, you can ask for changes to be made, but under the sex discrimination law (for more details see below). You need to explain what has changed and why it really is an issue, rather than you just not wanting to send your child to daycare.

For more details on making a request, check out the Maternity Action website. It is really important to show you have thought it all through: how it will work, what the challenges might be and how they could be overcome.

Employers must consider your request seriously, but they are allowed to say no for the following reasons:

- It would cost them more
- It would have a detrimental impact on customer demand or experience
- They cannot reorganise other staff to cover
- They cannot recruit more staff
- It would negatively affect their performance
- There is not enough work to do when you want to do it
- Planned structural changes

If your employer does say no and you think they have been unreasonable, you can appeal. For example, they cannot say that they don't employ people part-time or allow job share. They also can't say that you are too specialist or senior to job share. If they have said they cannot find anyone to replace you, they must show that they have genuinely put in the effort of trying to do so.

If they turn this down, you can appeal on grounds of sex discrimination. The Equality Act 2010 allows women with childcare responsibilities who have been refused flexible working to appeal. Notably, it also allows men to appeal if they have asked for flexible working for childcare reasons and have been refused, but women in their organisation have had their requests accepted.

The core rationale of such an appeal is to show you are being disadvantaged by not working child-friendly hours. For example:

- You can't find childcare for the hours you are required to work
- Childcare costs are too expensive
- You are experiencing stress or health issues from juggling care and your working hours

Returning full-time and dealing with working-mum guilt, especially if you're the main wage earner

The most common working pattern among partners in the UK is for a father to work full-time and a mother to work part-time. As we've seen, just 2 per cent of fathers are full-time stay-at-home dads. Yet women are increasingly earning more than their male partners, with around a quarter with a child under three now working full-time. Couples are slowly making changes where women are the main wage earners. Unfortunately, social attitudes, and the associated guilt and pressure directed at women who work full-time don't appear to be changing at the same rate.

We all know that there is no reason why couples shouldn't take an approach where the woman is working full-time or is the main wage earner. Whatever works best for you is best for your family. But that doesn't mean women in this position don't have a lot of doubts or worries. Research with mothers who are the breadwinner finds some really common concerns, including:[1,2]

- Dealing with cultural expectations that you should and will be the one at home caring for the child.
- Cultural judgement that 'good mothers' sacrifice everything for their children, including their job.
- Guilt at being away from children or following a career.
- Jealousy of your partner if their lower income meant you needed to make this decision.
- Guilt when you watch your partner caring for your children, feeling like you should be doing it.
- Feeling the need to make up for it at home, meaning you do much more childcare and housework than male colleagues.
- The assumption from others and cultural pressure to know all the details of your children's lives, like piano practice.

None of these are justified, but the emotions involved still make a lot of sense. Our society does still expect women to be the ones taking care of the children and home and doesn't deal well with those who for very logical reasons do otherwise. All I can say is ignore it. It's down to generations of thinking in a patriarchal society that struggles with women who 'have it all'. Especially powerful ones.

Guilt is a big deal. It nags away at us, telling us we are doing something wrong. But where does it come from? You know you are doing what is right for your family by going out to work and making sure the bills are paid and food is on the table. Why would that mean you have done something wrong? Why is a father who does the same praised?

The pressure to be the one caring for your children and home seems to reach even the most feminist women. Society tells us every day that a 'good

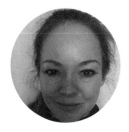

Being a breadwinner mother

Vicky Thomas, paediatrician and mother to Tom and Rose, returned to work full-time after her maternity leave ended when they made the decision for her husband Steve to be a full-time stay-at-home dad.

How did you initially feel after making the decision for you to go back to work and Steve stay home?

We had always anticipated me going back to work full-time or close to it after we had our first child, and maintaining that. The surprise was that when it came to it, it felt really hard. Before and during pregnancy, I had really no idea of what it was going to be like having an actual baby – ironic as I'm a paediatrician. When I was pregnant I remember a colleague, on hearing my plan to go back full-time at six months, saying 'Oh but Vicky! A baby needs a mummy!' – it was like a gut punch of guilt about a child who wasn't even born yet. I just smiled and nodded (a response I highly recommend in general), but in my head I replied 'A baby also needs the mortgage paid'.

What have the challenges been?

The first challenge was finding that, for us, not all of the work of mothering is transferable. My husband is an incredible, hands-on, nurturing father. But especially when the children were very little, they mostly wanted me if I was around. This could lead to exhaustion and frustration for both of us until we learned to accept it and find strategies that helped. I've also worried that Steve would find it emasculating and disempowering not being in paid work. He fortunately does not suffer from ego fragility and I think we work well as a team to support our family.

Another challenge is the workplace itself. I feel like a funny creature, neither fish nor fowl: I'm not quite full-time (I work between 30 and 60 hours a week, depending on our rota and how busy it is), but I'm also not working the same hours as many of my female colleagues who are parents. I often feel split between work and home, and like I'm doing both badly. There are days when I am booking dental check-ups and buying birthday presents in gaps in clinic, and then I come home and answer work emails and write presentations and papers on my phone while the kids are splashing in the bath. The boundaries are blurred and almost impossible to maintain.

Recently we recognised the issue of emotional labour. Steve has always been amazing at the domestic aspects, but until lately I still felt responsible for

World Book Day outfits, school shoes and birthday presents. This has changed in the last year, but it needed me to verbalise the stress I was feeling about these things as Steve is much more sensible and able to do an Elsa (let it go) than I am.

What is the stupidest assumption people make?
Stupid assumptions come Steve's way much more than mine – the one that made me laugh most was when the school mums assumed I was responsible for our four-year-old's immaculate Dutch plaits when they were all Steve's work. We couldn't decide if this was a sexist or 'hairist' assumption (Steve is follicularly challenged). I get annoyed when people say things like 'Well, my husband just couldn't do it' – why not? Men are just as capable of doing childcare and domestic work as women, but for centuries it's been undervalued, which has meant that lower-status people, usually women, have ended up doing it. If we valued this vital work properly, we would all appreciate the people who do it, regardless of their gender.

What advice would you give other women considering this?
My advice is born of the things we've found work for us:

- Be kind to each other. It helps if you've each had a go at both roles so you understand how the other one feels at 5pm on a Friday, whether you are the partner who's been at paid work all day or the partner waiting for the front door to open and the cavalry to arrive after 10 hours with a toddler or two.
- Have a good boss. When I got close to burn-out recently, my head of department recognised that I was carrying a parenting and paid workload. It felt so good to be seen.
- Never play the 'Who's the most tired' game. There are no winners.
- Separate out domestic chores and childcare if at all possible. Don't expect the person based at home to do the housework just because they are in the house. Stopping the children killing themselves is a full-time job in itself.
- If at all possible, find space to be individuals and a couple as well as parents. It's worth making time to do hobbies separately and together, to preserve your sense of self and to protect your relationship. Otherwise it can feel like all you do is soldier on in the trenches of childcare together.

mother' is the one sacrificing stuff for her children. This explains why research shows that when women work full-time and their partner less, they still on average do more housework and childcare. And we can feel guilt when we see partners doing their fair share. All I can repeat is that it's social conditioning at its finest. You know it doesn't make any logical sense.

Know that you are setting an amazing example to your children – they can see you working, earning and having that role and identity. Why does that matter? Well, it means there is less chance of them growing up with the same sort of guilt, either as women working or men staying home.

Finally, remember time with your children is about quality, not quantity. If you were at home all day you would not spend all day entertaining and educating them. And remember that there is no evidence to show that you returning to work has any negative consequences for them. Don't fall into the trap of idealising what you don't have. Focus on the time you do have with them – that's how positive attachments grow and are maintained.

Who is going to look after your baby?

If you're both returning to work or you're a single parent you'll need to consider who is going to look after your baby and what that might cost. Some common options include:

- **Family**

  If you are all happy and they are willing to do it this can be a great option as it can probably be more flexible, especially if you are working irregular hours. The benefits are that your child stays with someone you know, and in a home environment. The downside of this is – well, your child will stay with someone you know. It all really depends how closely your ethos and preferences around caring for your child are shared with family that might look after them. Will they care for your baby in the way you want? It can be difficult to argue your point if family are giving free childcare.

  It also depends on the age and fitness of family members, and things might change as your baby gets older. If your parents are going to care for your baby, will they still have the stamina or ability to chase them round when they're toddling?

  Things get a little complicated if you decide to pay family for this care. You won't be able to use childcare vouchers or claim the childcare element of tax credits or Universal Credit unless they register themselves as a childminder and look after at least one other child unrelated to yours.

- **Friends**

  Perhaps you and a friend both work part-time and your babies know each other. Helping each other out by caring for each other's baby when the other is working can seem like a great solution. However, there is a very strange rule (that I can't see any logical reason for) that if your friend looks after your child aged under eight for more than two hours a day during working hours they have to register legally as a childminder, which is not simple. Likewise, if you then looked after theirs you would too. However, if you both did manage to register, you could then pay each other for the care using childcare vouchers or the childcare element of tax credits or Universal Credit.

A daycare nursery

This type of nursery usually has regular opening hours from roughly 8am (or earlier if you are lucky) to 6pm from Monday to Friday. This is often tricky if you work irregular hours, although some rare places might have children later in the evening or even overnight if you are lucky. You can use any childcare vouchers you might be entitled to, but you may have to pay on the days your child is sick or you take holidays and your child doesn't attend.

Nurseries tend to have lots of children of different preschool ages and maybe even older children before and after school. They also tend to employ lots of different staff, which means they are less likely to be affected by one or two being off sick. You may view both these things either positively or negatively depending on your own preferences for your baby. And both views are very valid. Having lots of other children around is a great social experience, but it also means your baby is part of a much larger group.

Registered childminders

Childminders tend to look after children in their own homes. Depending on the individual they might offer more flexible hours than day nurseries, perhaps including overnight stays. When your child is a little older they may do school pick-ups and drop-offs which is really useful, as school is only 6.5 hours of the day. You can use childcare vouchers but may have to pay when your child is not there. Childminders are self-employed and offering you a service so you don't need to think about additional payments such as Income Tax or NI contributions.

The benefits and challenges of choosing a childminder for care are pretty much the opposite of those for daycare nurseries. If your childminder works alone you will need to find another option if they are sick, on holiday or close for whatever reason. However, your baby will consistently receive care from the same person. Likewise, there will be fewer children around - whether you see that as a positive or negative will depend on your baby.

- **A nanny**

  A nanny is a trained childcare worker who typically looks after your child in your home – some will come to you and some will live in. Nannies tend to be a more expensive option than your child going to a nursery or childminder because they may be caring only for your child (although some will do a nanny share). But if you have more than one baby, it might work out the same or even cheaper than day nursery.

  Your baby will be cared for by one person, in your home. Again, do you see that as a positive or a negative? There is no right answer. You will also be reliant on one person, although many areas will have emergency temporary nannies if needed. Nannies are not self-employed like childminders. You employ them, so you will need to draw up a contract, give them holidays and be responsible for sickness, maternity leave and so on.

Things you might like to consider when making your choice include:

- The location. A work-based childcare option is perfect, but in general the nearer to work the location, the shorter the hours your child is there, and the less difficult your commute between work and childcare. Think about the logistics between your work, your partner's work and home. Where would work best?

- If you have a partner and they're working too, think about who is going to do pick-up and drop-off. It often works well, if possible, for one of you to start early and pick-up from childcare, and the other start later and drop-off. Try to balance it so it's not just one of you doing both and having the pressure at each end of the day, unless there are major constraints such as location or timing of shifts.

Will my baby be harmed by putting them in childcare?

Nope.

You've probably seen loads of headlines about babies in childcare being more stressed or whatever it is they're trying to make parents feel guilty about today. Other days you'll see articles saying it's a great decision and they end up more intelligent or something. Take it all with a pinch of salt, because whatever the study found it was not looking at your baby. You will know at heart what is right for them and whether they are okay at whatever setting you choose.

There are some very strong voices in society about this. It feels like some would argue there is no harm to babies going from the womb to 24/7 daycare, while others would say just walking past a nursery harms your child forever. Some studies show that early daycare helps development and others show the opposite. As with everything, it's never as black or white as that and will depend on your circumstances. I mean, if it's a choice between you being able to keep a roof over your head or not (as it is for many families) then obviously that is something to take into consideration!

A number of studies show that babies in daycare settings have higher stress levels during the day compared to those babies who stay home. Now this isn't as straightforward or as scary as it sounds. Firstly 'more' does not automatically mean catastrophically high. Most studies simply measure levels – they don't categorise them as 'harmful levels' or not. Also, although our stress hormones do rise when we are feeling anxious or threatened, they also rise in relation to positive stimulation too – including novelty. So some proportion at least of that increase is probably due to the faster pace of the day in daycare and meeting new people and doing new things compared to the home environment.

There are, however, a number of factors that are associated with lesser increases in stress in children in daycare:

- **The quality of the care matters**
  This does not mean you need to find a daycare centre that promises to teach your baby quantum mechanics and three languages by the time they leave. It is more about the consistency, responsiveness and gentleness of the care they receive. Where babies are hugged and engaged with, receiving consistent attention and interaction, their stress levels are much lower – in fact some studies show as low as if they were at home.[3]

- **Who is caring for your baby**
  The turnover of staff who care for your baby. Research shows that babies can form close and loving attachments with their caregivers, which is really important. Good childcare workers can be just as engaging and loving as a parent at home, which makes a big difference to your baby.[4]

- **Your relationship with your baby**
  Research shows that babies who have a good attachment to their caregivers are far less stressed by childcare than those who are already in difficult circumstances at home. Even if your baby goes to nursery 50 hours a week, they are still home with you more than twice that. It's the bigger picture that matters and their relationship with you overrides other things.[5]

- **How many other children are there?**
  Research shows that in large settings, with more than 15 other babies, stress levels are higher. Now this figure is for the room your baby is in, not the whole nursery. Many nurseries split their children into different age ranges and have each in a different space. It's that space that matters, not the whole setting.[6]

- **How long your baby is there**

  There is some evidence that shorter periods in childcare are better for babies under one. Not all research is conclusive, but babies who are in childcare for 35 hours a week or less have the lowest stress levels, followed by under 45 hours, compared to those who are there longer.[7]

It's important not to get too worried about the research when you make your decision – use it to help you, but don't beat yourself up over it. You'll find studies that suggest harm is done, but it's important to look at them closely. What did they actually measure? When? Who with? In what settings? In what country?

Remember as well that research is about averages across populations. It can't tell you about your individual baby, and most babies are in fact just fine. When a study says 'an increased risk of' it simply means a high percentage, not all babies. As Jay Belsky, an academic specialising in the impact of childcare, says:[8] *When mothers come to me, and say, 'What should I do with my kid?' I say, 'The truth is these effects are small enough... I don't know if this is a decisive enough finding to tell you what to do with your kid. It's a probability not a certainty. The probability looks small, the effect is modest, not big. You might conclude therefore not to worry about it'.*

Financing childcare

Sadly, childcare is rarely cheap – although when you look at it properly, good quality childcare should never be inexpensive given that you are paying someone to look after something very precious to you. Cheap childcare also means low wages for the person looking after your child, and since childcare is still largely dominated by women, this further increases inequality and the gender pay gap.

The average childcare costs differ according to what sort of provider you use, where you live (London is much more expensive) and whether you have more than one child enrolled (you might get a discount). The average costs for a full-time place (per week based on 50 hours a week) for a child aged two or under are £221 for a registered childminder, £242 for a day nursery, and anywhere from £400–£800 plus other expenses for a nanny.[9] A nanny would likely become more cost-effective with more than one child, as they may charge for their time rather than per child. Bear in mind that these are average figures and it is certainly possible to pay a lot more and sometimes a lot less (remembering the importance of quality care).

That's so expensive – is it worth me going back to work?

Looking at those figures, it's easy to fall into a state of shock, especially the first time you read them. The costs are certainly more than many people's mortgages, even with the current housing market. So this is an important decision that will differ according to your family.

It is possible that childcare will cost more than one of your wages. Some couples therefore decide they don't want to pay out as a family to both be working. This is not the same as seeing childcare as solely being the woman's cost to bear, but if your costs are higher than your salary you might think twice.

It's not that simple though and will really depend on:

- How much you want to return to work – you are allowed to go back to work because you want to, or think you are an overall better parent with the balance.
- Whether you think your job has greater earning potential in the future – if you are earning a low wage now, but it might increase in the next few years, will the overall impact be a financial gain (assuming you can afford to take that hit now)?
- The stage of your career – are you on a career ladder that you are climbing? Will it have any impact if you pause?
- Your type of job – do you need to be regularly updated to keep on track, or will your job be there in the future without too much major retraining?

Remember as well there is the option to go part-time. This lets you keep one foot in the workplace. You might also decide that your current job is not for you and choose a different one. Maybe more highly paid, or indeed maybe less so, because you want something closer to home that can be easily done part-time or would be less stressful. You might also like to think about whether you have particular skills that could enable you to work from home while your baby naps (hopefully) or in the evenings, or could be done with less formal childcare.

It's also really important to take an honest and objective look at your long-term future, especially if you are not married. It might not be something you wish to think about right now, but if in the future, after you have given up work, you separate or divorce, what will your financial situation be? Will you be able to rejoin the workforce? What sort of income would you be able to have?

If you are not married, you have far fewer rights. If you are the main caregiver your child's other parent will need to pay you child maintenance for the children based on their salary. But they will not owe you any support legally. If the house is in their name alone – a common scenario if you are not working or they bought it before meeting you – then you would have a fight to prove entitlement to anything in it or part of a sale. Marriage legally entitles you to more, including a share in any house you are not named on and potentially spousal support depending on how long you have been married and not working. This is obviously deeply unfair if you have given your time to raising children, especially if it enables the other parent to work freely and without childcare costs. So think carefully before giving up work.

Can I get any help with childcare costs?

In the UK there are a number of different ways in which you might get support for childcare. The government website has details here **www.gov.uk/help-with-childcare-costs/childcare-vouchers** and I also recommend visiting **www.entitledto.co.uk** which will give you an estimate of the support you might get.

1. A work childcare voucher scheme (but only if you are already receiving these)

This scheme has now closed to new entrants but if you were registered before 4 October 2018 you can carry on using them until you either change jobs, your employer stops the scheme or you take an unpaid career break longer than a year.

2. Government Tax-Free Childcare scheme

This scheme applies if you have a child aged 11 and under and they usually live with you. You may be able to get money for older children if they receive Disability Living Allowance, Personal Independence Payment or Armed Forces Independence Payment – or are certified as blind or severely sight impaired. You can only apply if you are from within the European Economic Area or your partner is.

Here you set up a childcare account, through which you directly pay your childcare provider. For every £8 you put in, the government will add in £2. The cap on this is £2,000 per child per year. It must be used only for approved childcare, including childminders, nurseries, nannies, after-school clubs, play schemes and home care agencies. Your provider must be signed up to the scheme.

You and your partner (if you live with them) must both be working to apply for this scheme unless one parent at home is in receipt of Incapacity Benefit, Severe Disablement Allowance, Carer's Allowance or Employment and Support Allowance. You (and your partner if relevant) must also earn at least a set amount equivalent to the national minimum wage × 16 hours a week for at least the next three months. It can't be used, for example, if you are registered as self-employed but not really making any money – unless you only started your business in the last year. Also, if either of you has an adjusted net income (total taxable income minus personal allowances) including bonuses of over £100,000 a year you can't apply. If you are separated from your child's other parent, only one of you can access this scheme for a child.

Finally you won't be able to use this if you receive tax credits or Universal

Credit, which include childcare money. You can check on the website to see whether you would be better off **www.gov.uk/childcare-calculator**.

3. Childcare element of tax credits or Universal Credit

You may be eligible for childcare contributions under tax or Universal credits. If you are already claiming tax credits and have not been moved across to Universal Credit yet this will likely happen by 2023. All new claimants will need to apply for Universal Credit.

The rules are pretty similar, but under universal credit, depending on your income and circumstances, you may receive up to 85% of your childcare costs back up to a maximum of £646 for one child or £1,108 for two children or more. You and your partner (if you live with them) must be in work, although for the childcare element it does not matter how many hours you work. The more you earn the lower the percentage will be, but it does also take into account other financial information, so it's difficult to estimate here what you might get. You can apply online **www.gov.uk/apply-universal-credit** or just use it to take a look at what you might be entitled to before making a decision.

4. A subsidised workplace scheme

Your employer may offer a subsidised scheme privately to their employers or even money towards childcare. Check directly with them.

5. Free childcare for older children

When your baby reaches three years old (or two if you are on a low income) you'll be eligible for up to 30 hours a week of free childcare. However, the rules in each country in the UK are different and a bit complicated so it's best to look up what applies to you. The Money Saving Expert website has detailed information and links **www.moneysavingexpert.com/family/childcare-costs**.

Breastfeeding your baby on return to work

There are lots of reasons why you might want to continue breastfeeding on return to work, including simply because you want to. The World Health Organization recommends breastfeeding for two years and beyond – for as long as you and your baby want to, so you are certainly protected by public health policy encouraging you to do so.

Breastmilk still continues to offer so much nutrition to babies even when they have moved to solid foods. It also continues to deliver immune support to your baby, and in fact levels of immune properties in milk actually start to rise in the second year of life, probably because they're running around attempting to lick everything. This can be really handy, especially if they are going to childcare for the first time and mixing with lots of other children (and bugs).

Breastfeeding is also a lovely way to reconnect with your baby after a long day. You're shattered and they want you... feeding is a lovely way of getting that skin-to-skin connection and entertaining your baby while you sit down!

Some practical tips for combining breastfeeding and work

Your experience of breastfeeding and returning to work is likely to be different based on your personal circumstances. Some things that might affect it:

1. How old is your baby? A younger baby who has not been introduced to solid foods is going to need more feeds than an older baby who could drink water and eat some food during the day.

2. How many hours do you work and can they be flexible? If you work part-time you may not need to think about expressing so much compared to if you work full-time.

3. Your job. Do you work in an office-based job with flexibility? Or a more practical job such as the police, medicine or teaching? The latter is going to need a bit more planning.

Babies under six months old

Babies under six months old are going to need more milk feeds during the day than older babies, so think about how that might work for you. Some options include:

- Expressing milk for them to have in a cup or bottle
- Whoever is looking after your baby bringing them to you for feeds
- You going to the baby for feeds
- Them having formula milk during the day if expressing is too difficult

Remember, breastmilk isn't an either/or situation. If you decide you need to use formula milk in the day, that doesn't mean you have to stop breastfeeding altogether. Some milk will still give your baby all those immune properties over no milk. It also allows you to continue feeding at night and when you pick them up (or however you will fit feeds in around night shifts).

Your baby is older and eating solid foods

This will all depend on your individual baby and the factors above – essentially how long you need to leave them for. You have all the options above, but it is also possible with a baby who will eat solids and drink from a cup for them not to have any milk feeds during the day. This will be more feasible if you work fairly close to your place of childcare or relatively short days than if you have 12-hour shifts with a commute each end.

Some babies will simply refuse to have milk from anything other than a breast and as they are eating and drinking some food in the day they may not be hungry enough to bother accepting a bottle. The good news is that your baby will likely be fine in this scenario, although quite possibly will want to feed immediately on pick-up and more frequently over the next few hours. It is also possible that they do something called 'reverse cycling', where they start feeding lots during the night again. Perhaps that's not what you wanted on top of the exhaustion of returning to work, but at least it's a way of them getting lots of breastmilk.

If this happens, you might still want to think about expressing milk during work, even if just for your comfort. However, many women find that as their supply is well established after months of breastfeeding, they don't need to express during the day (apart from a little for comfort reasons) and their body adapts. If you're working part-time you might also find your body seems to get into a rhythm where on work days you don't need to express but on days home with your baby you have plenty of milk to feed them. Remember if you're reading this when your baby is tiny and feeding every two hours or more, that as your baby gets older and starts eating solid foods too, they won't feed as much.

All of this, however you decide to feed your baby, can feel overwhelming at the start. An important thing to remember is that it is not going to be like this forever. Once your baby starts to get a little older they won't need milk in the day in the same way. Remember, if they are over 12 months they can have cows' milk as a drink, so if you are finding expressing challenging there is no need to buy formula milk.

Expressing milk

A few things to think about when expressing milk outside the house include:

- How will you express it?
- Where will you express it and when?
- Where will you store it during the day?
- How will you get it home?

Some of the answers to these questions will depend on whether you plan to give the milk to your baby or not. If you are just expressing for comfort or to keep up your supply there is no need to carefully store and transport the milk. If you don't have a job where you have a private space and flexibility, it is a good idea to start talking to your employer before you return to work (see the following section on talking to your employer and your rights at work).

Hand-expressing

Hand-expressing is a great tool for every breastfeeding mother to have. It can be particularly useful once you've returned to work if you're feeling very full and just want to express enough to remain comfortable during the day. However, some women get a lot of milk out while hand-expressing and might prefer to express milk this way all the time. The best way to learn about hand-expressing if you're not familiar is to watch some videos. Some great ones can be found here: **med.stanford.edu/newborns/professional-education/ breastfeeding/hand-expressing-milk.html**.

Some quick tips:

- Wash your hands and if you're going to keep the milk for your baby, sterilise a container to catch it in.
- Work out where your milk ducts are – these will be in slightly different places in different women, but are around or just on your areola (the darker bit by your nipples). The idea is to put gentle pressure on these (the key word being gentle).
- Different positions can help. Some women find cupping their breast with one hand and making a C-shape with the other around their areola works. Others put both hands around their breast with thumbs pointing up and apply pressure that way.
- Once you have your hands in position, apply pressure by pushing gently into the chest wall. On the way 'in' you can also squeeze very gently – but don't pull on the way 'out'.
- Keep applying this pressure gently and release, repeating until you get a rhythm going.
- Try not to slide your fingers about as this could hurt.
- Milk should now start to appear.
- It's likely after a bit it will slow down – try moving your hand around to apply pressure in a different place.

Using a pump

There are lots of different styles of pump available. Some are hands-free, or have hands-free attachments allowing you to pump and work at the same time (although some people find that a bit overwhelming).

The important thing is to make sure you are not in any pain – if it hurts at any time stop (and seek help). It's important to make sure that the flange of the pump fits your breast – it should be snug, but with room for your nipple to move when the suction is applied, without rubbing against anything. Some pumps come with different-sized flanges you can buy to make sure you get one that is comfortable for you.

Most electric pumps have a feature allowing you to increase the suction force and some have automatic cycles built in. The most efficient way to pump is to start by using the maximum pressure you can without feeling pain, then ease it down once your milk starts flowing. Once you've got the hang of it, and if you need to express lots of milk, you can buy another pump and express from both sides at the same time.

Storing your milk

If you want to keep your milk for your baby (or to donate) then think about how you will store it. You can use any sterilised container, or breastmilk storage bags.

If you have a fridge on the premises you can store your milk in there. If you are working in a larger workplace with people you may not know or trust it might be worth placing it in another container in a way you will know it has not been tampered with (by tampered with I also mean looked at by the curious idiot). Even if you know everyone and they're great, it might be worth letting them know if it's going in the shared fridge so they don't accidentally move it/ throw it out/add it to their tea. If you cannot get access to a fridge, or prefer to keep your milk close, you can store milk in insulated bags with freezer blocks for up to 24 hours.

Once home, if you plan on feeding the milk to your baby in the next few days, it can be stored in your fridge for up to five days as long as your fridge is at 4 degrees Celsius or lower. If you want to save it for future use you can freeze it. Milk can be frozen for two weeks in the ice compartment of a fridge and for up to six months in a freezer. Label the milk with the date before you freeze it. Storing it in smaller amounts is useful, so that you can give your baby just a smaller feed if that's all they want.

Using your milk

Milk from the fridge can be taken out and used just as it is, depending on your baby. Some babies will drink it cool, while others will prefer it at body temperature. There is no need to boil the milk or heat it to over 70 degrees like you would to make up a bottle of formula. Never use a microwave to heat it as this can heat the milk unevenly, leading to very hot spots.

If you are taking frozen milk out of the freezer, it needs to be used as soon as possible. If you are taking it out with you, you can carry it for up to 24 hours in a cool bag with ice packs in it. If you need to defrost milk quickly for your baby you can run the bag under a warm tap or put the bottle in a jug of warm water.

As with formula, once your baby has drunk from a bottle of expressed breastmilk, it needs to be finished within the hour. Once this is up, throw the remaining milk away.

Tips for making expressing easier

Although stress itself doesn't interfere with milk production, there is some evidence that it can interfere with your 'let down reflex' – essentially the reflex that lets the milk out of your breast.

- Flick through some photos or videos of your baby. The 'old' advice used to be to look at a photo of your baby, but now many of us have so many photos and videos of our babies on our phones that these can be really useful for helping you feel closer to your baby.
- Try and relax as much as possible. Obviously this is more challenging if you're feeling stressed, rushed or awkward. What helps you relax? Listening to relaxing music or a podcast? Having a muslin cloth that reminds you of your baby? Distracting yourself by reading or colouring?
- Try gently massaging your breasts or placing a warm compress on them if feasible.
- If you are able to, trying a different style of pump might help. Some women find an electric pump easier, while others hate the sound.

Talking to your employer

There are many benefits for your employer of you continuing to breastfeed on your return to work. Research has shown that workplaces save money if they support breastfeeding women. In fact, a study in the USA found that for every $1 a company invested in making sure its breastfeeding women were well supported, they made back $3.[10] Why? Well if you are breastfeeding...

- Your baby is statistically less likely to get sick, meaning you need less time off work.
- You are less likely to have longer-term health issues.
- Your mental health on average will be better. This is helped by breastfeeding mothers actually getting more sleep (even if it might not feel like it).
- Employees who feel valued are more productive. Also, if you're feeling supported and have a good feeding plan in place you're also less likely to be worrying about your baby.
- You're more likely to return to your job after maternity leave and stay at the company if you feel valued. This is great for employers, not just because they still have you working for them, but because recruiting and training new people takes time and money.

Unfortunately, not all workplaces are supportive and in the UK we still don't have great protection under employment law. Here, on returning to work you have the right to:

- A risk assessment to check that your work would not put you at risk. This is highly unlikely unless you spend your day working with dangerous chemicals such as organic mercury, lead or radioactive material.
- A space to lie down and rest.
- The right to request flexible working hours, which might include, for example, a longer lunch hour to go and feed your baby.

Your workplace must take any requests you make seriously. If you ask them to consider your needs as a breastfeeding mother and they simply dismiss you, this may be a case for a complaint under unlawful sex discrimination. They must listen to you and take your concerns seriously, and if they cannot adapt to your requests give you a reasonable reason why. They must take your request as seriously as they would any other request for changes to working patterns, i.e. not laugh or dismiss you simply because the request is about breastfeeding.

Unfortunately, additional breaks to breastfeed or express are not a legal right. Some workplaces might tell you to use your current breaks. However, handily, the Equality Act 2010 states that you should not have your health or safety put at risk by your workplace. If, for example, you find yourself becoming very engorged, that would be a risk factor for developing mastitis.

Remember that any negative comments, no matter whether they are supposedly made in humour, also come under the Equality Act in terms of harassment. No one has the right to treat you badly because you are breastfeeding.

Best practice guidelines

Thankfully, ACAS has put together some best practice guidelines for supporting breastfeeding in the workplace. Although these are not legally binding, they are a great starting point for having a conversation with your workplace. It would be expected that most decent workplaces should try to follow these guidelines. They recommend that all workplaces make adjustments to ensure that all breastfeeding women are supported and that these adjustments are made into a workplace policy on breastfeeding. These adjustments include:

- A private space in which to feed or express milk. This space should be hygienic, safe and secure (or in other words, should not be a toilet). It is recommended that it has a lockable door.
- Access to a fridge where milk can safely be stored.
- Additional/amended breaks/flexible working.

It might be useful to send your employer the ACAS guidance, which can be found on their website archive.acas.org.uk/media/3924/Accommodating-breastfeeding-employees-in-the-workplace/pdf/Acas-guide-on-accommodating-breastfeeding-in-the-workplace.pdf.

Maternity Action has also developed a handy leaflet for employers, also found online, which has lots of references to research that shows the benefits to the employer. It also contains handy links showing why breastfeeding is important and how often babies need to feed/you might need to express. www.maternityaction.org.uk/wp-content/uploads/2014/11/BORTW-employer-leaflet-FINAL.pdf.

I feel absolutely overwhelmed by the thought of going back

Yup. Deep breaths! It feels overwhelming somehow condensing what you used to do with what you now do into just one role. But it will get easier and more manageable. Here are some practical considerations to make life easier:

- Consider whether you can have a phased return. One idea is to use some holiday (you'll have accrued it while on leave) to perhaps have a two-day return the first week, three days the next week and so on. Or take some random days off in the first months of being back and sit in the house/go to a spa all on your own.
- Be kind to yourself in the first few weeks. Expect to feel knackered, fraught and overwhelmed. If you feel better than this then great. But don't make any major decisions in the early days. Give it chance.
- Have everything ready the night before. Pretend you're 13 again and your mother is shouting at you to pack your bag the night before. But seriously, pack your bag the night before. For you, and make sure someone has packed one for your baby too.
- Keep spare clothes in your car, locker or office. A particular party trick for babies is to dribble over you or worse when you've dropped them off at childcare and there's no time to get home. Also, a box of cereal bars in your locker/drawer works wonders when you haven't had time for breakfast. And any spare other stuff that you'll forget and not want to waste time popping out or home for.
- Have a back-up childcare plan, even if it's just theoretical.
- If possible, buy in support (always paying more than the living wage). Or, pretend you have a small baby again and focus on meal delivery services, batch cooking and calling on family and friends for favours.
- Try and find the time to continue looking after yourself physically. Eat well. Be active. Get some rest. These are bigger priorities than a really tidy house. You matter. Invest in yourself.
- Talk to your partner to make sure any household chores are renegotiated if you have been doing more while on maternity leave. You do not want to fall into the trap of being back earning and taking the lion's share of domestic work too.
- Follow Vicki Psarias – 'the honest mum' on her website and social media. Her book *Mumboss* is a great guide to balancing work and parenting honestmum.com/buy-mumboss-book.

Workplace support packages
Another thing to explore is whether your workplace offers any support packages for new parents on return to work, not just in terms of flexible

working, but also looking after their health. We know that the first year in particular of adjusting to being a new parent can be tricky. You might still have physical complications after a difficult birth. Your back might be hurting from all the bending and lifting of a growing baby. You might be finding a transition to pumping milk tricky. Perhaps you need some relationship support with changing roles at home. And mental health challenges can crop up at any time.

Some workplaces recognise that looking after their employees on return to work and through major transitions isn't just about working hours or perks such as dress-down Fridays, free coffee or a fancy office chair. A number of larger employers in particular might have all sorts of further support you can access such as free counselling, support groups or access to free or reduced health-related services like physiotherapy or massages. It's certainly worth asking. It might be a self-referral or automatic perks that build up over time, or you might need the support of occupational health to get a referral. Never be afraid to ask. These services are there for a reason. Yes your employer might care for you, but they also recognise that when their employees are healthy and happy they're more likely to be productive and loyal to the company. See it as a win-win for everyone.

One recently developed scheme specifically for supporting the health and wellbeing of new and expectant parents that workplaces can sign up to is called 'Peppy Baby'. Peppy Baby was founded by a group of parents with significant experience in working in healthcare, digital economy and business management to meet a gap they saw in supporting new parents during pregnancy and on return to work. Partnering with the NCT, Peppy have brought together a brilliant group of practitioners such as lactation consultants, counsellors and physiotherapists to provide a holistic package of care free at point of access to new parents. The concept works through employers signing up to a package of support that their employees can access, working on the basis that investing in the physical and emotional wellbeing of their staff will bring long-term benefits. A recent trial of Peppy support outside of the workplace found that having access to such services had a really positive impact on maternal mental health among new mothers who were struggling. You can read more on their website and encourage your employer to sign up www.peppy.health/baby.

Getting further support

If you are really still feeling overwhelmed at decisions around work or balancing it all, it may be worth taking some time to pause and get some coaching around understanding your different options. Coaching doesn't tell you what to do, but it helps you work through your options, understanding them better and helping you feel more confident and empowered.

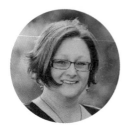

Working with a women's coach

Lisa Thompson, from Women Are Amazing, is a coach who works with women throughout the childbearing year and beyond, to help them feel more confident and in control of their lives. She talks about how coaching may help you with decisions around work and work-life balance.

What do you do as a women's coach?

I help women feel confident, powerful and excited by their life! Coaching is a wonderful extension of my work as a midwife and an IBCLC because I want women to have agency in their lives, to know just how amazing they are, and to step into leadership – whether that's in their families, their communities, their workplace or higher.

What sort of things do women come to see you about?

Many of my coaching clients are mothers, perhaps at the point of going back to work after maternity, or sometimes further on than that but feeling they need to explore how their various roles in life fit together. Sometimes becoming a mother highlights aspects of how they were mothered and they want to explore that.

What happens during sessions?

At a very basic level it's just talking and listening. But very special listening! Coaches don't tell you what to do, they help you discover what's right for you, so they might ask questions and point out things you hadn't noticed. Most of us also have tools and resources that we introduce to our clients to help make their lives easier or more satisfying. When I first start working with women most of them do a tailored three-month programme – it's a blend of coaching and teaching and is designed to make a significant improvement in whatever area of life the client is focusing on.

What are the benefits of coaching?

Working with a coach usually brings clarity on what you want in life and how to get it – that might be a career goal, easier relationships at home or a fitness target. Many of the women I work with discover increased confidence in asking for what they need (and getting it) and notice they still get plenty done but that it feels less like hard work – they usually have more fun.

One piece of advice for women going back to work?

Be kind to yourself – a lot of people rely on you, it's true, but you can't drive a car with no fuel in the tank so plan time to top yourself up somehow.

A final word

Drawing things to a close, I hope that you have found this book useful. Well, better than useful – I hope you now feel both informed and empowered. I want to leave you with my top 10 messages as a reminder of everything we've discussed in the book.

1. It's okay to put yourself first sometimes. It's okay to do things that help you feel happier, fitter or you simply enjoy doing. Nourish your body and your soul before you break.
2. Never be afraid to ask for support. We were never meant to do this alone. It is never a sign of failure. It's a sign of wanting to fix things.
3. Other people will always have opinions. That's fine. It's also fine to completely ignore them! You don't have to justify your decisions, especially not to people who haven't played a major role in creating or caring for your baby. Smile and wave – it's not just for penguins.
4. 'Good' parents have bad thoughts sometimes. It's normal to feel overwhelmed, frustrated or like getting in the car and driving away as fast as possible. You are not required to enjoy everything about this. People who tell you to savour the time when they are young have forgotten the intensity of having a baby. Is your baby cared for? Great. You're a good parent.
5. When asking questions or seeking professional support, look at qualifications and experience, not number of Instagram followers.
6. Waking at night, feeding frequently and wanting to stay close to you are normal baby behaviours. Exhausting, yes. But as long as your baby is healthy, don't listen to anyone who tells you to parent in a way you are not comfortable with.
7. A partner should be a partner. The load should be shared. The clue is in the name.
8. If motherhood and stay-at-home parenting was rewarded according to its true monetary and societal value you would be a millionaire. Don't let a capitalist society that has forgotten about the importance of nurturance, family and the next generation determine your worth.
9. If something hurts or doesn't seem to be working right, whether that's a physical part of your body or your soul, get help. You don't need to justify it, nor does the health of your baby indicate whether you deserve to feel a certain way or not. It's perfectly possible – common even – to have a healthy baby but be struggling yourself.
10. Whatever you are stressing about right now and thinking will never change, most probably will. It might be replaced by a different issue, but a change is as good as a rest. They will sleep one day.

Good luck, you've got this!

Acknowledgements

I had so many people in mind when writing this book. Talking to friends, colleagues and new parents on social media over the years I realised we were all pretty much experiencing the same thoughts, feelings and aches and pains – yet often not opening up and sharing these or even knowing there was support out there, let alone where to get it. I wanted to write this book for you, and myself. So, this book is for you all, thank you. I hope it's useful... well, more than useful – healing, empowering and most of all reassuring. I've had several requests to go back in time and publish it 10, 20 or even more years ago. I'm working on the time machine I promise.

To everyone who contributed – thank you a million times over. Your expertise, ability to connect with others through your writing, and willingness to write, often at speed, is amazing. For some of you, I am in awe of your positive response to a stranger who popped up in your social media inbox one evening asking for your wise words.

To my family as always, thank you for being you and supporting me in being me. I promise I'm most definitely not writing any more books... this week.

To everyone at Pinter & Martin – again as always, thank you. What book are we on now? I can't keep up. What's next?*

* *Let's talk about feeding your baby* x

References

Chapter 1: First things first, let's make sure you're supported

1. www.ippr.org/news-and-media/press-releases/one-third-of-mothers-in-working-families-are-breadwinners-in-britain
2. www.theguardian.com/lifeandstyle/2019/aug/01/birth-rate-in-england-and-wales-at-all-time-low
3. www.co-operative.coop/media/news-releases/shocking-extent-of-loneliness-faced-by-young-mothers-revealed
4. www.huffingtonpost.co.uk/entry/mums-feel-lonely-after-birth_uk_58bec088e-4b09ab537d6bdf9?ir=UK+Parents&utm_hp_ref=uk-parents
5. www.todaysparent.com/baby/postpartum-care/hey-new-mom-crying-in-public-i-see-you/
6. Blum, L. D. (2007). Psychodynamics of postpartum depression. *Psychoanalytic Psychology, 24*(1), 45.
7. Leger, J., & Letourneau, N. (2015). New mothers and postpartum depression: a narrative review of peer support intervention studies. *Health & social care in the community, 23*(4), 337-348.
8. McComish, J. F., & Visger, J. M. (2009). Domains of postpartum doula care and maternal responsiveness and competence. *Journal of Obstetric, Gynecologic & Neonatal Nursing, 38*(2), 148-156.
9. Edwards, R. C., Thullen, M. J., Korfmacher, J., Lantos, J. D., Henson, L. G., & Hans, S. L. (2013). Breastfeeding and complementary food: randomized trial of community doula home visiting. *Pediatrics, 132*(Supplement 2), S160-S166.
10. McLeish, J., & Redshaw, M. (2019). 'Being the best person that they can be and the best mum': a qualitative study of community volunteer doula support for disadvantaged mothers before and after birth in England. *BMC pregnancy and childbirth, 19*(1), 1-11.

Chapter 2: Managing the early days

1. Dennis, C. L., Fung, K., Grigoriadis, S., Robinson, G. E., Romans, S., & Ross, L. (2007). Traditional postpartum practices and rituals: a qualitative systematic review. Women's Health, 3(4), 487-502.
2. Lal, J. (2012). Turmeric, curcumin and our life: a review. *Bull Environ Pharmacol Life Sci, 1*(7), 11-17.
3. Kendall-Tackett, K. (2007). A new paradigm for depression in new mothers: the central role of inflammation and how breastfeeding and anti-inflammatory treatments protect maternal mental health. *International breastfeeding journal, 2*(1), 6.
4. Laroia, N., & Sharma, D. (2006). The religious and cultural bases for breastfeeding practices among the Hindus. *Breastfeeding Medicine, 1*(2), 94-98.
5. Posmontier, B., & Horowitz, J. A. (2004). Postpartum practices and depression prevalences: technocentric and ethnokinship cultural perspectives. *Journal of Transcultural Nursing, 15*(1), 34-43.

Chapter 3: Looking after yourself once everything goes back to normal

1. www.telegraph.co.uk/finance/personalfinance/11164040/How-much-is-a-housewife-worth.html
2. Smith, J. P. (2013). "Lost milk?" counting the economic value of breast milk in gross domestic product. *Journal of Human Lactation, 29*(4), 537-546.
3. www.todaysparent.com/blogs/opinion/self-care-is-a-bunch-of-bs/
4. Van Lith, T. (2016). Art therapy in mental health: A systematic review of approaches and practices. *The Arts in Psychotherapy, 47*, 9-22.

Chapter 4: Caring for your small baby mammal

1. Landry, S. H., Smith, K. E., & Swank, P. R. (2006). Responsive parenting: establishing early foundations for social, communication, and independent problem-solving skills. *Developmental psychology, 42*(4), 627.
2. Leifield, L., & Sanders, T. B. (2007). Responsive Infant Caregiving: Eight Proven Practices. *Dimensions of early childhood, 35*(1), 17-26.
3. Zeskind, P. S., & Marshall, T. R. (1988). The relation between variations in pitch and maternal perceptions of infant crying. *Child Development*, 193-196.
4. Leerkes, E. M., & Siepak, K. J. (2006). Attachment linked predictors of women's emotional and cognitive responses to infant distress. *Attachment & Human Development, 8*(01), 11-32.
5. Van Ijzendoorn, M. H., & Hubbard, F. O. (2000). Are infant crying and maternal responsiveness during the first year related to infant-mother attachment at 15 months?. *Attachment & Human Development, 2*(3), 371-391.
6. Hiscock, H., & Jordan, B. (2004). 1. Problem crying in infancy. *Medical journal of Australia, 181*(9), 507-512.
7. Ong, T. G., Gordon, M., Banks, S. S., Thomas, M. R., & Akobeng, A. K. (2019). Probiotics to prevent infantile colic. *Cochrane Database of Systematic Reviews*, (3).
8. Sung V, Hiscock H, Tang ML, Mensah FK, Nation ML, Satzke C, Heine RG, Stock A, Barr RG, Wake M. Treating infant colic with the probiotic Lactobacillus reuteri: double blind, placebo controlled randomised trial. Bmj. 2014 Apr 1;348:g2107.
9. Moore, E. R., Bergman, N., Anderson, G. C., & Medley, N. (2016). Early skin‐to‐skin contact for mothers and their healthy newborn infants. *Cochrane database of systematic Reviews*, (11).
10. Shorey, S., He, H. G., & Morelius, E. (2016). Skin-to-skin contact by fathers and the impact on infant and paternal outcomes: an integrative review. *Midwifery, 40*, 207-217.
11. Lozoff, B., & Brittenham, G. (1979). Infant care: cache or carry. *The Journal of pediatrics, 95*(3), 478-483.
12. www.naturalchild.org/articles/guest/claire_niala.html
13. Esposito, G., Yoshida, S., Ohnishi, R., Tsuneoka, Y., del Carmen Rostagno, M., Yokota, S., ... & Venuti, P. (2013). Infant calming responses during maternal carrying in humans and mice. *Current Biology, 23*(9), 739-745.
14. Reynolds-Miller, R. L. (2016). Potential therapeutic benefits of babywearing. *Creative nursing, 22*(1), 17-23.

Chapter 5: Understanding your baby's development and needs as they grow

1. www.stanfordchildrens.org/en/topic/default?id=newborn-reflexes-90-P02630
2. Lampl, M., Veldhuis, J. D., & Johnson, M. L. (1992). Saltation and stasis: a model of human growth. *Science, 258*(5083), 801-803.

Chapter 6: When your baby is premature or sick

1. www.firststepsnutrition.org/pdfs/Specialised_infant_milks_January_2018b.pdf
2. Boyd, C. A., Quigley, M. A., & Brocklehurst, P. (2007). Donor breast milk versus infant formula for preterm infants: systematic review and meta-analysis. *Archives of Disease in Childhood-Fetal and Neonatal Edition, 92*(3), F169-F175.
3. Andreas, N. J., Kampmann, B., & Le-Doare, K. M. (2015). Human breast milk: A review on its composition and bioactivity. *Early human development, 91*(11), 629-635.
4. Menon, G., & Williams, T. C. (2013). Human milk for preterm infants: why, what, when and how?. *Archives of Disease in Childhood-Fetal and Neonatal Edition, 98*(6), F559-F562.
5. Schanler, R. J. (2011, February). Outcomes of human milk-fed premature infants. In *Seminars in perinatology* (Vol. 35, No. 1, pp. 29-33). WB Saunders.
6. Underwood, M. A. (2013). Human milk for the premature infant. *Pediatric Clinics, 60*(1), 189-207.

Chapter 7: When your baby is developing differently

1. Emily Perl Kingsley - Welcome to Holland
2. Kirsten Groseclose - The Trouble with Welcome to Holland smithkingsmore.org/the-trouble-with-welcome-to-holland/

Chapter 8: Feeding your baby - making a decision

1. Eidelman, A. I., & Schanler, R. J. (2012). Breastfeeding and the use of human milk. *Pediatrics.*
2. Bartok, C. J., & Ventura, A. K. (2009). Mechanisms underlying the association between breastfeeding and obesity. *International Journal of Pediatric Obesity, 4*(4), 196-204.
3. Chowdhury, R., Sinha, B., Sankar, M. J., Taneja, S., Bhandari, N., Rollins, N., ... & Martines, J. (2015). Breastfeeding and maternal health outcomes: a systematic review and meta-analysis. *Acta paediatrica, 104*, 96-113.
4. Kendall-Tackett, K. (2007). A new paradigm for depression in new mothers: the central role of inflammation and how breastfeeding and anti-inflammatory treatments protect maternal mental health. *International breastfeeding journal, 2*(1), 6.
5. Doan, T., Gardiner, A., Gay, C. L., & Lee, K. A. (2007). Breast-feeding increases sleep duration of new parents. *The Journal of perinatal & neonatal nursing, 21*(3), 200-206.
6. Lawrence, R. M., & Lawrence, R. A. (2001). Given the benefits of breastfeeding, what contraindications exist?. *Pediatric Clinics of North America, 48*(1), 235-251.
7. McAndrew, F., Thompson, J., Fellows, L., Large, A., Speed, M., & Renfrew, M. J. (2012). Infant feeding survey 2010. *Leeds: health and social care information Centre, 2*(1).

Chapter 10: Giving your baby formula

1. www.unicef.org.uk/babyfriendly/wp-content/uploads/sites/2/2008/02/start4life_guide_to_bottle_-feeding.pdf
2. www.firststepsnutrition.org/pdfs/Statement_on_making_up_formula%20safely_Mar_2015_final.pdf

Chapter 11: Introducing solids

1. World Health Organization. (2005). Guiding principles for feeding non-breastfed children 6-24 months of age.
2. Brown, A., & Harries, V. (2015). Infant sleep and night feeding patterns during later infancy: Association with breastfeeding frequency, daytime complementary food intake, and infant weight. *Breastfeeding Medicine, 10*(5), 246-252.
3. www.gov.uk/government/publications/feeding-in-the-first-year-of-life-sacn-report
4. static1.squarespace.com/static/59f75004f09ca48694070f3b/t/5ceed06a15fc-c07f8822270b/1559154825802/Eating_well_first_year_April19_for_web.pdf
5. www.firststepsnutrition.org/babyfood-composition
6. Maier, A., Chabanet, C., Schaal, B., Issanchou, S., & Leathwood, P. (2007). Effects of repeated exposure on acceptance of initially disliked vegetables in 7-month old infants. *Food quality and preference, 18*(8), 1023-1032.
7. Coulthard, H., Harris, G., & Emmett, P. (2009). Delayed introduction of lumpy foods to children during the complementary feeding period affects child's food acceptance and feeding at 7 years of age. *Maternal & child nutrition, 5*(1), 75-85.
8. Bentley, A. (2014). *Inventing baby food: Taste, health, and the industrialization of the American diet* (Vol. 51). Univ of California Press.
9. Brown, A., Jones, S. W., & Rowan, H. (2017). Baby-led weaning: the evidence to date. *Current nutrition reports, 6*(2), 148-156.

Chapter 12: Your baby's sleep

1. Blair, P. S., Mitchell, E., Fleming, P. J., Smith, I. J., Platt, M. W., Young, J., ... & Golding, J. (1999). Babies sleeping with parents: case-control study of factors influencing the risk of the sudden infant death syndromeCommentary: Cot death—the story so far. *Bmj, 319*(7223), 1457-1462.
2. www.lullabytrust.org.uk/safer-sleep-advice/what-is-sids/
3. Paul, I. M., Hohman, E. E., Loken, E., Savage, J. S., Anzman-Frasca, S., Carper, P., ... & Birch, L. L. (2017). Mother-infant room-sharing and sleep outcomes in the INSIGHT study. *Pediatrics, 140*(1), e20170122.
4. Tully, K. P., & Sullivan, C. S. (2017). Parent-infant room-sharing is complex and important for breastfeeding. *Evidence-based nursing*, ebnurs-2017.
5. Fleming, P., Blair, P., & Pease, A. (2017). Why or how does the prone sleep position increase the risk of unexpected and unexplained infant death?.
6. McKenna, J. J., & McDade, T. (2005). Why babies should never sleep alone: A review of the co-sleeping controversy in relation to SIDS, bedsharing and breast feeding. *Paediatric respiratory reviews, 6*(2), 134-152.
7. Mosko, S., Richard, C., McKenna, J. (1997a). Infant arousals during mother-infant bed sharing: Implications for infant sleep and sudden infant death syndrome research. Pediatrics, 100(5), 841-9.
8. Salm Ward, T. C . (2015). Reasons for mother-infant bed-sharing: A systematic nar-

rative synthesis of the literature and implications for future research. *Maternal and Child Health Journal, 19*(3), 675-90.

9. Blair, P. S., Ball, H. L., McKenna, J. J., Feldman-Winter, L., Marinelli, K. A., Bartick, M. C., & Academy of Breastfeeding Medicine. (2020). Bedsharing and Breastfeeding: The Academy of Breastfeeding Medicine Protocol# 6, Revision 2019. *Breastfeeding Medicine.*

10. www.unicef.org.uk/babyfriendly/wp-content/uploads/sites/2/2016/07/Co-sleeping-and-SIDS-A-Guide-for-Health-Professionals.pdf

11. Thompson, J. M., Tanabe, K., Moon, R. Y., Mitchell, E. A., McGarvey, C., Tappin, D., ... & Hauck, F. R. (2017). Duration of breastfeeding and risk of SIDS: an individual participant data meta-analysis. *Pediatrics, 140*(5), e20171324.

12. Ball, H. L. (2006). Parent-infant bed-sharing behavior. *Human Nature, 17*(3), 301-318

13. Ball, H. L. (2003). Breastfeeding, bed-sharing, and infant sleep. *Birth, 30*(3), 181-188.

14. Rudzik, A. E., Robinson-Smith, L., & Ball, H. L. (2018). Discrepancies in maternal reports of infant sleep vs. actigraphy by mode of feeding. *Sleep medicine, 49*, 90-98.

15. Brown, A., & Harries, V. (2015). Infant sleep and night feeding patterns during later infancy: Association with breastfeeding frequency, daytime complementary food intake, and infant weight. *Breastfeeding Medicine, 10*(5), 246-252.

16. Perkin, M. R., Bahnson, H. T., Logan, K., Marrs, T., Radulovic, S., Craven, J., ... & Lack, G. (2018). Association of early introduction of solids with infant sleep: a secondary analysis of a randomized clinical trial. *JAMA pediatrics, 172*(8), e180739-e180739.

17. Nevarez, M. D., Rifas-Shiman, S. L., Kleinman, K. P., Gillman, M. W., & Taveras, E. M. (2010). Associations of early life risk factors with infant sleep duration. *Academic pediatrics, 10*(3), 187-193.

18. Doan, T., Gardiner, A., Gay, C. L., & Lee, K. A. (2007). Breast-feeding increases sleep duration of new parents. *The Journal of perinatal & neonatal nursing, 21*(3), 200-206.

19. Kendall-Tackett, K., Cong, Z., & Hale, T. W. (2011). The effect of feeding method on sleep duration, maternal well-being, and postpartum depression. *Clinical Lactation, 2*(2), 22-26.

20. Harries, V., & Brown, A. (2019). The association between use of infant parenting books that promote strict routines, and maternal depression, self-efficacy, and parenting confidence. *Early Child Development and Care, 189*(8), 1339-1350.

21. Blunden, S. L., Thompson, K. R., & Dawson, D. (2011). Behavioural sleep treatments and night time crying in infants: challenging the status quo. *Sleep medicine reviews, 15*(5), 327-334.

22. Mindell, J. A., Kuhn, B., Lewin, D. S., Meltzer, L. J., & Sadeh, A. (2006). 'Behavioral treatment of bedtime problems and night wakings in infants and young children': Erratum.

23. Bornstein, M. H., Putnick, D. L., Rigo, P., Esposito, G., Swain, J. E., Suwalsky, J. T., ... & De Pisapia, N. (2017). Neurobiology of culturally common maternal responses to infant cry. *Proceedings of the National Academy of Sciences, 114*(45), E9465-E9473.

24. Letourneau, N., Watson, B., Duffett-Leger, L., Hegadoren, K., & Tryphonopoulos, P. (2011). Cortisol patterns of depressed mothers and their infants are related to maternal-infant interactive behaviours. *Journal of Reproductive and Infant Psychology, 29*(5), 439-459.

25. Grant, K. A., McMahon, C., Austin, M. P., Reilly, N., Leader, L., & Ali, S. (2009). Maternal prenatal anxiety, postnatal caregiving and infants' cortisol responses to the still□ face procedure. *Developmental Psychobiology: The Journal of the International Society for Developmental Psychobiology*, 51(8), 625-637.

26. Hiscock, H., & Wake, M. (2002). Randomised controlled trial of behavioural infant sleep intervention to improve infant sleep and maternal mood. *Bmj*, 324(7345), 1062.

Chapter 13: Normal emotions on becoming a parent

1. Kerrick, M. R., & Henry, R. L. (2017). 'Totally in love': Evidence of a master narrative for how new mothers should feel about their babies. *Sex Roles*, 76(1-2), 1-16.

2. Nyström, K., & Öhrling, K. (2004). Parenthood experiences during the child's first year: literature review. *Journal of advanced nursing*, 46(3), 319-330.

3. Vanassche, S., Swicegood, G., & Matthijs, K.(2013). Marriage and children as a key to happiness? Cross-national differences in the effects of marital status and children on well-being. *Journal of Happiness Studies*, 14, 501-524.

4. Jenkins, J. M., Rasbash, J., & O'Connor, T. G.(2003). The role of the shared family context in differential parenting. *Developmental Psychology*, 39, 99-113.

5. Rich, Adrienne. 1976. *Of Woman Born: Motherhood as Experience and Institution*. New York: Norton.

6. Sevón, E. (2011). 'My life has changed, but my life hasn't': Making sense of the gendering of parenthood during the transition to motherhood. *Feminism & Psychology*, 22, 60-80

7. Wilcox, W. B., & Nock, S. L. (2006). What's love got to do with it? Equality, equity, commitment and women's marital quality. *Social Forces*, 84, 1321-1345.

8. Gibson, F. L., Ungerer, J. A., Tennant, C. C., & Saunders, D. M. (2000). Parental adjustment and attitudes to parenting after in vitro fertilization. *Fertility and sterility*, 73(3), 565-574.

Chapter 14: Am I a good enough parent?

1. www.oxfordclinicalpsych.com/page/winnicott-radio-bbc

2. www.psychologytoday.com/gb/blog/freedom-learn/201512/the-good-enough-parent-is-the-best-parent

3. Woodhouse, S. S., Scott, J. R., Hepworth, A. D., & Cassidy, J. (2020). Secure base provision: A new approach to examining links between maternal caregiving and infant attachment. *Child Development*, 91(1), e249-e265.

4. www.economist.com/graphic-detail/2017/11/27/parents-now-spend-twice-as-much-time-with-their-children-as-50-years-ago

5. www.sirc.org/publik/CFOM.pdf

6. Hays, S. (1996) *The Cultural Contradictions of Motherhood*. New Haven, CT: Yale University Press

7. DiBartolo, P. M., Li, C. Y., & Frost, R. O. (2008). How do the dimensions of perfectionism relate to mental health?. *Cognitive Therapy and Research*, 32(3), 401-417.

8. Lee, M. A., Schoppe-Sullivan, S. J., & Dush, C. M. K. (2012). Parenting perfectionism and parental adjustment. *Personality and individual differences*, 52(3), 454-457.

9. Djafarova, E., & Trofimenko, O. (2017). Exploring the relationships between self-presentation and self-esteem of mothers in social media in Russia. *Computers in Human Behavior*, 73, 20-27. doi.org/10.1016/j.chb.2017.03.021

10. Schoppe-Sullivan, S. J., Yavorsky, J. E., Bartholomew, M. K., Sullivan, J. M., Lee, M. A., Dush, C.M.K., & Glassman, M. (2017). Doing gender online: New mothers' psychological characteristics, Facebook use, and depressive symptoms. *Sex Roles, 76,* 276-289. doi.org/10.1007/s11199-016-0640-z

11. Dorethy, M. D., Fiebert, M. S., & Warren, C. R. (2014). Examining social network- ing site behaviors: Photo sharing and impression management on Facebook. *International Review of Social Sciences and Humanities, 6,* 111-116.

12. Padoa, T., Berle, D., & Roberts, L. (2018). Comparative social media use and the mental health of mothers with high levels of perfectionism. *Journal of Social and Clinical Psychology, 37*(7), 514-535.

13. Komiya, N., & Taniguchi, H. (2011). A study on the psychological effects of yoga practice. *Japanese Journal of Counseling Science.*

Chapter 15: Spotting the signs of postnatal depression

1. Leigh, B., & Milgrom, J. (2008). Risk factors for antenatal depression, postnatal depression and parenting stress. *BMC psychiatry, 8*(1), 24.

2. Matthey, S., Barnett, B., Kavanagh, D. J., & Howie, P. (2001). Validation of the Edinburgh Postnatal Depression Scale for men, and comparison of item endorsement with their partners. *Journal of affective disorders, 64*(2-3), 175-184.

3. Leigh, B., & Milgrom, J. (2008). Risk factors for antenatal depression, postnatal depression and parenting stress. *BMC psychiatry, 8*(1), 24.

4. acestoohigh.com /got-your-ace-score

5. Lanius, R. A., Vermetten, E., & Pain, C. (2010). *The impact of early life trauma on health and disease: The hidden epidemic.* Cambridge, UK.

6. Lee, C. H., & Giuliani, F. (2019). The role of inflammation in depression and fatigue. *Frontiers in immunology, 10,* 1696.

7. McDonnell, C. G., & Valentino, K. (2016). Intergenerational effects of childhood trauma: evaluating pathways among maternal ACEs, perinatal depressive symptoms, and infant outcomes. *Child maltreatment, 21*(4), 317-326.

8. Cipriani, A., Furukawa, T. A., Salanti, G., Geddes, J. R., Higgins, J. P., Churchill, R., ... & Tansella, M. (2009). Comparative efficacy and acceptability of 12 new-generation antidepressants: a multiple-treatments meta-analysis. *The Lancet, 373*(9665), 746-758.

9. Kendall-Tackett, K. (2007). A new paradigm for depression in new mothers: the central role of inflammation and how breastfeeding and anti-inflammatory treatments protect maternal mental health. *International Breastfeeding Journal, 2*(1), 1-14.

10. Milgrom, J., Danaher, B. G., Gemmill, A. W., Holt, C., Holt, C. J., Seeley, J. R., ... & Ericksen, J. (2016). Internet cognitive behavioral therapy for women with postnatal depression: a randomized controlled trial of MumMoodBooster. *Journal of Medical Internet Research, 18*(3), e54.

11. Buttner, M. M., Brock, R. L., O'Hara, M. W., & Stuart, S. (2015). Efficacy of yoga for depressed postpartum women: a randomized controlled trial. *Complementary Therapies in Clinical Practice, 21*(2), 94-100.

12. Erkkilä, J., Punkanen, M., Fachner, J., Ala-Ruona, E., Pöntiö, I., Tervaniemi, M., ... & Gold, C. (2011). Individual music therapy for depression: randomised controlled trial. *The British Journal of Psychiatry, 199*(2), 132-139.

13. Bodnar, L. M., & Wisner, K. L. (2005). Nutrition and depression: implications for improving mental health among childbearing-aged women. *Biological Psychiatry,*

58(9), 679-685.

14. Chan, K. P. (2015). Effects of perinatal meditation on pregnant Chinese women in Hong Kong: a randomized controlled trial. *Journal of Nursing Education and Practice*, *5*(1), 1-18.

15. Daley, A. J., Blamey, R. V., Jolly, K., Roalfe, A. K., Turner, K. M., Coleman, S., ... & MacArthur, C. (2015). A pragmatic randomized controlled trial to evaluate the effectiveness of a facilitated exercise intervention as a treatment for postnatal depression: the PAM-PeRS trial. *Psychological Medicine*, *45*(11), 2413-2425.

16. Miller, B. J., Murray, L., Beckmann, M. M., Kent, T., & Macfarlane, B. (2013). Dietary supplements for preventing postnatal depression. *Cochrane Database of Systematic Reviews*, (10).

17. Onozawa, K., Glover, V., Adams, D., Modi, N., & Kumar, R. C. (2001). Infant massage improves mother-infant interaction for mothers with postnatal depression. *Journal of Affective Disorders*, *63*(1-3), 201-207.

Chapter 16: Coping with anxiety and intrusive thoughts

1. Wu, A., Noble, E. E., Tyagi, E., Ying, Z., Zhuang, Y., & Gomez-Pinilla, F. (2015). Curcumin boosts DHA in the brain: Implications for the prevention of anxiety disorders. *Biochimica et Biophysica Acta (BBA)-Molecular Basis of Disease*, *1852*(5), 951-961.

2. Lindseth, G., Helland, B., & Caspers, J. (2015). The effects of dietary tryptophan on affective disorders. *Archives of Psychiatric Nursing*, *29*(2), 102-107.

3. Al Sunni, A., & Latif, R. (2014). Effects of chocolate intake on perceived stress; a controlled clinical study. *International journal of health sciences*, *8*(4), 393.

4. Lawrence, P. J., Craske, M. G., Kempton, C., Stewart, A., & Stein, A. (2017). Intrusive thoughts and images of intentional harm to infants in the context of maternal postnatal depression, anxiety, and OCD. *Br J Gen Pract*, *67*(661), 376-377.

5. Murray, L., & Finn, M. (2012). Good mothers, bad thoughts: New mothers' thoughts of intentionally harming their newborns. *Feminism & Psychology*, *22*(1), 41-59.

Chapter 17: Postnatal anger and rage

1. Ou, C. H., & Hall, W. A. (2018). Anger in the context of postnatal depression: An integrative review. *Birth*, *45*(4), 336-346.

2. Kim E, Hogge I, Ji P, Shim YR, Lothspeich C. Hwa-Byung among middle-aged Korean women: family relationships, gender-role attitudes, and self-esteem. *Health Care Women Int*. 2014; **35**: 495-511.

Chapter 18: Birth trauma

1. Dikmen Yildiz P, Ayers S, Phillips L. The prevalence of post-traumatic stress disorder in pregnancy and after birth: a systematic review and meta-analysis. *J Affec Disord*. (2017) 208:634-45. doi: 10.1016/j.jad.2016.10.009

2. Simkin P. Just another day in a woman's life? Women's long-term perceptions of their first birth experience part 1. *Birth* 1991; 18(4)203-210

3. Kilpatrick, D. G., Resnick, H. S., Milanak, M. E., Miller, M. W., Keyes, K. M., & Friedman, M. J. (2013). National estimates of exposure to traumatic events and PTSD prevalence using DSM-IV and DSM-5 criteria. *Journal of traumatic stress*, *26*(5), 537-547.

4. Beck, C. T. (2006). Pentadic cartography: Mapping birth trauma narratives. *Quali-*

tative Health Research, 16(4), 453-466.

5. www.ppsupportmn.org/resources/Documents/Image_1_Development%20 of%20a%20Measure%20of%20Postpartum%20PTSD_%20The%20City%20 Birth%20Trauma%20Scale.pdf

6. Ayers, S., & Ford, E. (2009). Birth trauma: Widening our knowledge of postnatal mental health. *European Health Psychologist, 11*(2), 16-19.

7. Beck, C. T. (2004). Birth trauma: in the eye of the beholder. *Nursing research, 53*(1), 28-35.

8. Beck, C. T. (2005). Benefits of participating in Internet interviews: Women helping women. *Qualitative health research, 15*(3), 411-422.

9. Daniels, E., Arden-Close, E., & Mayers, A. Be Quiet and Man Up: A Qualitative Questionnaire Study into Men Who Experienced Birth Trauma.

10. Etheridge, J., & Slade, P. (2017). 'Nothing's actually happened to me.': the experiences of fathers who found childbirth traumatic. *BMC pregnancy and childbirth, 17*(1), 80.

Chapter 19: Partners' mental health

1. Darwin, Z., Galdas, P., Hinchliff, S., Littlewood, E., McMillan, D., McGowan, L., & Gilbody, S. (2017). Fathers' views and experiences of their own mental health during pregnancy and the first postnatal year: a qualitative interview study of men participating in the UK Born and Bred in Yorkshire (BaBY) cohort. *BMC pregnancy and childbirth, 17*(1), 45.

2. Matthey S, Barnett B, Howie P, Kavanagh D (2003) Diagnosing postpartum depression in mothers and fathers: whatever happened to anxiety? *J Affect Disord* 74:139-147

3. Wilhelm K, Parker G (1993) Sex differences in depressiogenic risk factors and coping strategies in a socially homogenous group. *Acta Psychiatr Scand* 88:205-211

4. Isacco, A., Hofscher, R., & Molloy, S. (2016). An examination of fathers' mental health help seeking: A brief report. *American journal of men's health, 10*(6), NP33-NP38.

5. Dudley M, Roy K, Kelk N, Bernard D (2001) Psychological correlates of depression in fathers and mothers in the first postnatal year. *J Reprod Infant Psychol* 19(3):187-202

6. Ramchandani P, Stein A, O'Connor T, Heron J, Murray L, Evans J (2008) Depression in men in the postnatal period and later child psychopathology: a population cohort study. *J Am Acad Child Adolesc Psychiatry* 47(4):390-398

7. Giallo, R., D'Esposito, F., Cooklin, A., Mensah, F., Lucas, N., Wade, C., & Nicholson, J. M. (2013). Psychosocial risk factors associated with fathers' mental health in the postnatal period: results from a population-based study. *Social psychiatry and psychiatric epidemiology, 48*(4), 563-573.

8. Kumar, S. V., Oliffe, J. L., & Kelly, M. T. (2018). Promoting postpartum mental health in fathers: Recommendations for nurse practitioners. *American journal of men's health, 12*(2), 221-228.

Chapter 20: I wish I'd never had a baby

1. Newport, F., Wilke, J. (2013, September 25). Desire for children still norm in U.S. Gallup News. Retrieved from news.gallup.com/poll/164618/desire-children-norm.aspx

2. Bartholomaeus, C., Riggs, D. W. (2017). Daughters and their mothers: The reproduction of pronatalist discourses across generations. Women's Studies International Forum, 62, 1-7.

3. Donath, O. (2015). Regretting motherhood: A sociopolitical analysis. Signs: Journal of Women in Culture and Society, 40, 343-367

4. Garncarek, E. (2020). 'Living with Illegal Feelings'—Analysis of the Internet Discourse on Negative Emotions towards Children and Motherhood. *Qualitative Sociology Review, 16*(1), 78-93.

5. Moore, J., & Abetz, J. S. (2019). What do parents regret about having children? Communicating regrets online. *Journal of Family Issues, 40*(3), 390-412.

6. en.wikipedia.org/wiki/Pat_Sharp

7. McMahon, Martha. 1995. *Engendering Motherhood: Identity and Self-Transformation in Women's Lives*. New York: Guilford.

Chapter 21: Pains, posture and pelvic floors – recovering physically from your birth

1. www.nhs.uk/conditions/caesarean-section/recovery/

2. Thurston, R. C., Luther, J. F., Wisniewski, S. R., Eng, H., & Wisner, K. L. (2013). Prospective evaluation of nighttime hot flashes during pregnancy and postpartum. *Fertility and sterility, 100*(6), 1667-1672.

3. Patel, R. R., Peters, T. J., & Murphy, D. J. (2007). Is operative delivery associated with postnatal back pain at eight weeks and eight months? a cohort study. *Acta obstetricia et gynecologica Scandinavica, 86*(11), 1322-1327.

4. Bozkurt, M., Yumru, A. E., & Şahin, L. (2014). Pelvic floor dysfunction, and effects of pregnancy and mode of delivery on pelvic floor. *Taiwanese Journal of Obstetrics and Gynecology, 53*(4), 452-458.

5. Harvey, M. A. (2003). Pelvic floor exercises during and after pregnancy: a systematic review of their role in preventing pelvic floor dysfunction. *Journal of Obstetrics and Gynaecology Canada, 25*(6), 487-498.

Chapter 22: Eating for strength, health and wellbeing

1. World Health Organization. (2001). *The optimal duration of exclusive breastfeeding: a systematic review* (No. WHO/NHD/01.08). World Health Organization.

2. Breymeyer, K. L., Lampe, J. W., McGregor, B. A., & Neuhouser, M. L. (2016). Subjective mood and energy levels of healthy weight and overweight/obese healthy adults on high-and low-glycemic load experimental diets. *Appetite, 107*, 253-259.

3. Strasser, B., Gostner, J. M., & Fuchs, D. (2016). Mood, food, and cognition: role of tryptophan and serotonin. *Current Opinion in Clinical Nutrition & Metabolic Care, 19*(1), 55-61.

4. Galland, L. (2010). Diet and inflammation. *Nutrition in Clinical Practice, 25*(6), 634-640.

5. Tramullas, M., Finger, B. C., Dinan, T. G., & Cryan, J. F. (2016). Obesity takes its toll on visceral pain: high-fat diet induces toll-like receptor 4-dependent visceral hypersensitivity. *PLoS One, 11*(5).

6. Veronese, N., Koyanagi, A., Stubbs, B., Cooper, C., Guglielmi, G., Rizzoli, R., ... & Notarnicola, M. (2019). Mediterranean diet and knee osteoarthritis outcomes: a longitudinal cohort study. *Clinical Nutrition, 38*(6), 2735-2739.

7. Kunnumakkara, A. B., Sailo, B. L., Banik, K., Harsha, C., Prasad, S., Gupta, S. C., ... & Aggarwal, B. B. (2018). Chronic diseases, inflammation, and spices: how are they linked?. *Journal of translational medicine, 16*(1), 14.

8. Johnson, F., Pratt, M., & Wardle, J. (2012). Dietary restraint and self-regulation in eating behavior. *International Journal of Obesity, 36*(5), 665-674.
9. Hicks, S., & Brown, A. (2016). Higher Facebook use predicts greater body image dissatisfaction during pregnancy: The role of self-comparison. *Midwifery, 40*, 132-140.
10. Bravi, F., Wiens, F., Decarli, A., Dal Pont, A., Agostoni, C., & Ferraroni, M. (2016). Impact of maternal nutrition on breast-milk composition: a systematic review. *The American Journal of Clinical Nutrition,104*(3), 646-662.
11. www.nhs.uk/conditions/pregnancy-and-baby/breastfeeding-alcohol/
12. Little, R. E., Northstone, K., Golding, J., & ALSPAC Study Team. (2002). Alcohol, breastfeeding, and development at 18 months. *Pediatrics, 109*(5), e72-e72.
13. Dorea, J. G. (2007). Maternal smoking and infant feeding: breastfeeding is better and safer. *Maternal and child health journal, 11*(3), 287-291.
14. Soltanian, H. T., Liu, M. T., Cash, A. D., & Iglesias, R. A. (2012). Determinants of breast appearance and aging in identical twins. *Aesthetic surgery journal, 32*(7), 846-860.

Chapter 23: Exercising again (or just exercising)

1. Sharma, G., Lobo, T., & Keller, L. (2014). Postnatal exercise can reverse diastasis recti. *Obstetrics and gynecology, 123*, 171S-171S.
2. Cramp, A. G., & Bray, S. R. (2010). Postnatal women's feeling state responses to exercise with and without baby. *Maternal and child health journal, 14*(3), 343-349.
3. Armstrong, K., & Edwards, H. (2004). The effectiveness of a pram⬚walking exercise programme in reducing depressive symptomatology for postnatal women. *International journal of nursing practice, 10*(4), 177-194.
4. Currie, J. (2001). Pramwalking as postnatal exercise and support: An evaluation of the stroll your way to well-being® program and supporting resources in terms of individual participation rates and community group formation. *The Australian Journal of Midwifery, 14*(2), 21-25.
5. Doran, F., & Hornibrook, J. (2013). Women's experiences of participation in a pregnancy and postnatal group incorporating yoga and facilitated group discussion: A qualitative evaluation. *Women and Birth, 26*(1), 82-86.
6. MacDonald, C. (2013). Mother and baby yoga is good for you. *The practising midwife, 16*(5), 14-16.

Chapter 24: Postnatal deficiencies and disorders

1. Souberbielle J-C, Body J-J, Lappe JM, Plebani M, Shoenfeld Y, Wang TJ, et al. Vitamin D and musculoskeletal health, cardiovascular disease, autoimmunity and cancer: Recommendations for clinical practice. Autoimmun Rev. 2010;9:709-15.
2. Wuertz C, Gilbert P, Baier W, Kunz C. Cross-sectional study of factors that influence the 25-hydroxyvitamin D status in pregnant women and in cord blood in Germany. Br J Nutr. 2013;110:1895-902.
3. Cavalier, E., Delanaye, P., Morreale, A., Carlisi, A., Mourad, I., Chapelle, J. P., & Emonts, P. (2008). Vitamin D deficiency in recently pregnant women. *Revue médicale de Liège, 63*(2), 87-91.
4. Nair, R., & Maseeh, A. (2012). Vitamin D: The 'sunshine' vitamin. *Journal of pharmacology & pharmacotherapeutics, 3*(2), 118.

5. www.nhs.uk/live-well/healthy-body/how-to-get-vitamin-d-from-sunlight
6. www.nhs.uk/conditions/vitamins-and-minerals/vitamin-d
7. www.nhs.uk/conditions/vitamin-b12-or-folate-deficiency-anaemia/causes
8. World Health Organization. (2016). Guideline: Iron supplementation in postpartum women.
9. www.nhs.uk/conditions/iron-deficiency-anaemia
10. Ngo, S. T., Steyn, F. J., & McCombe, P. A. (2014). Gender differences in autoimmune disease. *Frontiers in neuroendocrinology*, *35*(3), 347-369.
11. Gaberšček, S., Zaletel, K., Glinoer, Burrow, Abalovich, Laurberg, ... & Kurioka. (2011). Thyroid physiology and autoimmunity in pregnancy and after delivery. *Expert review of clinical immunology*, *7*(5), 697-707.

Chapter 25: Your new relationship with your partner – what's normal?

1. Keizer, R., & Schenk, N. (2012). Becoming a parent and relationship satisfaction: A longitudinal dyadic perspective. *Journal of Marriage and Family*, *74*(4), 759-773.
2. Stanca, L. (2012). Suffer the little children: Measuring the effects of parenthood on well‐being world‐wide. *Journal of Economic Behavior & Organization*, **81**, 742-750.
3. www.relate.org.uk/relationship-help/help-family-life-and-parenting/new-parents/top-4-reasons-couples-argue-after-having-baby
4. Nomaguchi, K. M., & Milkie, M. A. (2003). Costs and rewards of children: The effects of becoming a parent on adults' lives. *Journal of Marriage and Family*, **65**, 356-374.
5. Gjerdingen, D. K., & Center, B. A. (2004). First-time parents' postpartum changes in employment, childcare, and housework responsibilities. *Social Science Research*, *34*, 103 – 116. doi:10.1016/ j.ssresearch.2003.11.005
6. Feeney, J., Peterson, C., & Noller, P. (1994). Equity and marital satisfaction over the family life cycle. *Personal Relationships*, **1**, 83-99.
7. Richter, D., Krämer, M. D., Tang, N. K., Montgomery-Downs, H. E., & Lemola, S. (2019). Long-term effects of pregnancy and childbirth on sleep satisfaction and duration of first-time and experienced mothers and fathers. *Sleep*, *42*(4), zsz015.
8. Sloan, E. P. (2011). Sleep deprivation and postpartum mental health. *Archives of women's mental health*, *14*(6), 509-511.
9. Meltzer, L. J., & Mindell, J. A. (2007). Relationship between child sleep disturbances and maternal sleep, mood, and parenting stress: a pilot study. *Journal of Family Psychology*, *21*(1), 67.
10. Mills,M., & Täht, K. (2010). Nonstandard work schedules and partnership quality: Quantitative and qualitative findings. *Journal of Marriage and Family*, *72*, 860 – 875. doi:10.1111/j.1741-3737. 2010.00735.x
11. Dew, J., & Wilcox, W. B. (2011). If momma ain't happy: Explaining declines in marital satisfaction among new mothers. *Journal of Marriage and Family*, *73*, 1 – 12. doi:10.1111/j.1741- 3737.2010.00782.x
12. www.ons.gov.uk/employmentandlabourmarket/peopleinwork/earningsandwork-inghours/articles/womenshouldertheresponsibilityofunpaidwork/2016-11-10
13. McMunn, A., Bird, L., Webb, E., & Sacker, A. (2020). Gender divisions of paid and unpaid work in contemporary UK couples. *Work, Employment and Society, 34*(2), 155-173.

14. www.pewsocialtrends.org/2013/03/14/chapter-6-time-in-work-and-leisure-patterns-by-gender-and-family-structure/

15. Schneider, D. (2012). Gender deviance and household work: The role of occupation. *American Journal of Sociology, 117*(4), 1029-1072.

16. Chesley, N. (2017). What does it mean to be a 'breadwinner' mother?. *Journal of Family Issues, 38*(18), 2594-2619.

17. www.independent.co.uk/life-style/men-women-parenting-housework-childcare-a9098091.html

18. www.nytimes.com/2020/05/06/upshot/pandemic-chores-homeschooling-gender.html

19. www.pewsocialtrends.org/2015/11/04/raising-kids-and-running-a-household-how-working-parents-share-the-load/

20. Walzer, S. (1996). Thinking about the baby: Gender and divisions of infant care. *Social problems, 43*(2), 219-234.

21. Barrett, G., Pendry, E., Peacock, J., Victor, C., Thakar, R., & Manyonda, I. (2000). Women's sexual health after childbirth. *BJOG: An International Journal of Obstetrics & Gynaecology, 107*(2), 186-195.

22. Duffin, C. (2005). Lack of breaks leaves nurses burnt out: many nurses experience loss of libido, poor sleep and constant exhaustion, a Nursing Standard survey has shown. *Nursing Standard, 20*(6), 16-17.

23. Gettler, L. T., McDade, T. W., Agustin, S. S., Feranil, A. B., & Kuzawa, C. W. (2013). Do testosterone declines during the transition to marriage and fatherhood relate to men's sexual behavior? Evidence from the Philippines. *Hormones and Behavior, 64*(5), 755-763.

24. Impett, E. A., Kogan, A., English, T., John, O., Oveis, C., Gordon, A. M., & Keltner, D. (2012). Suppression sours sacrifice: Emotional and relational costs of suppressing emotions in romantic relationships. *Personality and Social Psychology Bulletin, 38*(6), 707-720.

25. Egbert, N., & Polk, D. (2006). Speaking the language of relational maintenance: A validity test of Chapman's Five Love Languages. *Communication Research Reports, 23*(1), 19-26.

Chapter 26: When things can't be fixed - spotting the signs of relationship breakdown and domestic abuse

1. www.womensaid.org.uk/information-support/what-is-domestic-abuse/domestic-abuse-is-a-gendered-crime/

2. www.independent.co.uk/news/uk/home-news/domestic-abuse-victims-pregnant-support-service-england-a8846831.html

3. www.womensaid.org.uk/information-support/what-is-domestic-abuse/how-common-is-domestic-abuse/

4. McDonnell E, Holohan M, Reilly MO, Warde L, Collins C, Geary M. Acceptability of routine enquiry regarding domestic violence in the antenatal clinic. *Ir Med J.* 2006;99:123-4

5. Johnson JK, Haider F, Ellis K, Hay DM, Lindow SW. The prevalence of domestic violence in pregnant women. *BJOG.* 2003;110:272-5

6. Bacchus L, Mezey G, Bewley S. A qualitative exploration of the nature of domestic violence in pregnancy. *Violence against women.* 2006 Jun;12(6):588-604.

7. Ellsberg M, Jansen HA, Heise L, Watts CH, Garcia-Moreno C, WHO Multi-country Study on Women's Health and Domestic Violence against Women Study Team. *Lancet*. 2008 Apr 5; 371(9619):1165-72.

8. Jeyaseelan L, Sadowski LS, Kumar S, Hassan F, Ramiro L, Vizcarra B *Inj Control Saf Promot*. 2004 Jun; 11(2):117-24.

Chapter 27: Thriving as an LGBTQ parentcouples

1. www.ons.gov.uk/peoplepopulationandcommunity/birthsdeathsandmarriages/families/bulletins/familiesandhouseholds/2018#number-of-families-continues-to-grow-with-large-increases-for-same-sex-couple-families

2. www.independent.co.uk/news/uk/home-news/lgbt-gay-relationships-britain-acceptance-social-attitudes-survey-bsa-a8998596.html

3. Chan, R. W., Brooks, R. C., Raboy, B., & Patterson, C. J. (1998). Division of labor among lesbian and heterosexual parents: Associations with children's adjustment. *Journal of Family Psychology, 12*(3), 402.

4. Ross, L., Steele, L., & Sapiro, B. (2005). Perceptions of predisposing and protective factors for perinatal depression in same-sex parents. *Journal of Midwifery Womens' Health, 50*, 65-70.

5. Dunne, G. (2000). Opting into motherhood: Lesbians blurring the boundaries and transforming the meaning of parenthood and kinship. *Gender and Society, 14*, 11-35

6. Crouch, S. R., Waters, E., McNair, R., Power, J., & Davis, E. (2014). Parent-reported measures of child health and wellbeing in same-sex parent families: A cross-sectional survey. *BMC public health, 14*(1), 635.

7. Heaphy, B. (2018). Troubling traditional and conventional families? Formalised same-sex couples and 'the ordinary'. *Sociological Research Online, 23*(1), 160-176.

Chapter 30: Deciding to be a stay-at-home parent

1. www.ons.gov.uk/employmentandlabourmarket/peopleinwork/employmentandemployeetypes/articles/familiesandthelabourmarketengland/2017

2. Rubin, S. E., & Wooten, H. R. (2007). Highly educated stay-at-home mothers: A study of commitment and conflict. *The Family Journal, 15*(4), 336-345.

3. Pöllänen, S., & Voutilainen, L. (2018). Crafting Well-Being: Meanings and Intentions of Stay-at-Home Mothers' Craft-Based Leisure Activity. *Leisure Sciences, 40*(6), 617-633.

4. Zimmerman, T. S. (2000). Marital equality and satisfaction in stay-at-home mother and stay-at-home father families. *Contemporary Family Therapy, 22*(3), 337-354.

5. fullfact.org/education/childcare-costs-england/

6. metro.co.uk/2018/10/19/getting-kids-ready-for-school-is-like-working-an-extra-day-8054433/

7. abcnews.go.com/Lifestyle/stay-home-parent-luxury-spouse/story?id=26022052

8. Chesley, N. (2011). Stay at home fathers and breadwinning mothers: Gender, couple dynamics, and social change. Gender & Society, 25, 642-664.

9. Merla, L. (2008). Determinants, costs, and meanings of Belgian stay-at-home fathers: An international comparison. *Fathering: A Journal of Theory, Research & Practice about Men as Fathers, 6*(2).

Chapter 31: Returning to work

1. Chesley, N. (2017). What does it mean to be a 'breadwinner' mother?. *Journal of Family Issues, 38*(18), 2594-2619.
2. Meisenbach, R. (2010). The female breadwinner: Phenomenological experience and gendered identity in work/family spaces. Sex Roles, 62, 2-19. doi:10.1007/ s11199-009-9714-5
3. Gunnar MR, Kryzer E, Van Ryzin MJ, Phillips DA. The rise in cortisol in family day care: Associations with aspects of care quality, child behavior, and sex. *Child Development.* 2010;81:851–869.
4. Dettling AC, Parker SW, Lane S, Sebanc A, Gunnar MR. Quality of care and temperament determine changes in cortisol concentrations over the day for young children in childcare. *Psychoneuroendocrinology* 2000;25:819–836
5. Ahnert L, Gunnar MR, Lamb ME, Barthel M. Transition to child care: Associations with infant-mother attachment, infant negative emotion, and cortisol elevations. *Child Development.* 2004;75:639–650
6. Legendre, A. (2003). Environmental features influencing toddlers' bioemotional reactions in daycare centers. *Environment and Behavior*, 35, 523–549.
7. Sylva, K., Stein, A., Leach, P., Barnes, J., Malmberg, L. E., & FCCC-team. (2011). Effects of early child-care on cognition, language, and task-related behaviours at 18 months: An English study. *British Journal of Developmental Psychology, 29*(1), 18-45.
8. www.theguardian.com/lifeandstyle/2010/oct/02/nurseries-child-care-pre-school-cortisol
9. www.moneyadviceservice.org.uk/en/articles/childcare-costs#how-much-does-childcare-cost
10. M.Gettas & A.Morales, 2013, 'Breastfeeding in the Workplace', *ICAN: Infant, Child, & Adolescent Nutrition* 2013 5: 197

Index